The Truth About Children's Health

The Comprehensive Guide to Understanding, Preventing, and Reversing Disease

"Even if you are a minority of one, the truth is still the truth."
—Ghandi

"Genius is the ability to recognize the truth."
—Bernardini

by Robert Bernardini, M.S.

Reproduction or translation of any part of this work beyond that permitted by Section 107 or 108 of the 1976 United States Copyright Act without permission of the copyright owner is unlawful. Requests for permission or further information should be addressed to PRI Publishing, P.O. Box 74, Clifford, VA 24533.

This publication is designed to provide accurate and authoritative information in regard to the subject matter covered. It is sold with the understanding that the publisher is not engaged in rendering medical, legal or other professional services. If such advice or other expert assistance is required, the services of a competent professional person should be sought.

Disclaimer: The ideas and suggestions contained in this book are not intended as a substitute for the appropriate care of a licensed health care practitioner. Qualified medical assistance should always be sought before beginning any treatments. The following is intended for educational purposes only. Suggestions are not made to treat a specific condition.

Publisher's Cataloging-in-Publication
(Provided by Quality Books, Inc.,)
Bernardini, Robert.
    The truth about children's health : the comprehensive guide to understanding, preventing, and reversing disease/ by Robert Bernardini - 1st ed.
        p.cm.
        Includes bibliographical references and index.
        ISBN 0-9703269-6-3

    1. Children--Health and hygiene--United States.
    I. Title.

RJ102.B47 2003   362.1'9892'000973
                                 QBI03-200152

Printed in Korea
3rd Printing

Table of Contents

"The ultimate cure must rest with the children."

—Harold E. Buttram, M.D.

Introduction
(Please read first.)

Health care professionals have called this book "one of the best books of the millenium," "one of the finest resources on the market," and "absolutely one of the most important books of our time. Not just for children, but for adults, our society, and our very survival." If you read it from beginning to end, which is highly recommended, you will see the development of some intriguing and somewhat shocking concepts that until now have not been well publicized.

Those concepts apply to all of us, no matter the age. So don't let the title mislead you. This book is much more than just a book about children's health. It is an expose on the fundamental reasons people get sick.

When you learn the causes underlying illness and disease, you will not only have the opportunity to use that knowledge to get and stay healthy, but you will also free yourself from the shackles of confusion and misunderstanding that are so prevalent these days in the area of health. You will feel liberated because you will know and feel in your heart the truth of health. And the truth will set you free. You will no longer fear the unknown and dread "coming down with something." You will know that if you follow some simple guidelines, you will be impenetrable to disease. And as you'll see, doing so is not that complicated.

These guidelines are suitable—if not critical—for the health of everyone, no matter their age. They are basic and fundamental practices that everyone responds to. Whether you're a newborn or ninety, this book, its knowledge, and its guidelines are for you. My recommendations will help you to overcome and even reverse virtually any health problem you may now have and head off any other diseases you may be fearing for the future.

I originally wrote this book was to explain how and why diseases occur in human beings. While researching that topic, I made some startling discoveries. One worth noting here is that most adult diseases actually get started due to conditions the person experienced earlier in his or her life – not just earlier as an adult, but as far back as childhood, infancy, while in the womb, and even before conception! (There is actually more to it than that, but I will leave you to discover it as you read.)

Cancer, heart disease, diabetes, arthritis, depression, and other maladies just don't appear out of nowhere. There must be a cause for them to manifest. Nearly all conditions (even the common cold or seemingly transient sickness) result from conditions building up in an individual over time. Eventually the bad overtakes the good, and the disease manifests.

For you to better and fully understand disease, why it happens and how you can avoid it, it is best to understand it from the very beginning. Once you know why, then you can take the necessary steps for healing or prevention with a clear conscience, *knowing* that you are doing the right things—the things that will stop your pain and keep you healthy for the rest of your life.

And besides, who doesn't have a child in his or her life? If you are a parent and your children are grown, they may be thinking of starting a family. You may even have grandchildren. Think of your siblings' children, and your friends'. Wouldn't it be nice for you to be able to help them get and stay healthy for the rest of their lives? What good parent or grandparent wouldn't? Think of the pain, suffering, and expense you'll be saving them!

And the children. What is happening to them? All across America many parents are looking up to heaven and asking "why?" Why is their child sick? Why did their little loved one develop cancer, Attention Deficit Disorder, diabetes, or autism? Why did their child lash out and become hostile and aggressive or blatantly disrespectful and totally out of control? And why, in some extreme cases, did their child commit an act of such horrible violence that a person gets sick just thinking about it? How could a youngster, who should be experiencing the happiest times of his or her life, be so off track that he or she could become so seriously compromised of mind, body, emotions, and soul?

Parents hold their heads in frustration. "What did I do wrong? How can this be happening? What did I do to deserve this?" And mixed with that frustration are anger, confusion, and shame.

And as a parent, or if you're soon to be one, you wonder if it's possible to rescue your child from the pain and misery of sickness and protect them from becoming frustrated, difficult to handle, or even violent. The intent of this book is to show you that these misfortunes can be avoided or conditions reversed if certain simple guidelines, or "laws," if you will, are followed.

We live in a universe of laws. Laws that don't care if you're black or white, Japanese or Mexican, ninety years old or still a fetus. Those laws are fundamental to the nature of matter and energy and determine how life progresses. If we live in harmony with those laws, we will as consequence live in harmony. If we break the laws, we will become discordant. Enough of that discord will create sickness, disease, and aberrant behavior.

To find a solution to a problem, we must first recognize what the problem truly is. All the knowledge and technology in the world are of little help if we apply them in the wrong direction. To arrive at a healthy, happy state of being, we must first determine not just what the symptoms are and how to alleviate them (what modern Western medicine is good at doing), but what the true underlying causes of these symptoms are (where modern medicine falls short). Once we know that, it's much easier to find the solutions that will not only alleviate the symptoms, but also eliminate the problem all together.

If you are an adult reading this who is older than about 40 years of age, I'd like you to think back to your childhood. How many kids did you know who had leukemia, asthma, diabetes, attention deficit/hyperactivity disorder (ADHD), arthritis, multiple sclerosis, cancer, or autism or were obese? Chances are, you may have known a few. Perhaps the kid down the street had asthma. Maybe

The Truth About Children's Health

there was a distant relative who had juvenile diabetes. Or you heard on the news about some rare child with leukemia.

Today? It seems like everywhere you turn, you read or hear about a child with a serious health problem. How many kids do you know who are on Ritalin or have been diagnosed with a learning disability? There are whole hospitals devoted to children's cancer. Asthma and diabetes are now considered epidemics. And when as a child growing up did you ever, ever hear of another child or adolescent shooting, stabbing or killing someone else? Now it seems like the news reports such events almost daily. In my own life as a youngster, the most serious act of violence I can remember was a fellow sixth grader hurling a chair across the room toward a teacher. The boy was suspended from school immediately and the school was in an uproar for days afterward. These days, that act sounds relatively mild.

Harold E. Buttram, M.D., sums up this disturbing trend:

American children today may be confronted with the greatest difficulty and danger that can be placed on any generation, that of a subtle deterioration in health, largely the result of an increasingly hostile and toxic environment. Considering the circumstances, the marvel is that many do turn out well... Children are much more vulnerable to toxic exposures than adults... In the present case, the ultimate cure must rest with the children... Increasing health problems in children today largely involve two closely related and interacting systems of the body, the immune system and the brain and nervous system. Health problems involving these systems express themselves as various manifestations of crippled immune systems, delayed development, and "minimal brain dysfunction."... Allergic disorders such as asthma are rapidly increasing, both in frequency and severity. Although more difficult to quantify statistically, susceptibility to common viral infections and their complications appears to have increased on a scale largely unknown in earlier generations, as indicated by the increasing numbers of children who are becoming dependent on frequent or prolonged courses of antibiotics.... Corresponding increases have taken place in behavioral disorders, attention deficit hyperactive disorder (ADHD), and learning disabilities. ADHD, with its long-term consequences in terms of impaired learning capacity and social adjustment difficulties that commonly ensue in later adolescence, is arguably one of the foremost health problems of our times. Although statistics confirm the increasing prevalence of ADHD and related problems among children, statistics alone do not tell the entire story. Many factors involved are subtle and intangible and are difficult to measure statistically.

Perhaps the best way to gain insight into the pervasiveness of the problem is to talk with veteran teachers with a perspective of 20 or

30 years teaching experience. In our office we have asked a number of these teachers, inquiring if they have observed a change in children during their teaching careers. Without exception, they have replied there has been a dramatic change, most notably since the 1970s. Steadily increasing numbers of children, they report, are restless, impulsive, less focused, less able to maintain sustained concentration, and therefore, less able to learn....

We believe that meaningful progress will best come about through public education. Large portions of the public are already seeking sound guidance in this area. Above all, there should be freedom of choice in matters pertaining to health. Those seeking health for themselves and their families must return to more natural patterns of living. This requires effort and, very often, the braving of public opinion. This cannot come about in a society where basic freedoms in the health field are denied. (1)

Developmental disabilities such as autism, attention deficit/hyperactivity disorder (ADHD), dyslexia, and uncontrollable aggression currently affect an estimated 12 million children under age 18 in the United States – almost one child in five. Furthermore, the incidence of some of those disabilities has increased dramatically in recent decades. (2)

It appears that:

1. The health of our children in just about every area is degenerating, and

2. Behavioral problems and serious violence by the young are escalating.

Is it possible that the two things – children's health and acts of violence by the young -- are related? Could it be that the state of sickness in the body contributes to or even leads to unstable mental health – even in our young? Is there any evidence to support these theories?

Or are these dual epidemics just a "blip on the radar screen" that is serious, yes, but more a function of probability than causality?

Statistics from a variety of sources and over long periods of time have been used to identify the deteriorating health trends in our children and validate their existence. The prudent thing to do is to recognize these trends and attempt to figure out why they are occurring. We must not ignore these warning signs with denial or a Pollyanna attitude. If we do, we might witness in the not too distant future many diverse and widespread tragedies affecting our children, ourselves, and our society.

But as useful and helpful as statistics are, we must not allow them to usurp our own common sense. We must evaluate everything with our own keen eye and judgment and use scientific information as a guideline, but not a rule. *Always* ask yourself these two questions when given information: "Does this make sense to me?" and, "Is this what I'm seeing or experiencing in my own world?" After looking at all sides of a problem and keeping these questions in mind, then you will be able to make the decision that is best for you.

You must scrutinize closely the information you receive from the government and the mass media. Policy decisions, guidelines, and laws are oftentimes made not so much for the preservation of our health, but for the preservation of profits. Big money can do big things, including influencing our government. A 1980 study showed that almost half of the leading officials at the Food and Drug Administration (FDA) had at one time worked for organizations the agency is mandated to regulate. (3) Similarly, many FDA officials quit to go work for a company in the field they were once regulating. The battle lines between the *regulated* and the *regulator* are not as clear as one is led to believe.

As you read these pages, again I urge you to take the information presented and think about it on your own and for yourself. Ask yourself if it makes sense to *you*. Is it consistent with natural law?

Look around you. See what's happening in our world. Compare it with what you used to see. Do some research and ask some questions. Don't necessarily believe somebody just because he or she is on the nightly news, in the papers or is a so-called "expert." Make yourself the expert. Learn to *seek* answers, not just accept what is foisted upon you – for the truth is often quiet and the truth is often hidden. Truth is not in it for the money, it just is. Truth doesn't advertise.

As a society, we have amassed literally millions of volumes of medical information. We have the most sophisticated testing equipment and medical devices the world has ever seen. It's really incredible how far technology has come in just the past few decades.

That's all well and good, but has it solved the problem? Have all these devices made us healthier? Has all that knowledge kept your kid from having an attention deficit or from coming down with juvenile diabetes? There are more doctors in our society now than ever before. And yet, we are sicker than ever. And our children are in the worst shape in history. Why?

Will throwing more money at those problems really solve them? Are more potent drugs, lasers, transplants, genetic engineering, and cloning really the answer? Some seem to think so. But these technological solutions cannot, because of the simple laws of nature and what I call "The Ancestry Factor" (explained later) give us long-term lasting solutions.

If you have a child who is sick, has attention deficit disorder, is violent or "acting out," you want answers. And you want solutions that will solve the problem - permanently, so you never have to worry about it again. ·

We need to do more than just alleviate the symptoms – we need to discover the causes and correct them at their root. For example, putting a child on Ritalin may calm him or her down, but it does nothing to balance brain chemistry. It may look like a solution to the immediate problem of hyperactivity, but has been shown to merely delay more serious problems that show up later in life.

We will be examining the reasons for this and many other problems through-out these pages, and you will be provided strategies for handling them and improving your and your child's life.

A better life awaits you and your child when you let the power and truthful-ness of nature prevail.

CHAPTER I
Children of the USA

To understand the scope of our subject, let's first consider who they are, how they live and how they are changing. The following information comes from *America's Children: Key National Indicators of Well-Being, 2001.* (1)

- In 2000, there were 70.4 million children under age 18 in the U.S., or 26 percent of the population. This is down from a peak of 36 percent at the end of the baby boom (1964). They are expected to comprise 24 percent of the population in 2020.

- The racial and ethnic diversity of America's children continues to increase. In 2000, 64 percent of U.S. children were white, non-Hispanic; 15 percent were black, non-Hispanic; 4 percent were Asian or Pacific Islander; and 1 percent were American Indian or Alaska Native. The number of Hispanic children has increased faster than that of any other racial or ethnic group, growing from 9 percent of the child population in 1980 to 16 percent in 1999.

- The family structures for children have become more varied. The percentage of children living with one parent increased from 20 percent in 1980 to 26 percent in 2000. Most children living with single parents live with a single mother. However, the proportion of children living with single fathers doubled over this time period, from 2 percent in 1980 to 4 percent in 2000. Some children live with a single parent who has a cohabiting partner: 16 percent of children living with single fathers and 9 percent of children living with single mothers also lived with their parents' partners.

- In 1999, 54 percent of children from birth through third grade received some form of childcare on a regular basis from persons other than their parents, up from 51 percent in 1995.

- The poverty rate for children living with family members dropped from 18 percent in 1998 to 16 percent in 1999.

- Many children live in households that have housing problems, such as physically inadequate housing, crowded housing, or a high cost burden. The percentage of households with children living with these difficulties has been increasing since 1978; 35 percent had one or more housing problems in 1999, up from 30 percent in 1978.

- The percentage of children living in households experiencing food insecurity was 3.8 percent in 1999. However, nearly one third of children in poverty experienced food insecurity.

- The percentage of children born with low birth weight (less than about 5.5 pounds) or very low birth weight (less than about 3.3 pounds) has steadily increased since 1984. About 7.6 percent of infants were low birth weight in 1999, and 1.4 percent were very low birth weight. The increase in the proportion of low birth weight infants is partly due to the rising number of twins and other multiple births. (It is the opinion of many health professionals that a high percentage of multiple births are an indication of reproductive and fertility abnormalities within the population.)

- The leading cause of death in ages one to four and five to 14 was unintentional injuries, with most of these fatal injuries resulting from car crashes. Birth defects, cancer, and homicide were also leading causes of death for children ages one to 14.

Unfortunately, this data paints a picture that is less than ideal for our children. Although we live in the richest and most technologically advanced civilization on earth, many of our children are living in less than tolerable conditions. Could these conditions be responsible in part for the trends in youth violence?

The American Psychological Association reports:

Some people mistakenly believe that violence in the United States is on the downswing because crime overall has decreased since its peak year in 1981. But much of the decrease in crime has been due to the aging of the baby boom generation and the consequent reduction in the number of teenagers; it is this demographic group that contributes disproportionately to crime in general. In addition, violent crime is up, especially among juveniles, and this trend is likely to continue. The Office of Juvenile Justice and Delinquency Prevention reports that between 1985 and 1994, there was a 40 percent increase in murders, rapes, robberies, and assaults reported to law enforcement agencies across the nation. And despite their relatively low numbers in the population, our youth were responsible for 26 percent of this growth in violence.

According to the Federal Bureau of Investigation, the years between 1985 and 1995 saw a 249 percent increase in gun-related murders committed by juveniles. By the year 1992, when murder became the second leading cause of death among males 15 to 24 in the United States, three quarters of the killings already involved guns. Indeed, for black and white older adolescents, firearm murders are the most rapidly increasing cause of death.

In 1994 alone, for example, juveniles were responsible for 14 percent of all violent crimes solved by the law enforcement system. They committed:

- 20 percent of robberies
- 14 percent of rapes
- 13 percent of assaults
- 10 percent of murders

Thus, even if arrest rates recorded in 1992 remain constant, we could still see a 22 percent increase in violence arrests for youths age 10 to 17 until the year 2010.

Worse, the National Center for Juvenile Justice reports that the number of youths age 10 to 17 who are arrested for violent crimes could more than double by the year 2010 if arrest rates continue to increase as they did between 1983 and 1992.

This projected growth between 1992 and 2010 is expected to vary among categories as follows:

- Murders, up 142 percent
- Rapes, up 66 percent
- Robberies, up 58 percent
- Assault, up 129 percent. (2)

According to the FBI, while the U.S. population increased by 40 percent from 1960 through 1991, violent crime increased 560 percent, murders increased 170 percent, rapes 520 percent, and aggravated assaults 600 percent. (3) As we will see in the following chapters, there are many factors that could be responsible for these increases, and our young are not exempt from them. In fact, they are even more susceptible to them than adults.

The New York Times seems to think youth violence is a real problem also. It stated on December 7, 1990, that "In some areas of the country, it is now more likely for a black male between 15 and 25 to die from homicide than it was for a United States soldier to be killed on a tour of duty in Vietnam." (4)

By these accounts, it's evident that the incidences of youth violence are happening more often, especially within the last few years. Some serious events have shocked the country, not just because of where and how they occurred, but the because of the age of the offenders. Consider:

- On March 5, 2001, a high school student shoots and kills two fellow students at Santana High School in Santee, California. A week later, just a mile away, a student at Granite High School in El Cajon opens fire on his classmates.

- On April 20, 1999, two students storm into Columbine High School in Littleton, Colorado, at lunchtime, killing 13 people and wounding 23 with guns and explosives during a six hour siege.

- Exactly one month later, a student goes on a rampage at his high school in Conyers, Georgia, shooting six schoolmates.

- On May 21, 1998, a 15-year-old boy opens fire in his high school in Springfield, Oregon, killing two teenagers and injuring 20 others. On a police videotape, he is asked why. He responds: "I had no other choice."

- On May 19, 1998, in Fayetteville, Tennessee, an 18-year-old honor student uses a firearm in the parking lot three days before graduation, killing a classmate who was dating his ex-girlfriend.

- On May 24, 1998, a 14-year-old student shoots to death a science teacher in front of fellow students at an eighth-grade dance in Edinboro, Pennsylvania.

- On March 24, 1998, two boys, 11 and 13, go on a shooting rampage at a middle school in Jonesboro, Arkansas. Four girls and a teacher are killed.

- On December 1, 1997, three students are killed and five others wounded in a hallway at Heath High School in West Paducah, Kentucky. One girl is left paralyzed. The 14-year-old murderer, when asked why he did it, says he doesn't know.

- On October 1, 1997, a 16-year-old boy in Pearl, Mississippi, kills his mother and then shoots nine students at his high school soon after.

From all these reports, it's clearly evident something is terribly wrong. Just watching the news at home in rural Virginia, I hear acts of violent crimes, murders, rapes, and other acts of violence by our youth reported with alarming frequency. Is juvenile violence just a short-term trend? Perhaps like the sniper attacks and assassinations in the 1960s, is it just a phase we're going through? Let's hope so.

On the other hand, it could get worse. Our world is becoming more and more complex, more and more stressful, and more and more difficult to handle – for adults and children alike. In all this stress and confusion, we need to find some answers. To point to one or two factors and say they are the cause would be simplistic. There are a myriad of factors influencing our health and well being. But let's face it, if those kids were happy and content, they would not go on shooting sprees. They would not to turn to cults. They would not turn to drugs.

And even though there are seemingly countless reasons why our kids are going crazy, there is really one underlying cause: they're not happy. And they're not happy because they're not healthy. They're stressed out and on the edge. They're pressured, barraged with too much information and acts of violence, carted off to day care at a vulnerable age, fed junk food from infancy, poisoned by drugs, affected by environmental pollutants, raised by only one parent (or parents who are never around because they work two jobs each), plopped in front of the TV or video games because they keep them quiet, not taught well in school, and treated with disrespect. It's almost a wonder that there are any normal kids at all. On the following pages we will explore the reasons for all this insanity. I believe most of them stem from physiological stresses caused by improper lifestyles. The varied and often horrifying sociological abnormalities we have identified in this chapter arise from the problems that result. But as numerous and varied are the causes, the solutions are surprisingly simple. Not easy perhaps, but simple. To save our children we must correct those problems as soon as possible. Then this downward spiral into decay and violence will end.

Why Our Children Are Especially Vulnerable

Children are not just "little adults." Their exploratory behavior, increased biological sensitivity, and different diet make them more vulnerable and susceptible to environmental contaminants. Keep in mind that most if not all studies of exposures to and possible health effects of environmental toxins have used adults. The same exposure to children would magnify their health risks.

The National Research Council states:

The data strongly suggest that exposure to neurotoxic compounds at levels believed to be safe for adults could result in permanent loss of brain function if it occurred during the prenatal or early childhood period of brain development. This information is particularly relevant to dietary exposure to pesticides, since policies that established safe levels of exposure to neurotoxic pesticides for adults could not be assumed to adequately protect a child less than four years of age. (5)

The National Academy of Sciences says that infants are likely to be 10 times more sensitive to any *single* pesticide than an adult. But the *additive* effects of pesticides consumed in combination are not considered when regulating pesticides. Nor are multiple routes of exposure (food, water, household use). There are 275 pesticides allowed on food and 102 of these were detected by the FDA from 1990 through 1992 on just 22 different fruits and vegetables. (6) So the additive effect of simultaneous exposure to multiple pesticides presents a real-world risk to infants and children.

Yet, there are no standards to protect infants, children or anyone else from the effects of multiple pesticides on food, around the house or from any other source, for that matter. Indeed, the EPA has just begun to consider the combined effects of certain groups of pesticides, but once again, the studies focus on adults, not children. The likely effect of multiple pesticide exposure is probably synergetic (similar to adding 2 plus 2 and getting 5), and may even be exponential (similar to adding 2 plus 2 and getting 20). There are so many chemicals in our environment these days, there is no way studies could be performed to determine the health risks of every combination. What's more, different people may have different levels of sensitivity to various chemicals or combinations of chemicals "generally considered safe," and these may not apply to you or your child. The only way to eliminate the risks is to completely eliminate the chemicals.

Children are more sensitive and more easily harmed, placing them at special risk for adverse effects from toxic exposure. Their metabolic mechanisms for processing and excreting toxic substances are not fully developed. Children are especially sensitive because of their different pathways of absorption, tissue distribution, ability to biotransform and eliminate chemicals, and the manners in which they respond to chemicals and radiation.

Children go through various stages of development – fetal, newborn, infant, school age, adolescent – and each stage may be particularly vulnerable to specific toxins. For example, infants are more vulnerable to the effects of secondhand smoke because their lung capacity is still increasing. Toddlers' respiratory rates are more rapid, so they are more vulnerable to air pollutants than an adult might be. Several organ systems, including the nervous, immune, reproductive, and endocrine systems, which are not fully developed at birth, may "demonstrate particular sensitivity during the postnatal [newborn] period." (7)

The reproductive system is also vulnerable to the toxic effects of chemical pollutants and pesticides – whether exposure occurs in the womb or in early childhood – which can interfere with normal sexual development. That exposure may also be contributing to declining male reproductive health in general in the industrialized world. (8,9)

In many cases infants and children suffer far more serious damage than adults do. Aspirin, for example, can cause Reye's syndrome (a condition that kills 80 percent of its victims) in children and teenagers, but it does not cause this condition in adults. Lead causes permanent loss of mental capacity when infants and children are exposed at levels of little consequence to adults. Phenobarbital, a sedative in adults, produces hyperactivity in most children. Ritalin produces hyperactivity in most adults but is a sedative in children. Infants under six months of age suffer methemoglobanemia, or "blue baby syndrome," from nitrate exposure at levels that are safe for older children and adults. Radiation treatment for brain cancer in children under four can cause major cognitive problems later in life, but causes almost no cognitive problems if performed after age eight. (10)

A study in the journal *Cancer Research* reported a sevenfold increase in cancer rates when animals were exposed to carcinogens starting in infancy, as compared with exposure only during adulthood. (11) A review of the scientific literature in 1992 (we've known for that long) found that exposure to chemicals early in life (dosing animals in utero, in infancy, and in adulthood), increases the rate of cancer in the exposed population and that *these cancers generally occur earlier in life.* (12)

This is an important point. Exposure to toxins (and other stressors such as deficient diet, emotional stress, and physical inactivity) is taking its toll on people earlier and earlier in life. Once only older people got cancer – and not many of them at that. Then, middle-aged people started getting it. Now, our children are getting it and dying from it. Cancer is just one manifestation of ill health. There are many others such as ADHD, autism, childhood diabetes, asthma, and so on. Some of those conditions were not even defined in the scientific and medical literature until very recently since they were either so rare or they simply did not exist. People are getting sicker younger and younger – physically, mentally and emotionally. And it's not by chance – it's because our bodies are not being treated and cared for the way nature intended.

Not only can children suffer devastating effects from environmental toxins that go unnoticed or are relatively harmless for adults, they may also respond more acutely to these toxins at much smaller exposures simply because their bodies are smaller and not fully developed.

That sensitivity is present even before a baby is born. Many environmental toxins can cross the placenta, thus exposing the fetus. Air pollutants and toxins from secondhand smoke, or if the mother smokes herself, can impact the fetus. A pregnant mother who had been overexposed to lead would have stored it in her bones, from which it could escape and be potentially harmful to the fetus as well.

The risk of exposure more than multiplies at birth. Infants spend much time exploring their world through touch, taste, and movement. Their curiosity puts them at greater risk to exposure from environmental hazards. They put their fingers and objects they find in their mouths and spend their time crawling on the floor, where household chemicals, pesticides, and other environmental toxins accumulate. And, since they spend more time outdoors, have an increased respiratory rate and high levels of activity, they have increased exposure to air pollution. (Yet keeping them in deprives them of sunlight – important, as we shall see.)

A child's rapid growth during the first years of life requires proportionally more food and liquid consumption than an adult needs. And their bodies naturally absorb more of what they eat and drink. So any pesticides or chemicals in their food will be taken in more fully and at higher levels and do more harm faster and more permanently.

A growing child will typically eat more of certain foods such as apples and bananas per unit body weight than adults. But produce (if not organically grown) may be more highly contaminated than the foods adults typically eat. Children also drink more water, thus increasing their potential exposure to any toxins in it – including those such as chlorine added to sanitize it.

Safe levels of pesticides and food additives are calculated for lifetime exposure to adults. Those may be grossly underestimated or even just erroneous for a child, however.

A faster and more responsive metabolism and rapid growth and development are the basic reasons for an infant's increased vulnerability to any toxic substance. After birth the most pronounced period of growth is the first year of life, during which the human infant triples in weight. Different organs grow at different rates as the infant matures, creating a roulette of infant organ susceptibility. For instance, the brain of a newborn child grows rapidly and is particularly sensitive to toxic substances. Not only that, but where an infant's brain weighs about 33 percent what an adult brain weighs, the infant body weighs about 4 percent of an adult body. That relatively large brain grows rapidly in the newborn child, achieving 50 percent of its adult weight by six months of age, with 75 percent of all brain cells present by age two. (13,14) In contrast, children do not attain even 50 percent of adult weight in the liver, heart, and kidneys until age nine. (15)

During puberty, there are rapid metabolic and physiological changes that increase the impact of environmental toxins. And as adolescents enter the work force through summer jobs or jobs after school, or start smoking, drinking, or experimenting with drugs, any harmful effects of exposures are magnified.

In general, rapid growth increases the risk of cancer from toxic exposure. The NAS Committee on Pesticides in the Diets of Infants and Children concluded that in the absence of other factors, "Direct carcinogens are more potent in rapidly growing animals," adding that "infants and children are subject to rapid tissue growth and development, which will have an impact on cancer risk." (16) Does this have an effect on their health? It appears so. The incidence of childhood brain cancer and childhood leukemia has increased 33 percent since 1973. (17) Cancer now kills more children under age 14 than any other disease.

Hazardous substances such as lead, Polychlorinated Biphenyls (PCBs), asbestos, radon, solvents, pesticides, food additives, and air pollution have found their way into the schools, homes, food and playgrounds. Resultant exposures to these toxins can have significant impacts on children's health, putting them at risk of developing learning disabilities, chronic and acute respiratory diseases,

Children of the USA

neurological problems, asthma, bronchitis, and cancer. Consider this: Dr. Roger D. Masters says that children absorb up to 50 percent of the lead they ingest, compared with only 8 percent for adults. And even low exposures to toxins in early childhood and even in the womb can have permanent effects on intelligence and behavior. (18)

Our children are underprotected. There are very few data banks that have information on children's exposures, and again, risk assessments do not routinely differentiate between adults and children. However, the Federal government has officially recognized the vulnerability of children. On April 21, 1999 an Executive Order was issued by the White House titled *Protection of Children From Environmental Health Risks and Safety Risks*. Part of this order is quoted below:

> A growing body of scientific knowledge demonstrates that children may suffer disproportionately from environmental health risks and safety risks. These risks arise because: children's neurological, immunological, digestive, and other bodily systems are still developing; children eat more food, drink more fluids, and breathe more air in proportion to their body weight than adults; children's size and weight may diminish their protection from standard safety features; and children's behavior patterns may make them more susceptible to accidents because they are less able to protect themselves. Therefore, to the extent permitted by law and appropriate, and consistent with the agency's mission, each Federal agency:
>
> (a) shall make it a high priority to identify and assess environmental health risks and safety risks that may disproportionately affect children; and
>
> (b) shall ensure that its policies, programs, activities, and standards address disproportionate risks to children that result from environmental health risks or safety risks. (19)

In the words of Dr. Lynn Goldman, Assistant Administrator for the EPA: "We can no longer behave as though all environments were created equal. Children especially bear the brunt of environmental pollution in our most polluted environments, and they must be protected." (20)

CHAPTER II
Hazards Our Children Face

Kermit the Frog sings a song "It's Not Easy Being Green." Well, in today's world, it's not easy being a kid. They're faced with a seemingly endless number of factors that make growing up healthy, smart, and emotionally stable a real challenge. In this chapter we're going to examine some agents that can have a big impact on a growing child.

Lead

The American Journal of Public Health called lead poisoning an epidemic among American children. The U.S. Department of Health and Human Services referred to it as "the most important environmental health problem facing young children." [1]

The EPA report *Lead in Your Home: A Parent's Reference Guide* (a free government publication) says, "In the United States, about 900,000 children ages one to five have a blood-lead level above the level of concern."

The report goes on to discuss the health effects of lead:

Lead is poisonous because it interferes with some of the body's basic functions. A human body cannot tell the difference between lead and calcium, which is a mineral that strengthens bones. Like calcium, lead remains in the bloodstream for a few weeks, then it is absorbed into the bones, where it can collect for a lifetime.

Although children are especially susceptible to lead exposure, lead can be dangerous for adults too. In adults, high lead levels can cause:

- Increased chance of illness during pregnancy.
- Harm to a fetus, including brain damage or death.
- Fertility problems (in men and women).
- High blood pressure.
- Digestive problems.
- Nerve disorders.
- Memory and concentration problems.
- Muscle and joint pain.

Lead can affect anyone, but children ages six and younger face special hazards. In part, this is because the bodies of children in this age group develop rapidly. It is also because young children tend to put things in their mouths... It is important to know that even exposure to low levels of lead can permanently affect children. In low levels, lead can cause:

- Nervous system and kidney damage.
- Learning disabilities, attention deficit disorder, and decreased intelligence.
- Speech, language, and behavior problems.
- Poor muscle coordination.
- Decreased muscle and bone growth.
- Hearing damage.

While low-level exposure is most common, exposure to high levels of lead can have devastating effects on children, including seizures, unconsciousness, and in some cases, death.

Lead poisoning is not easy to detect. Sometimes no symptoms occur, and sometimes the symptoms are the same as those of more common illnesses. Some of the early signs and symptoms of lead poisoning in children are:

- Persistent tiredness or hyperactivity.
- Irritability.
- Loss of appetite.
- Weight loss.
- Reduced attention span.
- Difficulty sleeping.
- Constipation. (2)

The report goes on to say: "The only way to know if you have lead poisoning is to get a blood test from your doctor. Many people mistake the symptoms of lead poisoning for other common illnesses... Sometimes there are no symptoms at all."

Food for Thought

Would it surprise you to learn that the symptoms of lead poisoning in children are all classic signs of ADHD? I have two comments about this: One is that I wonder how many doctors prescribe a blood test be done on the hyperactive children they see before they prescribe Ritalin? I think every pediatrician in the country should be mailed the above referenced publication and be required to read it. Philip Landrigan, chair of the department of community and preventive medicine at Mount Sinai School of Medicine in New York City, says that any evaluation of a child suspected to have ADHD should start with screening for lead. My other comment is that since lead stays in the blood only a couple weeks or so, before it is

---

The Truth About Children's Health

absorbed into the bones, a blood test may not catch the fact that the child was previously exposed to lead. A better test would be a tissue mineral analysis, which tests hair or fingernail samples. It is a long-term picture of a person's exposure, not just a snapshot of a blood test that might miss something. Really, both should be done. (You may be wondering if there are any treatments available to help children combat lead poisoning. There are, and they will be discussed in the Chapter XIV.)

According to the American Academy of Pediatrics, between two million and four million American children have sufficient lead in their blood to reduce their physical stature, damage their hearing, decrease hand-eye coordination, and shorten their attention span enough to impair their ability to learn in school and diminish their IQ. Sad thing is, this damage is thought to be permanent. (3,4)

About 400,000 babies are delivered each year with toxic levels of lead already in their blood. Interestingly, the fetus acts as a "sink" for lead (and cooper, aluminum, cadmium, and other toxic metals) that is difficult for the mother to eliminate. Of the children living below the poverty level, some 55 percent have toxic levels of lead and one child in six is exposed to toxic levels of lead from the environment. Even low levels of lead are associated with hyperactivity, attention deficit/hyperactivity disorder (ADHD) and developmental failures. Again, any evaluation of a child suspected to have ADHD should start with screening for lead. (5)

In fact, the American Academy of Pediatrics showed that in 18 scientific studies, lead diminished a child's mental abilities. "The relationship between lead levels and IQ deficits was found to be remarkably consistent," they report. "A number of studies have found that for every 10 mcg/dL increase in blood lead levels, there was a lowering of mean (average) IQ in children by four to seven points." An average IQ loss of five points puts 50 percent more children into the IQ 80 category, which is borderline for normal intelligence. (6)

The academy says these IQ losses are permanent and they translate into reduced educational attainment, diminished job prospects, and decreased earning power, as was evident in a study in which groups of children with different blood levels of lead were tracked through high school. The high-lead children had higher absenteeism in school, lower class rank, poorer vocabulary, and longer reaction times with poorer hand-eye coordination. The high-lead group also was seven times less likely to graduate from high school and had reading scores two grades below expected.

It's interesting to note just what "excessively high levels" of lead actually are. In 1960, it was said that it was safe for a child to have 60 micrograms of lead in each deciliter (a tenth of a liter) of blood (i.e., 60 mcg/dL). In 1975 the medical community determined that this in fact was too high, and lowered it to 30 mcg/dL. By 1985, it was determined that 25 mcg/dL was the safe limit. But that was found to be too high too. In 1991, the safe limit was lowered again to 10 mcg/dL. Now, the National Research Council believes this level is still too high.

The Centers for Disease Control (CDC) says, "Blood lead levels at least as low as 10 mcd/dL can adversely affect the behavior and development of children." What this means is that the federal government has set an "acceptable" level of lead in blood (10 mcd/dL) that it acknowledges *does not protect children*. Damage to children has been documented at blood-lead levels considerably below 10 mcg/dL. The federal Agency for Toxic Substances and Disease Registry cites studies showing that children's growth, hearing, and IQ can be diminished by blood-lead levels as low as 5 mcg/dL. (7)

Between 1991 and 1994, the CDC tested the blood of a representative sample of the U.S. population for lead poisoning. They report that 4.4 percent of children ages one to five have at least 10 mcd/dL. That 4.4 percent represents about 890,000 children in the U.S. In some cities of the northeastern United States, it's estimated that 35 percent of preschool children have 10 mcg/dL or more of lead in their blood. (8)

Yet both the federal Department of Housing and Urban Development (HUD) and the U.S. EPA have set standards for lead in dust that, if met, essentially guarantee that childhood lead poisoning at the level of 10 mcg/dL will continue. Even if the current government standard for lead in dust were reduced to one tenth its present level, it would still allow children to be poisoned by lead in dust. (9)

It seems the whole philosophy behind all these safety standards is not one of "How do we prevent lead poisoning?" but more of "How much lead is safe for us to put into our children?" This even though there is convincing evidence that lead is a poison even at extremely low levels and that it has been poisoning people for many thousands of years.

Food for Thought

Ancient Greeks and Romans mined lead, and its toxicity was well established, even back then, long before the birth of Christ. Roman miners sometimes died from what the medical literature of the time called "lead colic." One of the reasons the Roman Empire fell, according to some historians, was that they used lead pipes for water (they abandoned their stone aqueducts) and had lead in their pottery. The accumulation of lead in their tissues would have led to mental problems. Could the crazy act of Nero playing a fiddle on the balcony as Rome burned below him have been because he had lead poisoning?

In 1989, the EPA reported that more than one million elementary schools, high schools, and colleges were still using lead-lined water storage tanks or lead-containing components in their drinking fountains. The EPA estimates that 20 percent of human exposure (including children) is attributed to lead in drinking water. (10)

Lead has also been implicated in aggressive behavior (in addition to delinquency and attention disorders) in boys between the ages of seven and 11. In the

Journal of the American Medical Association (JAMA), Herbert Neeleman examined 301 boys in public schools in Pittsburgh, Pennsylvania, measuring the lead in their bones and relating it to their behaviors as reported by the boys' teachers and parents and by the boys themselves. Boys with more lead in their bones consistently had more reports of aggressive and delinquent behavior and problems paying attention. The boys' behavior was measured at age seven and again at age 11. The behavior of the boys with more lead in their bones got worse as they grew older. On the other hand, behavior did not change among boys with less lead in their bones. The study also examined nine other variables in addition to lead (i.e., parents' socioeconomic status, mother's age, presence or absence of a father in the home, etc.) But even with all those variables taken into account, the relationship between lead and behavior was still statistically significant. (11)

Other studies have made the correlation between lead and aggressive behavior as well. In 1975 in Virginia, researchers compared 67 lead-exposed 11-year-olds to 70 nonexposed children to see if lead exposure was related to behavior problems. Nineteen of the lead-exposed children were described as "hyperactive, impulsive, and explosive, and as having frequent temper tantrums." Only five among the nonexposed group were described that way. (12) One year later, the group was re-evaluated. Fourteen of the lead-exposed children were described as having problems with lying, stealing, running away, and setting fires. Six of the non-exposed children were described this way.

In a study in 1994 in Boston, 1,782 children were examined for the amount of lead in their teeth and whether they had behavioral problems. Problem behaviors increased as lead levels in the children's teeth increased. (13)

In 1982 in Tennessee, a study was done examining the level of lead in children's hair. The lead levels in hair of 26 "problem children" were nearly twice as high as a control group of 29 students who had no behavioral problems. (14)

One scientific paper observed that as the concentration of lead in children increases, so does the incidences of violent crimes approximately 20 years later, when the children are grown. Bernard Weiss said in an article in the *International Journal of Mental Health* that the connections between brain-damaging lead and destructive behavior at least partially explained the increases in crime. (15)

As early as 1943, the correlation between levels of lead in children and behavioral problems was documented. In a study by Randolph Byers and Elizabeth Lord, 20 children who had recovered from "mild lead poisoning in infancy" were examined. Although none of the children had exhibited overt signs of lead poisoning, the growth and development of their nervous systems had been seriously impaired. Of the 20 children examined, only one had progressed normally in school. Many of the children were emotionally impaired. Byers and Lord said many of the children had "unreliable impulsive behavior, cruel impulsive behavior, short attention span, and the like." Three of the children were expelled from school – one for setting fires, one for repeatedly dancing on the desks, and the third for sticking a fork into another student's face. One of these lead-exposed children was reported to have attacked teachers with knives and scissors. (16)

Roger D. Masters, Ph.D., and his coworkers at Dartmouth College say that pollution causes people to commit violent crimes (homicide, aggravated assault, sexual assault, and robbery). Masters has developed what he calls the neurotoxicity hypothesis of violent crime, which holds that the toxic metals lead and manganese cause learning disabilities and increase in aggressive behavior and the loss of control over impulsive behavior. These traits combined with poverty, social stress, alcohol, and drug abuse, individual character, and other social factors can produce individuals who commit violent crimes. (17) In the largest study of its kind, of 1,000 black children in Philadelphia, showed that both lead levels and anemia were predictors of the number of juvenile offenses, the seriousness of juvenile offense, and the number of adult offenses for males.

Environmental sources of lead are everywhere. The main source of lead for children is house dust from paint that is disintegrating. Aside from remnants of the paint laced with lead in our homes, house dust also contains lead tracked into homes from soil outside. Forty-two million families live in housing that contains an estimated three million tons of lead in the paint. That's equivalent to about 140 pounds of lead per household. As that paint slowly disintegrates into house dust, it becomes available for a child to get on his hands and into his mouth and lungs. If a child ingests just 150 micrograms per day, the National Research Council says, the child is poisoned.

Manufacturers used to put lead pigments in paint because the pigments made the paint last longer and cling to surfaces better. They no longer do so, but some significant risks remain since as the paint breaks down with age, the dust it sheds contains significant amounts of lead. In 1978 the Consumer Product Safety Commission (CPSC) banned its use in paints for sale for use in residences, on children's toys or on household furniture. (18)

Food for Thought

If you think that the United States is on the cutting edge of health care, consider this: Australia passed a law curbing lead in paint in 1920. But they were behind the times. France and Austria had banned the use of lead in interior paint all the way back in 1909. I guess they thought centuries of known health problems from lead were enough proof of its toxicity. But the U.S.? We banned it in 1978. Maybe we're just plain old dumb from all the lead we've been ingesting all these years.

Drinking water is another source: the EPA estimates that over 800 municipal water systems serving some 30 million people have lead levels that exceed federal guidelines. The FDA estimates that a significant amount of lead exposure comes from food that's been in contact with ceramic hollowware, including coffee mugs with a ceramic glaze. Frequent use of them can contribute to elevated lead levels. Lead poisoning was often referred to as "the potter's disease" because those who made pottery with lead glazes often contracted it.

Should you worry about this with your everyday dishes? Probably not. Modern ceramics made by commercial firms are usually harmless. And major importers of pottery such as Pier One and William-Sonoma voluntarily prohibit the sale of lead-glazed items in their stores. The FDA has also mandated those imported items not safe for food-use must have a permanent stamp stating so. But you do need to be wary of pottery made by artisans or folk-potters in other countries that are brought into the U.S., or old heirlooms that have been in the family for years and passed on from generation to generation. And, there is concern that using a glazed mug for coffee or other acidic beverages may leach lead out of the glaze. If you don't know where you got a piece of ceramic ware, don't use it with anything you would consume.

Oil companies used to add lead to gasoline to stop engine knocking, but dangerous lead particles escaped into the air through auto exhaust systems. In 1978, the EPA reduced the amount of lead allowed in gasoline, hence the term "unleaded."

Lead was also used in fixtures, pipes, and pipe soldering and can leach into water that flows through the pipes. In 1986, and again in 1988, Congress changed the Safe Drinking Water Act to restrict the use of lead in pipes, solder, and other components used in public water systems and residential and nonresidential plumbing. However, lead may still be found in pipes manufactured prior to 1986 that are still in use today.

In 1995, the United States banned the use of lead solder in food cans. It was found that the lead solder which was used to seal the food cans leached into the food. Although it has been banned in the U.S. for this use, lead solder may still be found in cans imported here from other countries.

Most people would think that since lead has been eliminated from some products, it's no longer a problem. It's true that changes in the law have greatly reduced the amount of lead released into our homes, air, and environment. And the average blood level in U.S. children has gone down from 16 mcg/dl to 5 mcg/dL during the last 15 years. But remember, lead does not go away. It persists in the soil, gets into our food chain, and gets tracked into our houses. There is still an estimated 30 million tons of lead in our soils as a result of using lead in gasoline and industry. The lead problem will be with us for many years. That's why the Academy of Pediatrics says, there are still many children at high risk of exposure.

The National Research Council, in its 1993 book on lead, states:

> Once lead is mined and introduced into the environment, it persists. Over time, lead in various forms becomes available to the body as small particles. Most of the 300 million metric tons of lead ever produced remains in the environment, largely in soil and dust. That explains, in part, why background concentrations of lead in modern North Americans are higher by a factor of 100 to 1,000 than they were in pre-Columbian Americans. Today's production levels turn into tomorrow's background exposure, and despite reductions in the use of lead for gasoline, overall lead production continues to

grow and federal agencies have not addressed the impact of future increases of lead in the environment. (19)

The National Research Council says modern humans are estimated to have total body burdens of lead approximately 300 to 500 times those of our prehistoric ancestors who had blood lead level of only 0.016 mcg/dL (micrograms per deciliter) (determined from measurements of human bones). This, if considered the "background level," is 625 times lower than the 10 mcg/dL now established as "safe" for our children. (20)

Lead in the brain damages glia cells, a special kind of cell associated with inhibition (impulse control) and detoxification (eliminating poisons from the body). Manganese, another potential toxin, has the effect of lowering levels of serotonin and dopamine, which are neurotransmitters associated with impulse control and planning. Masters notes that low levels of serotonin in the brain are known to cause mood disturbances such as depression, poor impulse control, and increases in aggressive behavior.

Let's take a closer look at manganese. Children who are raised from birth on infant formula and who are not breastfed will absorb five times as much manganese as breastfed infants, Masters reports, and the absorption of manganese is *increased* when there is a *calcium deficiency*.

Food for Thought

Soft drinks increase the amount of calcium excreted in the urine, possibly leading to a calcium deficiency, possibly leading to higher blood levels of manganese, possibly leading to a loss of impulse control, possibly leading to... ?

Because of the increased manganese absorption by babies who drink infant formula and who are not breastfed, Masters considers infant formula toxic. Surprisingly, impoverished mothers are less likely to breastfeed their babies. Seventy-three percent of infants born to mothers with more than 12 years of education were breast fed, compared with 31 percent of infants born to mothers with less than 12 years of education. "The effects of manganese toxicity associated with infant formula are thus greatest for the poor, for ethnic minorities and for those with little education," Masters says.

Masters also says that toxic metals affect an individual in complicated ways. For example, because lead diminishes a person's normal ability to detoxify poisons, lead may heighten the effects of alcohol and drugs.

He also points to studies showing a synergistic (multiplier) effect between toxic metals and poor diet. It's been thoroughly documented that the uptake of lead is greatly increased in individuals who have a diet low in calcium, zinc, and essential vitamins. The amounts of lead and manganese that wouldn't harm a well-nourished individual may poison undernourished children. (21) Federal studies of nutrition make the point that black teenage males consume, on average, only about 65 percent as much calcium as whites; it follows that their risk of metals toxicity would be higher.

To explore the link between metals toxicity and the propensity to violence, Masters acquired data from the FBI for violent crimes in all counties of the United States. He correlated those with data on industrial releases of lead and manganese, and on alcohol consumption which has been shown to increase the uptake of toxic metals. He found that counties having all three measures of neurotoxicity – lead, manganese, and high alcohol consumption – had rates of violent crime *three times the national average*. He says that the highest levels of lead uptake are reported in precisely the demographic groups most likely to commit violent crimes (i.e., inner-city minority youths).

Masters notes that neurotoxicity is only one of many factors contributing to violence, but adds that he believes it may be especially important in explaining why violent crime rates differ so widely among geographic areas and by ethnic group. He says that traditional sociological approaches to crime cannot explain why the availability of handguns or drugs triggers violent behavior in only a small proportion of the population, a proportion that varies greatly from place to place. Part of the explanation may be the way the physical environment affects brain chemistry and behavior. "The presence of pollution is as big a factor as poverty," Masters says in an interview in the *New Scientist* magazine. "It's the breakdown of the inhibition mechanism that's the key to violent behavior." When our brain chemistry is altered by exposure to toxins, he believes, we lose the natural restraint that holds our violent tendencies in check. (22)

It is well established that lead poisoning occurs mainly in poor neighborhoods. In 1998, 13.5 million children (about 18.9 percent of all children in the U.S.) lived in poverty. Children living in low-income families are eight times as likely to be lead-poisoned as children who are not poor. Black children are five times as likely to be lead-poisoned as white children. One researcher said that "the homes of black children [in the study] had higher levels of lead-contaminated dust and their interior surfaces were in poorer condition." (23)

The General Accounting Office (an investigative branch of Congress) stated in 1999 that "hundreds of thousands of children exposed to dangerously high levels of lead are neither tested nor treated" because state governments are refusing to comply with the law. (24) That law was passed in 1989 and requires all infants (12 months old) and toddlers (2 years old) in the Medicaid program to be tested for lead poisoning. (Medicaid is a federally funded medical insurance program for economically disadvantaged people.) But this guideline is not being followed and it is it not being enforced.

"In sum," the Environmental Research Foundation states:

> ...we have a federally mandated blood-lead standard (10 mcg/dL) that permanently dumbs down any children who meet it, which is nearly a million children at any moment, and roughly 200,000 new dumbing-downs are occurring each year. Medical authorities agree that the only real solution is primary prevention – keeping lead contaminated dust away from children. Credible estimates show that

the federal government could make a profit of $1.08 billion by undertaking primary prevention in federally owned or assisted housing, but instead the government requires the dead-canary approach, blood-lead testing, which the states then refuse to carry out. We know... that public policies that put the onus on the private sector can make a big difference – but most states have failed to adopt such policies. (25)

Food for Thought

How could the federal government make a profit on lead abatement? It's estimated that the first-year cost of reducing lead hazards in federally owned and federally assisted housing would be $458 million. However, the calculated benefits from lead – abatement, such as reduced costs for medical care and for special education, plus increased salaries and resulting economic boost that go with higher IQs, would be $1.538 billion – a net benefit of $1.08 billion. (26) Seems that monetarily, there should be no excuse.

Can you do anything about lead exposure and poisoning? See Chapter XIV and the Resource Guide for recommendations.

Mercury

Mercury contamination may also be responsible for behavioral problems, learning disabilities, and ADHD. As early as the 1860s, a clinical disorder from mercury exposure was identified among "felters" (people who made the felt linings of hats and clothes). The term "mad as a hatter" was even coined to denote the strange behavior of people who did this kind of work. In the 19th century, mercury was known to be a deadly poison and back then it was known as Quick Silver (taken from the German phrase *Quak Silber*). People who put mercury, or Quak Silber, into other people's mouths were known as "quacks" – a term now used to denote a person who practices questionable medical procedures. Some believe it's no great surprise that dentists have a high rate of suicide. Mad Hatter's Disease may have become Mad Dentist's Disease.

Mercury exposure can come from seafood intake, environmental exposures at work and home (especially from mercury fungicides used in farming), and yes, from the silver fillings in a person's mouth. These "silver" fillings contain approximately 52 percent mercury. In a study reported in the *Journal of Dental Restoration*, those people in the study (including children) who had amalgam fillings had significantly greater levels of mercury in their blood. The authors concluded, "These examinations show that amalgam restorations contribute... to the origins of mercury in the organism [in children as well as adults]." (27) Another study, reported in the same journal, confirmed that blood concentrations of mercury are higher in people with amalgam fillings, and that the "...blood mercury concentrations were positively correlated to the number and surface area amalgam restorations and were significantly lower in the group without dental amalgams." (28) Also, levels of mercury in the brain are directly proportional to the number of amalgam fillings in the mouth.

But other sources of mercury abound. Prior to the 1990s household latex paints routinely contained mercury as an antifungal agent. Other possible sources include batteries, dyes, electronics, fluorescent lights, plastics, and many others. (A more complete list is in Chapter XIV.)

Another major source of mercury contamination comes from incinerating garbage. Approximately 187 incinerators nationwide emit almost 70,000 pounds of mercury each year. Originally, incinerators were thought to be a solution to keep mercury out of landfills and hence away from ground water. But studies have shown that the scrubber and filter technology that cleans smoke of toxic gasses fails to work on mercury. One of the biggest sources of contamination of mercury in some parts of the country is from coal-burning energy plants. There are no plans to limit mercury from these plants. Gary Glass, an EPA mercury research in Duluth, Minnesota, said, "In the past, we would take our mercury wastes and bury them so they would contaminate the ground water in just one place. Now we've gotten smarter – we're blowing it into the air so it can go everywhere." (29)

Although safety standards for mercury exposure are based on clearly visible signs of neurological problems, researchers point out that this is outdated thinking that doesn't take into account possible behavioral, biochemical, carcinogenic or other subtle effects such as lowered intelligence and premature senility. It accumulates in fish in its most toxic form, methyl mercury. The EPA estimates that 1.16 million women of childbearing age "eat sufficient amounts of mercury-contaminated fish to pose a risk of harm to their future children." (30) Joan M. Spyker and colleagues at the Minnesota Medical School and Johns Hopkins School of Public Health also reports, "...attention should be directed to the fetus since the unborn organism is much more susceptible to the toxic effects of methyl mercury. Methyl mercury easily crosses the placental barrier and is concentrated in fetal tissues; it has a greater affinity for the embryonic central nervous system than for that of the adult." (31) Methyl mercury arises (in the mouth especially) when it combines with a methyl molecule which is nothing more than carbon and hydrogen. Mercury is very reactive chemically and this reaction is likely to occur. Methyl mercury is 100 times more toxic than plain, elemental mercury and "is especially toxic to the brain and nerve tissue, which may explain amalgam's relationship to multiple sclerosis, epilepsy, and emotional disturbances." (32)

Children with attention deficit disorder are shown to have altered dopamine levels in their brain (dopamine is a neurotransmitter in the central nervous system). One study at Duke University Medical School has shown that even very low levels of methyl mercury result in dopamine and norepinephrine (a hormone) brain neurotransmitter changes. The researchers conclude that mercury exposure could produce both short-term and long-term effects on behavior and the growth of the organism exposed. (33)

Workers chronically exposed to mercury are shown to consistently have behavioral weaknesses along with short-term memory problems and mood-state problems. In a study in Singapore, 94 dentists and 54 people who were not dentists were evaluated. The dentists who had elevated mercury concentrations in the air in their office were found to have poorer scores in mood, finger tapping (reaction skills), logical memory, and visual reproduction. (34)

In a landmark study at the Rocky Mountain Research Institute, it was shown that amalgam mercury – from fillings – affects the neurotransmitters' uptake of dopamine, serotonin, acetylcholine, and norepinephrine. This points to a biochemical basis for why people who have silver amalgam dental fillings experience significantly higher levels of depression, excessive anger, and anxiety than those without such fillings. Low levels of serotonin are implicated in a lack of control, which may manifest as irritability, loss of temper, and explosive rage. The leader of the study, Robert L. Siblerud, suggests that in using amalgam, dentistry unwittingly may be contributing to this country's growing epidemic of depression, anger, anxiety, violence, alcoholism, the need to smoke, and other impulse disorders. (35)

Food for Thought

Dentists, although allowed to put silver amalgams into people's mouths, must dispose of scrap amalgam as a toxic waste following strict governmental guidelines and alert their dental hygienists of it's toxicity. It's illegal to put it in the garbage, sewer or down the drain. But it's okay to fill our children's cavities with it! If you want to get on your dentist's bad side, just ask him what he has to do with his scrap mercury fillings. Then ask him why.

Just to show you how far-reaching the effects of amalgams can be, consider the case of one woman who had hers removed: "With time, everything improved. Her complexion cleared, the bloating decreased, and she felt connected to her body again. Her thyroid became normal, she no longer felt pain in menstruation, her heart didn't hurt, and the schizophrenia was gone." (36)

At low doses, mercury exposure can produce impairments in language ability, attention, and memory; at high doses it can cause mental retardation, vision problems, and problems walking.

Hal Huggins, D.D.S., is a world-renowned expert on mercury, its use in dentistry and its effects on biological systems. He discovered many of the problems with mercury while working as a dentist himself. Although the American Dental Association says that silver amalgam fillings are safe, Huggins vehemently disagrees... "Does mercury pose a health problem? I can give you an unequivocal 'yes'..." He goes on to say that it's been proven that as mercury comes out of fillings, it forms a toxic compound in the mouth, methyl mercury, which is mercury's most poisonous form. Enough of this compound can cause illnesses. Those illnesses have been reduced or eliminated by amalgam removal.

An article in the *Journal of Orthomolecular Medicine* echoes his conclusions:

> The findings presented here suggest a correlation between many health complaints and mercury amalgam fillings. Removal of amalgam fillings results in significant improvement of these symptoms. These same symptoms which are improved or eliminated in amalgam-removal patients are present but undiagnosed in the general population. (37)

Of particular note is a section on mercury and how it can affect the unborn fetus, which may result in birth defects:

> It's bad enough that methyl mercury destroys our adult tissues, but it can also cross the placental barrier and do chromosomal damage early in life. The mechanism is simple. Mercury is attracted to what are called active sites on genetic code molecules called deoxyribonucleic acid (DNA). Chemicals react with other chemicals in the body by coming together in a docking mechanism, similar to a spacecraft at a space station. When mercury is in the vicinity, it can twist a molecule a few thousandths of a degree. Now when the molecule tries to dock with another molecule, it can't because the docking points no longer match... This defect can also prevent molecular reactions from taking place. The mercury sits on a spot where other specific molecules are supposed to park. It is impossible for two things to occupy the same space at the same time, so interference in molecular reactions occurs, causing a birth defect. (38)

Mercury stops the normal cellular division in mitosis of the developing fetus, causing an abnormal cell. If this new, abnormal cell is capable of reproduction, the abnormality may show up as a birth defect. Chromosomes can also be altered by mercury, since mercury is good at cleaving off segments of chromosomes so they don't contain the appropriate number of genes. If the chromosomal damage is in the heart or brain, a spontaneous abortion is probable. (39)

Dr. Huggins says:

> Just what could be the source of this mercury? The first three months of pregnancy is the time a baby is most susceptible to mercury-produced birth defects. Mercury from the mother's fillings can cross the placental barrier and do its damage within seconds. Enough animal research has been done over the years to indicate on exactly which day of pregnancy an exposure to mercury will produce a cleft palate in test cases. Why not share this information with pregnant women? While you should check with your obstetrician before you have any dental work done, I recommend having mercury fillings removed as soon as possible. (40)

Mercury in a filling not only gets into the bloodstream directly, but mercury vapor emitted from the filling can penetrate the mucousal lining of the mouth. A number of scientific studies indicate that from 20mcg/m3 to 150mcg/m3 (micrograms per cubic meter of air) may be found in the mouth of a person with amalgam fillings. One hundred mcg of mercury vapor is 500 times greater than the level the EPA says is safe and 3,300 times greater than the level regarded as an acute exposure by the Agency for Toxic Substances and Disease Registry (the ATSDR). In 1991, the World Health Organization stated that there is no known "no-observable-effect level" (NOEL) for mercury vapor. That means that any and all levels of mercury vapor are considered harmful. The ATSDR lists mercury as one of the top 20 most hazardous substances known to man. (41) And yet, we fill our babies' (and our own) teeth with it.

Huggins says it takes but a few atoms of mercury to create a birth defect and only one microgram to create other disturbances. One 16-year-old boy was chronically fatigued and could barely function. The removal of one small filling resulted in full teenage activity. One 11-year-old girl was having seizures every 15 minutes. Neurologists were baffled as to why. She had her amalgams removed, and within five days, her seizures stopped.

He also points out that mercury can deactivate zinc, which can not only contribute to birth defects, but also affect the development of children. Zinc is important for intelligence, bone growth and healing and, along with magnesium, is vital in the healing process. Zinc is also a key element in the insulin molecule, and a deficiency of it may contribute to diabetes (in children as well as adults). Zinc levels can also be decreased by the consumption of caffeine and alcohol.

Other symptoms of suspected reactions to dental materials include unexplained irritability, constant or very frequent periods of depression, unexplained chronic fatigue, difficulty with short-term memory, sudden unexplained or unprovoked anger, jumpiness, jitteriness, and nervousness, constant death wish or suicidal intent, frequent insomnia, and other behavioral and physiological problems. (42)

Food for Thought

In a recent development, on November 15, 2000, the judge of the Superior Court of California in San Francisco signed a consent decree that states there's a link between birth defects and silver-mercury dental fillings. A new law says this will have to be disclosed to California dental patients. This is a 180-degree turnaround from the American Dental Association's policy – still current – that silver mercury amalgams are safe and that any dentist who suggests otherwise to his patients can have his license revoked. In California, dentists with more than 10 employees must post this warning starting February 15, 2001:

WARNING:
Amalgam Fillings Contain a Chemical Element
Known to the State of California to Cause
Birth Defects or Other Reproductive Harm.

The Truth About Children's Health

(Interestingly, the California Dental Association refused to allow the word "mercury" to be used in this warning sign or while informing their patients of the risks.) (43)

Let's hope this awareness will spread across the country and new laws will be enacted in each state requiring similar warnings. Considering there are about 250,000 mercury fillings put into our mouths per day (down from one million per day in the 1970s due to the controversy over mercury toxicity), it's important not just for our own health, but the health of future generations. We need to promote awareness of this problem and how to avoid it. Sweden no longer allows mercury amalgams, and Germany has stated that no mercury should be placed in pregnant women or even in women who could become pregnant. It's a shame to think that a baby may be born deformed simply because some company wants to maintain its profit margin. I have had my fair share of work on my teeth, and I can tell you without hesitation that what goes on in your mouth has a big impact on your total health. My suggestion is to not have amalgams put into your teeth or the teeth of your child. There are many new materials that can be used instead that are just as effective and a lot less toxic. Find a dentist who understands the hazards of amalgams – these informed professionals are growing in number every day and it should not take you long to find one. If your child has amalgams already, have them removed by a dentist who is experienced and knows how to do it correctly. Some insurance companies will pay for this if you can justify it. Remember, mercury is a cumulative poison, and is not easily excreted from the body. Every bit of exposure to it builds up in your child's tissues and will have long-term effects.

Women are oftentimes encouraged to have their cavities filled (usually with mercury fillings) when they are pregnant. This is so they will be less likely to have the discomfort of an abscessed tooth during the final weeks just prior to delivery. This is tantamount to encouraging women to expose their fetus to mercury, which as we now know can cause birth defects.

See the Resource Guide and Chapter XIV for recommendations on how to get mercury, lead, and other heavy metals out of the body and how to find an informed dentist.

Mercury is also used in the preservative "thimerosal" in many vaccines. Huggins comments: "Thimerosol is the preservative in immunization shots, so anytime you get an immunization shot you are undergoing the same procedure that in the University Lab that we used to give animals auto-immune disease – give a little tiny injection of mercury. And when you get an immunization shot you are getting a little tiny dose of mercury there." (44) (Thimerosal is covered in more detail in the chapter on vaccines.)

PCBs

Polychlorinated biphenyls (PCBs) came on the scene in 1929 and are a class of toxic chemicals widely used in industry. They are known poisons and can have serious health effect on your child. They are so widespread that it's estimated that everyone living on this earth now has them in their systems.

A study published in the *New England Journal of Medicine* confirms that children exposed to low levels of PCBs in the womb grow up with poor reading comprehension, difficulty paying attention, memory problems, and low IQs. This study reports on a group of 11-year-old children whose mothers ate two to three meals per month of fish from Lake Michigan for at least six months prior to giving birth; Fish from Lake Michigan typically are contaminated with PCBs, mercury, and chlorinated organic chemicals. The researches analyzed PCB levels in the blood of the babies' umbilical cords providing a reliable measure of prenatal exposure. The overall fish consumption and the PCB level in the baby's blood both correlated with the baby's birth size. More fish consumed was linked to babies with reduced head size, diminished girth in the chest, shorter gestation periods, abnormally weak reflexes, less responsiveness to stimulation, and more jerky and unbalanced movement. These babies were clearly different from normal ones. The 242 children were followed from birth to age four. Upon testing at seven months, the babies with high exposure were determined to have memory problems that correlate with lower intelligence later in life. At four years of age, the more highly exposed children were uncooperative and balky when tested again, and refused to complete the exam. These were the children whose mother's had the highest levels of PCBs in their breast milk. Again, these children had the poorest memories. (45,46,47)

At age 11, the children were tested again. The 11 percent of the children whose mothers had the highest exposures had IQs 6.2 points lower than average. The highest exposed children were twice as likely to be at least two years behind their peers in word comprehension. The report stated: "Our IQ results indicate deficits in general intellectual ability, short-term and long-term memory, and focused and sustained attention."

It was determined that the children were harmed most by PCBs passing to them from their mothers prior to birth, and the mothers lifetime exposure to PCBs was more important than her fish-eating habits during pregnancy. Essentially, the exposure of females to PCBs at any time in their lives prior to having children may eventually cause mental deficits for their offspring. Other studies have reported similar results from PCB exposures, ranging from small size at birth to developmental disorders. The result is children with reduced attention span, diminished ability to handle stress, memory problems, and reading disabilities. (48,49,50,51)

Researcher Helen Daly of the Center for Behavioral Effects of Environmental Toxins at the State University of New York at Oswego has been studying humans and lab animals exposed to PCBs. She found that when rats were fed contaminated salmon from Lake Ontario, they overreacted to negative events such as mild electric shocks or disappointment at feeding time. Interestingly, the offspring of those rats showed the same pattern of altered responses to stress even though the offspring themselves were not fed contaminated fish. She wonders whether rats and children don't develop similar overreactions to stress after being exposed to PCBs while in the womb. (52)

The total world production of PCBs (excluding the Soviet Union) was 3.4 billion pounds or about 57 million pounds per year – between 1929 and 1989. Even after the U.S. banned PCBs in 1976, *world* production continued at 36 million pounds per year from 1980 to1984 and 22 million pounds per year from 1984 to 1989. And it is still being produced today.

PCBs are very stable in the environment and fat-soluble in the human body. They tend to move into the oceans over time, though only 1 percent of all PCBs have reached the oceans so far. Between 30 percent and 70 percent of PCBs manufactured over the years are still in use. And 30 percent of all PCBs in existence (about a billion pounds) are "lost"; that is, they cannot be accounted for. Another 30 percent are in landfills, in storage or in the sediments of lake, rivers, and estuaries. Considering that no one is trying to find the "lost" PCBs, it's likely that future generations will continue to be poisoned, at some level, by PCBs. (53)

Fluoride

Fluoride has been added to public water supplies since the 1940s in the belief that ingesting fluoride helps prevent cavities. It all started in 1939 when a dentist named H. Trendley Dean, working for the U.S. Public Health Service, said that high concentrations of fluoride in the water in certain areas of Texas corresponded to a high incidence of mottled teeth. (Mottled teeth are teeth with whitish flecks or spots, particularly the front teeth, or in severe cases, dark spots or stripes on the teeth.) Dean also said that there was a lower incidence of dental cavities in the communities having about 1 part per million (ppm) fluoride in their water supplies. Dean's report led to the fluoridation of drinking water at 1 ppm in order to supply the "optimal dose" of 1 mg fluoride per day if four glasses of water were drunk.

But Dean's original study suggesting fluoride ingestion was beneficial was flawed. When other scientists investigated Dean's data, they didn't reach the same conclusion. Dean was forced to state in court under oath that his data were invalid. In 1957 he admitted at an American Medical Association hearing that even waters containing a mere 0.1 ppm (0.1mg/l) could cause dental fluorosis, which is the first visible sign of fluoride overdose. And there has not been one single double-blind study indicating that fluoridation is effective in reducing cavities. (54)

Food for Thought

The EPA's Dr. William Hirzy says, "Clear back in 1934... the American Dental Association plainly treats the subject very matter-of-factly. It calls fluoride a general protoplasmic poison." And a 1944 article in the Journal of the American Dental Association said, "With 1.6 to 4 ppm fluoride in the water, 50 percent or more past age 24 have false teeth because of fluoride damage to their own." (55)

These do not sound like ringing endorsements for the fluoridation of drinking water. In fact, the idea of fluoride being good for people's teeth originated with the atomic bomb's Manhattan Project – the U.S. Military program to produce the first atomic bomb (prior to World War II there was no U.S. commercial production of fluorine). The fact that fluoride was beneficial constituted the government's cardinal defense against lawsuits stemming from an environmental contamination that took place from the DuPont chemical factory in Deepwater, New Jersey, in 1944. The factory was then producing millions of pounds of fluoride for the Manhattan Project. And one thing left over from manufacturing nuclear weapons and nuclear power is fluoride compounds. Instead of disposing of it properly, which costs money, our beloved government saw fit to turn a profit instead by promoting its use in water supplies.

Suddenly, fluoride was proclaimed as the "wonder nutrient" that stops cavities. As more and more industries found uses for fluorides, its wastes increased. Hirzy guesses that if fluoride were required to be disposed of properly as a waste product, the administrative costs of that disposal would exceed $100 million a year – for the fertilizer industry alone! Now you know why they want it in our water instead! John R. Lee, M.D., says of fluoride, "It's a toxic waste product of many types of industry; for instance, glass production, phosphate fertilizer production, and many others. They would have no way to dispose of the tons of fluoride waste they produce unless they could find some use for it, so they made up this story about it being good for dental health. Then they can pass it through everyone's bodies and into the sewer." (56)

It's interesting how the quest for better ways to kill and maim people can be turned on their heads and used for our "benefit." The production of deadly chemicals for chemical warfare in World War I and World War II led to our chemical pesticide industry. And the production of the atomic bomb has lead to fluoridation of our drinking water (same reason). Isn't mankind resourceful? Seems to me that if it kills, we shouldn't use it. But I always have had radical ideas (and I don't work for the government!).

There's evidence that suggests that fluoride in the water actually *increases* tooth decay. A study of 39,000 children ages five to 17 years conducted by the National Institute of Dental Research showed that children living in cities with fluoridated water had more tooth decay. And, when 1.0 ppm fluoride was added to the water supply there was a 5.4 percent increase in pediatric tooth decay. Another study examining 400,000 students showed that decay increased 27 percent when 1.0 ppm fluoride was increased in drinking water. (57) And it doesn't stop there as far as the health effects can go. Fluoride as sodium fluoride is another "cumulative toxin." That means it accumulates in the tissues and is not easily excreted by the body.

"Dental fluorosis" is the technical term for mottled teeth. Currently up to 80 percent of U.S. children have some degree of dental fluorosis, which has been shown to increase the likelihood of tooth decay.

Fluoride is added to toothpaste and public drinking water supplies for its supposed cavity- fighting property, but researchers have found that the ability of fluoride to prevent dental caries (cavities), if it exists at all, comes from using it topically, as in toothpaste. It has no identifiable beneficial effect when ingested. The Centers for Disease Control said in a 1999 report, "... laboratory and epidemiological research suggests that fluoride prevents dental caries predominately after eruption of the tooth into the mouth, and its actions primarily are topical for both adults and children." *Even the CDC* acknowledges that the effects of fluoride are "topical" and not "systemic," meaning that the addition of fluoride to drinking water supplies does not help prevent cavities. (58)

What exactly is fluoride and how can it affect your child? Its health effects can be profound and far-reaching and, as we shall see, it can contribute to ADHD, learning disabilities, lower IQs, along with other health problems.

Fluoride is actually a generic term given to a wide variety of substances that contain the element fluorine. Fluoride substances are used in a wide variety of industries including agricultural, pharmaceutical, ceramic and glass manufacturers, metallurgy, breweries and wineries, aluminum manufacturing, computer chip manufacturing, petroleum products, military, drugs (especially mood-regulating drugs such as Prozac), and others. In agriculture, fluoride is the key ingredient in the world's most widely used insecticides and pesticides and is used as a fumigant for termites.

Sodium fluoride is registered with the EPA as a rat poison and is also a powerful roach killer. Fluoride is used in the military in the production of nuclear warheads and in certain types of nerve gas, one of which – sarin gas – is 15 hundred times more deadly than cyanide. (59) According to the *Clinical Toxicology of Commercial Products, 5th Edition,* fluoride is rated as more toxic than lead. The U.S. Agency for Toxic Substances and Disease Registry (ATSDR) ranks fluoride compounds as among the top 20 of 275 substances that pose the most significant threat to human health. (60) So toxic is the raw fluoride added to drinking water that, according to William Hirzy, Ph.D., of the EPA, if you were to take a dose of it about half the size of a 500 milligram (mg) vitamin tablet, "you'd be long dead before the sun went down." (61)

The so called "cosmetic" defect of mottled teeth predisposes the person to tooth decay. But the health effects go much further than that. Dental fluorosis is merely the first visible sign of fluoride poisoning. Since fluoride is a cumulative poison, U.S. law requires that the Surgeon General set a Maximum Contaminant Level (MCL) for fluoride in public water supplies as determined by the EPA. That MCL is 4 parts per million (ppm) or 4 mg per liter, with the consideration that the body will retain half of this amount (2mg). They set this limit to avoid crippling skeletal fluorosis (CSF), which becomes severe when there's more than 4 mg/l in the water. A daily dose of 2mg to 8 mg of fluoride is known to cause severe CSF. (62,63) But did the EPA know this when they set the (too high) MCL?

Yes they did. In 1998 *EPA scientists* declared that this 4 ppm level was fraudulently set in a decision that omitted 90 percent of the data showing the mutagenic properties of fluoride. (64) Robert Carton, Ph.D., who worked for the EPA for 20 years, says that "on July 7, 1997, the EPA scientists, engineers and attorneys who assess the scientific data for the Safe Drinking Water Act standards and other EPA regulation have gone on record against the practice of adding fluoride to public drinking water." (65) And why is the EPA Maximum Contaminant Level (MCL) for fluoride 266 times greater than that of lead (4.0 parts per million for fluoride and 0.015 parts per million for lead)? Could it be that in order to add fluoride to drinking water they must make it appear less toxic?

William Hirzy explains that the negative health effects of fluoride are far more than just cosmetic: "What's going on in the teeth is a window to what's going on in the bones. What fluoride does in the hydroxyapatite structure in teeth it does to the same structure in bone. It is well known now that fluoride produces faulty bone, more brittle, basically mimicking in the bone what is clearly visible in the teeth." (66) Osteoporosis can result.

Food for Thought

You may hear, possibly from your dentist or other proponent of fluoridation, that fluoride is found in nature and nothing to be afraid of. The ADA slogan has been, "Nature thought of it first!" It's true that fluoride is found in nature in some waters – in the form of calcium fluoride, not the sodium fluoride we're talking about here. They are totally different in their chemistry and biological effects. Calcium fluoride does not readily dissolve in water; sodium fluoride does. Calcium fluoride is not retained in the body in great amounts; sodium fluoride is. Calcium fluoride is not toxic; and sodium fluoride is very toxic. The hydrofluorosilicic acid that is the direct byproduct of pollution scrubbers in the phosphate fertilizer and aluminum industries is even more toxic – and that is what's directly added to water supplies by our government. It has never been tested for safety even though it's listed as a Class I hazardous waste by the California Code of Regulations.

Phyllis Mullenix, Ph.D., conducted a detailed study of the neurological effects of fluoride. Her results were published in the Journal *Neurotoxicology and Teratology* in 1995. She discovered a pattern of behavioral problems associated with ingestion of fluoride that "... matches up with the same results of administering radiation and chemotherapy [to cancer patients]. All of these really nasty treatments that are used clinically in cancer therapy are well known to cause IQ deficits in children. That's one of the best studied effects they know of. The behavioral pattern that results from the use of fluoride matches that produced by cancer treatment that causes a reduction in intelligence." (67) This was the first study to show that the central nervous system output is vulnerable to fluoride, that it accumulates in the brain and that the effects on behavior depend on the age at exposure. Consequently, IQ, learning ability, and motor function may all suffer.

Mullenix's findings also showed that the developmental effects of fluoride affected the fetus as well: Doses of fluoride administered before birth produced marked hyperactivity in offspring. Postnatal administration caused the infant rats to exhibit what she calls the "couch potato syndrome" – the absence of initiative and activity.

Food for Thought

Phyllis Mullenix's ground breaking fluoride study was done on rats, not humans, but that's the best testing agent we have. Many scientific decisions are made using lab animals, particularly rats, as suitable subjects because their reactions mirror human ones. If we take this as possible in humans then, women who drink fluoridated water and ingest fluoride from other sources are more likely to have hyperactive children. And I wonder how much adults are affected by it, causing us to become a generation of "couch potatoes." It's very interesting that many drugs used to treat brain activity have fluoride as the primary active ingredient. Prozac (fluoxetene) is one of these and is used to treat depression in adults. As it's doing that, however, is it also making the person less intelligent and less likely to have initiative? More of a couch potato?

A 1995 study in China found attention deficit disorders in adults developed if sublingual drops containing 100 ppm (parts per million) of sodium fluoride were administered. Toothpastes typically contain 1,000 to 1,500 ppm fluoride and mouth rinses contain 230 to 900 ppm fluoride, well above the 100 ppm shown to be a problem in the Chinese study. This study also showed that at levels of 3 ppm to 11 ppm, fluoride can affect the nervous system without first causing physical malformations. (68) So you could be suffering from this poison with no telltale teethmarks.

Fluoride has also been implicated in hypothyroidism (low thyroid function) and in fact has been used in antithyroid medications prescribed when the thyroid is too active. It has an antagonistic effect on iodine and may even cause iodine deficiency. Iodine deficiency causes brain disorders, cretinism, miscarriages, and goiter and is considered to be the world's single most important and preventable cause of mental retardation, which affects 740 million people a year. (Good sources of iodine are the edible sea vegetables kelp and dulse found at health food stores. Iodized salt is *not* a good source.)

Robert Carton, the former EPA scientist, says there's research showing that a specific antibody (immunoglobulin - IgM) that is missing from patients with certain types of brain tumors is also missing from the blood of those who test as having elevated blood fluoride levels. This evidence leads to the theory that brain tumors are much more likely among individuals consuming fluoride compounds in their diet. (69)

You won't just get fluoride from your water and toothpaste. Hundreds of products on the market have significant levels of fluoride in them – partly because the water they use in processing and manufacturing is laden with fluoride, which gets into the mix. Among products with significant levels of fluoride are juices, colas, cereals, and baby juices. Most juice concentrates, including orange juice, are processed with fluoridated water. Almost every product with white grapes contains extremely high concentrations of fluoride because of the fluoride pesticide residues and processing with fluoridated water. Since many pesticides contain fluoride (because it's so deadly), it gives us another good reason to eat organic food.

When considering fluoride exposure, it's important to remember that you and your child can get it from a number of sources, not just drinking water. Eliminating all potential sources can only do good, since these toxic fluoride products are certainly not needed in any amounts by anyone, especially young and developing children.

Chlorine and Other Drinking Water Contaminants

Another chemical added to drinking water is chlorine, which eliminates or reduces the presence of bacteria and other microorganisms that may cause health problems if left unchecked. According to the Centers for Disease Control, about 940,000 Americans get sick and 900 die each year from waterborne microbial illness caused by contaminated tap water. (70) Another estimate by Tufts University Medical School and the EPA estimate that there are over seven million cases of waterborne diseases a year. (71) However, there is a growing concern that our water treatment methods are no longer adequate. Most treatment plants use pre-World War I technology, which employs sedimentation, filtration, coagulation, and chlorine disinfection. But the many byproducts of our modern chemical age such as synthetic organic industrial chemicals and pesticides often pass through these treatment plants unabated. A growing body of evidence indicates that a number of chemicals commonly found in tap water could be associated with cancer, reproductive effects, and developmental effects. The addition of chlorine to drinking water can also contribute to hardening of the arteries, can destroy proteins in the body, irritates the skin and sinuses, and can aggravate asthma, allergies, and respiratory problems. It's well documented that the levels of chlorine in tap water have been shown to present numerous serious health challenges.

The most common byproduct of drinking water treatment practices is the class of chemicals called "trihalomethanes" (THMs). They arise from the interaction of chlorine used to kill bacteria in the treatment plant and decomposing plant matter, naturally occurring humic and fulvic acids and other organic chemicals in the water. The federal drinking water regulations limit the total THMs in tap water to 100 parts per billion (ppb) in systems serving 10,000 people or more. (72)

Especially relevant for our discussion is that infants, children and pregnant women may be more susceptible to the effects of contaminants in drinking water than normal healthy adults. A recent study conducted in Norway indicated that byproducts in drinking water treated with chlorination may raise risks for birth defects. The report said the overall risk for birth defects rose by 14 percent in towns with both chlorinated water and water with a high amount of organic material (which would encourage the formation of THMs). Especially high were the risks for urinary tract birth defects: babies born in areas of high THMs had double the risk of urinary tract malformations. Also, there was a 26 percent rise in the risks for serious neural tube defects. (Neural tube defects are defects such as spina bifida, potentially paralyzing in which the spinal cord is not properly enclosed by the bone of the spine.) (73) The Agency for Toxic Substances and Disease Registry published a study in January 1998 showing that serious birth defects (neural tube defects) are associated with THM ingested from drinking water. (74) Chlorination byproducts (THMs) are also implicated strongly for causing bladder cancer and may cause colon and rectal cancer and brain tumors as well. (75)

In a study by the California Department of Health, 5,144 pregnant women were tracked and their drinking water habits studied. The outcomes of their pregnancies were compared with the amount and type of water they drank along with the total amount of THMs in the water. Sixteen percent of women drinking five or more glasses of water per day containing more than 75 ppb THMs had miscarriages. Only 9.5 percent of women who were drinking water with lower concentrations of THMs miscarried. The likelihood of spontaneous abortions was 1.8 times greater in the high-THM consumption group than the low-THM consumption group. In a similar study in central North Carolina, women were 2.8 times more likely to have a miscarriage if they had high exposure to THMs during pregnancy. (76)

Contamination by THMs can occur not only from drinking the water, but from indoor air pollution as well. Since THMs are volatile, they readily evaporate into the air. When you shower, flush the toilet, wash dishes and clothes, and so on, you can introduce these THMs into the household air. And even THMs in the *air* can contribute to neural tube defects in babies whose mothers had a high exposure. (77)

Hazards Our Children Face

These studies looked at long-term exposures to THMs. But according to Erik Olson, a water quality expert with the Natural Resources Defense Council (NRDC), short-term exposures may be very important too and can also contribute to spontaneous abortions, fetal deaths, and serious birth defects. He says, "We may be totally overlooking the risk of short-term exposure." (78)

EPA officials admit they have no idea how many U.S. water systems exceed the federal limit of 100 ppb. But they do say that THMs increase during the summer months, sometimes to twice their normal level. So it's best not to take chances. Chlorine can be removed by a simple filtration unit on your faucet and shower. For drinking, letting the water stand for several minutes allows the THMs to evaporate.

Fluoride and chlorine byproducts are not the only thing in drinking water that may cause health problems. As already discussed, pesticides may pollute a municipal water supply or drinking water well. In addition, Volatile Organic Chemicals (VOCs) found in solvents, degreasers, adhesives, gasoline additives, and such may contain benzene, trichloroethylene (TCE), toluene and vinyl chloride which have been shown to cause cancer, central nervous system disorders, liver and kidney damage, reproductive disorders, and birth defects. (79)

In Woburn, Massachusetts, in the 1980s, 21 children contracted leukemia (cancer of the blood) because the town's drinking water was contaminated from a shallow industrial injection well and dump, allowing VOCs to enter the reservoir. (The families' struggles were documented in the movie A Civil Action.) It's been shown that brain, nervous system cancers, and acute lymphocytic leukemia represent the majority of cancers attacking children – and clusters of higher than normal incidences of these diseases have been shown in areas with high VOCs in the drinking water. (80)

Philip Landrigan, chair of the department of community and preventive medicine at Mount Sinai School of Medicine in New York City, says, "I have no doubt certain VOCs in drinking water can cause cancer in children." Carolyn Poppell, program coordinator on safe drinking water for the Physicians for Social Responsibility concurs: "The concern we have is that drinking water standards are not protective of the public's health, particularly children." (81)

Oftentimes industries will get rid of their wastes by deep well injection. Sometimes they do it right, sometimes they don't. Also, ground water aquifers are very unpredictable, and leakage from one to another is possible. Dumps can also accept waste from industries, municipalities, and homes. A 1997 federal Agency for Toxic Substances and Disease Registry report noted that there are over 1,300 Superfund sites (waste dumps that are so toxic, they have to be cleaned up using masks and special clothing and equipment). The report stated that over 41 million Americans live within four miles of these toxic land dumps and are more susceptible to an increase of these toxic chemicals in their drinking water. There are over 436,000 hazardous waste sites nationwide. (82) Many dangerous chemicals can leach into the ground water from these also, not to mention pollution due to agricultural practices.

Just because you may get your water from a well does not mean it's clean water. It's always best to get it checked and treat it if needed. After all, your body is more that 70 percent water. If you give it the wrong kind, you cannot get healthy. Neither can your children. Consider this: The EPA monitors 80 substances and has drinking water limits for some of these. However, there are over 75,000 chemicals produced in the U.S. and data exists for only *7 percent* of the 2,700 most widely used chemicals on health effects on humans. The EPA's drinking water limits are not designed to protect children, because they are extrapolated from animal studies and based on an adult male's body weight and water consumption. As I've mentioned several times, children are more sensitive and vulnerable than adults since their enzyme systems and organs of detoxification are not fully developed. Play it safe and get a water filter or other water treatment system.

Inorganic contaminants may also be present in drinking water. They may include arsenic, barium, chromium, lead, mercury, and silver, which can cause acute poisoning, cancer, learning disabilities, and other health problems. (83) In a 1999 study by the National Academy of Sciences, arsenic in drinking water can cause bladder, lung, and skin cancer and may also cause kidney and liver cancer. The EPA estimates that in 25 states, more than 34 million Americans drink tap water which contains arsenic levels that pose unacceptable cancer risks. The Natural Resources Defense Council (NRDC) considers it likely that in those 25 states, as many as 56 million people have been drinking water with arsenic at unsafe levels.

The current national standard for arsenic in drinking water is 50 parts per billion (ppb). That standard was set in 1942 *before it was discovered that arsenic causes cancer.* The National Academy of Sciences estimates that 1 person out of 100 drinking water with this amount of arsenic in it will develop cancer (based on drinking 2 liters of water a day). This is an extremely high risk considering that standards are usually set so that the risk is 1 in 10,000. And although Congress ordered the EPA to update the arsenic standard in 1974 and again in 1986, they failed to do so. (84) The new proposed arsenic standard of 10 ppb is scheduled to go into effect in 2006.

Many filters can remove arsenic. Be sure the filter is certified by NSF International (800-NSF-MARK). Distillation also removes arsenic, as does reverse osmosis.

Another common contaminant in drinking water is nitrate. Nitrate (NO3) is a naturally occurring form of nitrogen found in soil and essential for plant growth. It is very soluble and easily leaches into ground water. Nitrogen compounds are used in most fertilizers, can come from animal feedlots, municipal wastewater and sludge, and septic systems. With the intensive agricultural practices used these days, nitrates can easily contaminate drinking water supplies. The National Pesticide Survey in 1992 detected nitrates in 57 percent of domestic wells and 52 percent of community wells. It was reported that some 22,500 infants drinking domestic well water were estimated to be exposed to levels of nitrates exceeding the EPA safe drinking water limits; for community systems, the number was estimated to be 43,500 infants. (85)

Nitrate is associated with "blue baby syndrome" in infants. This syndrome was far more common in and before the 1940's, but is still possible today. "Blue baby syndrome," the common name for methemoglobinemia, occurs most often in infants under six months of age whose stomach acid is not as strong as older children's and adult's. This allows a higher level of bacteria in their stomach that can easily convert nitrate to nitrite. Nitrite causes hemoglobin to be converted to methemoglobin, which does not carry oxygen well, and which babies cannot convert back to hemoglobin. This results in a reduced oxygen supply to vital tissues and organs such as the brain. When this happens, the infant will look blue (even indigo) – especially around the eyes and mouth. Methemoglobin can be changed back to hemoglobin in adults, potentially stopping this from happening, but again, not in infants. Severe cases of methemoglobinemia can cause brain damage and death.

A study in the Britain suggested that high nitrate levels also can cause juvenile diabetes. In rural areas where the nitrate levels in water were high, so were the incidences of juvenile diabetes. Nitrosamine, a breakdown product of nitrates, is known to cause diabetes in animals and has been linked to cancer, thyroid problems, and birth defects. Again, infants and young children are believed to be especially vulnerable to nitrate exposure.

There are other, less severe symptoms of methemoglobinemia: headaches, dizziness, weakness, and difficulty in breathing. The condition can be easily treated with an injection of methylene blue at a hospital emergency room.

Pregnant women, adults with reduced stomach acid and people deficient in the enzyme that converts methemoglobin back to normal hemoglobin are especially susceptible to nitrate-induced methemoglobinemia. Infants should not be allowed to consume drinking water or any other drink (including formula preparations) with a nitrate concentration above 10 mg/l NO3-N or 45 mg/l NO3 (these are two different ways to report nitrates, so when you have your water tested, be sure you know which value is being reported). (86)

Although infant deaths from "blue baby syndrome" are now quite rare (only one reported between 1960 to 1972), decreased oxygen in the blood cannot be beneficial to your baby – especially to its vulnerable, developing brain. You can remove nitrates from your water using distillation, reverse osmosis, and ion exchange methods or blending with non-contaminated water to get the concentration down to acceptable levels (use this method only in emergency situations). Charcoal filters and water softeners don't remove nitrates from water that well. Boiling the water does not make it better either, and actually *increases* the concentration of nitrates.

Since public water supplies – and many private water supplies such as wells – have become so contaminated, many people have been buying bottled water thinking it is cleaner. This is not necessarily the case, however, according to a four-year study by the NRDC. Their study included testing more than 1,000 bottles of 103 brands of bottled water. Most of the water was found to be of high quality, but about one third of the waters contained levels of contamination exceeding allowable limits. And realize bottled water products are not subject to the same rigorous testing and purity standards as those that apply to city tap water.

Here are some findings of the study:

- 25 percent to 40 percent of the bottled water produced in the U.S. comes directly from municipal water systems (even though the advertising and bottle label may claim otherwise).

- 33 percent of the bottled water tested contained bacteria (bottled water is not required to be disinfected).

- 25 percent of bottled water samples contained known carcinogens.

- 20 percent of the bottled water samples contained harmful industrial chemicals.

- Bottled water can cost between 240 and 10,000 times more per gallon than tap water.

The NRDC concluded that bottled water regulations are inadequate to assure consumers of either purity or safety, and buying bottled water is not necessarily safe. (87) It's best to buy bottled water that is "bottled at the source," such as Perrier.

Pesticides

In 1993 the National Academy of Sciences released its long-awaited report on the health hazards of pesticides to infants and young children. They stated that pesticides are harmful to the environment and are known or suspected to be toxic to humans. They are neurologically toxic, and can cause cancer, reproductive dysfunction, and dysfunction of the immune and endocrine systems. (88)

No allowable daily intakes have been calculated for infants, but recall that infants are much more susceptible to toxic chemicals than adults because their kidneys, liver, enzyme system, and blood-brain barrier are not fully developed. In addition, a newborn has very little body fat available for storage, so any fat-soluble chemicals are circulated in the blood throughout the body for longer periods, thus possibly impacting other organs.

Pesticides have been used for centuries. They were mostly natural ones until World Wars I and II, when synthetic chemicals were first manufactured for warfare. This proved to be the watershed for the modern agri-chemical industry since these chemicals later ended up on the farm to control pests. Why? Because these chemicals kill. In fact, one of the reasons the use of chemical pesticides were encouraged and touted was because the chemical companies wanted to find a use for all the leftover chemicals used for warfare after the wars. Instead of having to dispose of these poisons, they found a way to make a profit from them. (As we shall see, not only do they do this with pesticides and fluoride, but also with irradiating foods.)

German scientists, while experimenting with nerve gas during World War II, synthesized parathion, the first organophosphorous insecticide. It was first marketed in 1943 and is still widely used today. In the 1950s and 1960s, these kinds of chemicals became major pest control agents. By 1996, an estimated $26 billion worth of pesticides were used around the world. In 1939 Swiss chemist Paul Muller discovered the deadly properties of DDT (he later won a Nobel Prize for this). (89)

The term "pesticide" includes more than just insecticides, which is what most people think of when they hear the term. Actually, a pesticide refers to not only insecticides but many other kinds of chemicals. A pesticide is any substance intended to control, destroy, repel or attract a pest. They may be natural (for example, a living, pest-destroying organism such as Bacillus thuringiensis) or synthetic – like most of the pesticides we are familiar with.

Pesticides, due to their widespread use and mobility in the environment, are a major player in the toxic chemical debacle. A National Institute of Health Sciences research project found that in a large random sample of the general population, DDT was evident in 100 percent of the blood samples at an average level of 3.3 ppb (parts per billion). Chlordane (used for termite control, which seeps up into the living airspace) was found in 95 percent of the population. Other pesticides were also found in significant amounts, many of the type used on food. (90) Each year some 3.5 billion pounds of industrial toxins and one billion to two billion pounds of pesticides are released into the environment in the United States alone, according to the EPA.

Millions of Americans are being exposed to chemicals whose effects are unknown. Eighty percent of the chemicals now in use have never been tested for their carcinogenic, neurotoxic, immunotoxic or other toxic effects. (91)

Considering the lethal properties of such chemicals, pesticides being a major player, you would think their use might decline in inverse proportion to what we learn about them. But consider:

- There are 400 pesticides currently on the market that were registered before being tested to determine if they caused cancer, birth defects or wildlife toxicity.

- The amount of time it takes to ban a pesticide in the U.S. using present procedures is 10 years.

- There are 107 active ingredients in pesticides found to cause cancer in animals or humans. Of these, 83 are still in use today.

- There are 14 pesticides found to cause reproductive problems in animals.

- Thirty-eight percent of all food samples the FDA tested in 1980 contained pesticide residues. Of the 496 pesticides identified as likely to leave residues on food, the percentage the FDA tests can routinely detect is only 40 percent.

- Nationally, the EPA estimates that one out of every 10 public drinking water wells contains pesticides, as well as over 440,000 rural private wells. At a minimum, 1.3 million people drink water contaminated with one or more pesticide.

- Fifty percent of the U.S. population gets its water supply from ground water. Some 14 million people in the U.S. routinely drink water contaminated with carcinogenic herbicides. Seventy-four different pesticides documented by the EPA were present in ground water in 1988, in 32 states. Forty-six percent of all U.S. counties containing ground water are susceptible to contamination from agricultural pesticides and fertilizers.

- The highest rate of chemical-related illnesses of any occupational group in the U.S. is among farm workers, with approximately 300,000 cases reported each year. There are an estimated 10,400 cancer deaths related to pesticides each year. (92,93)

In April 1999, researchers in Switzerland reported that the rain falling on Europe contained such high levels of pesticides that the rainwater would be illegal if it were supplied as drinking water. It's contaminated with atrazine, alochlor and other common agricultural poisons sprayed onto crops. (94)

Atrazine is a weed killer used on 96 percent of the corn grown in the U.S. It was introduced in 1958 and some 68 million to 73 million pounds were used in 1995 alone, making it the best-selling pesticide in the nation. But it may kill more than pests. It interferes with the hormone systems of mammals, and two studies have suggested that it causes ovarian cancer in humans. The EPA lists it as a "possible human carcinogen." Atrazine is found in much of the drinking water in the Midwestern U.S. and is measurable in corn, milk, beef, and other foods. (95)

Childhood leukemias, lymphomas, neuroblastomas, and brain cancers have all been linked to pesticides as dozens of studies have shown. Considering this fact, there is a conspicuous absence of information on pesticide exposures and toxicity relating to children. (96)

Consumer Report magazine announced in February 1998 that many fruits and vegetables in the U.S. carry pesticide residues that exceed the limits that the EPA considers safe for children and that even one serving of some fruits and vegetables can exceed safe daily limits for young children. The U.S. Department of Agriculture took 27,000 food samples from 1994 to 1997 and looked at foods children are most likely to eat. Almost all the foods tested for pesticide residues were within legal limits, but were frequently well above the levels the Environmental Protection Agency says are safe for young children. (97)

Organophosphates (such as methyl parathion) are neurological poisons and work the same on humans as they do on insects. This insecticide accounts for most of the total toxicity on the foods that were analyzed, particularly peaches, frozen and canned green beans, pears, and apples – many foods children commonly eat. Late in 2000 the EPA stated that methylparathion posed an "unacceptable risk" but that it had not taken any action to ban it or reduce its use.

Another interesting point the *Consumer Report* study found was that U.S.-grown foods had, in almost every case, higher pesticide levels than imported foods and more toxic ones at that.

Food for Thought

Some say that pesticides are needed to feed the world. If it weren't for them, they argue, we couldn't grow enough food for everyone, and farming would be too labor-intensive, thus making food too expensive. One researcher estimates that if it weren't for pesticides, we would still have 10 percent to 12 percent of the population working on farms rather than the mere 2 percent now needed to produce enough food to sustain the U.S. population. (I wonder what would be wrong with that?) But consider that since the early 1930s the federal government has maintained a "price support" program, paying farmers not to grow certain crops, with the intent of keeping the price of food artificially high. The logic here is that since American agriculture is so productive that, without price supports, the abundance of crops which are reaching record yields, coupled with the law of supply and demand, would drive the price of food so low that many farmers couldn't survive, which ultimately might endanger the nation's food supply. Price supports started in the 1930s, a decade or two before chemical pesticides ever made the scene in any significant amount. Seems to me that if we were producing so much food back then without pesticides, so much so that we had to pay farmers not to grow food to keep the prices high, the crops must have been doing just fine without the "help" of toxic chemicals. Also, there are now many farmers that use strictly "organic" methods to grow food. Yes, the "organically raised food" is a bit more expensive. But if all the farms operated this way, would not competition and the law of supply and demand bring down the price of the food?

It's ironic that the manufacturers and sellers of pesticides say that there would not be enough food were it not for pesticides. Mass starvation might result, they tell us. But in a few years (and I mean a few), if we keep going in the same direction, we're all going to starve anyway because while there may be plenty of food, none of it will be edible because it will all be poisoned! Do you doubt this? Then why is it that the occupation with the highest rate of chemical poisonings is farmers?

Children are exposed to pesticides in many ways besides from food: pet collars; shampoos for pets for fleas, ticks and lice; pesticides used on lawns; in the garden; and around the home. And pesticides tend to settle on the floor, where children mostly play. A recent study revealed a strong relationship between brain cancers and compounds used to kill fleas and ticks. (98)

One study of chlorpyrifos (trade name Dursban) residues in a home showed that after treatment and a recommended ventilation period (on the government-approved label), pesticide residues were detected on the surfaces of children's plastic and cloth toys for two full weeks. Chlorpyrifos is one of the most commonly used pesticide in the United States. It is a potent nerve poison. One fifth of an ounce is all that's needed to kill an adult. (99)

In a study published in the November 1996 issue of *Environmental Science and Technology* (a monthly journal of the American Chemical Society), it was reported that outdoor pesticides, once carried inside on shoes and pets, can linger for long periods. The pesticides attach to house dust and accumulate in carpets, upholstered furniture, draperies, and on household surfaces. Since they are now protected from sun, rain, wind, and temperature extremes, the outdoor pesticides, which only last days or weeks outdoors, can persist for years. And, while exposure levels may be below the limit established by the World Health Organization for adults, the risk levels for children have not been established. And vacuuming only eliminates about one third of the contamination. If you use these products, it's good to remove your shoes at the door, and leave the pets outside. (100) The best thing is to avoid exposing your beloved pet to chemical pesticides – use natural products.

Chlorpyrifos (Dursban) is the common pesticide for flea treatment. Richard A. Fenske, Ph.D. and assistant professor at Rutgers University, conducted a study that showed that after recommended procedures were followed in applying the pesticide to carpets in an unoccupied apartment, levels of the pesticide in the "infant breathing zone" were ten times above the legal limit after seven hours and over three times the legal limit after 24 hours. Pesticide applicators typically state it is safe to return home "several hours" after the application. Please consider that the "legal limit" is not necessarily the actual limit at which adverse effects would not occur. (101)

According to the *Journal of the National Cancer Institute,* pet dogs exposed to the weed killer 2,4-D are dying of cancer at twice the normal rates. Dogs walk across or roll in herbicide-treated lawns and then ingest these toxic chemicals when they lick their coats or paws. The most popular lawn-care products contain 2,4-D. (102) Of course, children play on lawns too. So they will come in contact with the chemicals outside, and also track them into the house.

About 600 million pounds of 2,4-D are spread on American soil each year by homeowners and farmers. (Interestingly, federal law does not allow exact data to be gathered.) (103) It's used by homeowners to control crab grass and dandelions and by farmers on potatoes, tomatoes, rice, corn, sorghum, and other crops to keep weeds down.

Again, this deadly chemical has a wartime connection: 2,4-D was mixed with 2,4,5-T to create "Agent Orange" and was used from 1962 to 1971 during the Vietnam War to defoliate the jungle where the Vietcong were living. But they were not its only victims. *The American Journal of Public Health* reports that Vietnam veterans are 70 percent more likely to father children with one or more major birth defects compared with men with no military service. The article fails to say if exposure to the herbicide was the most important cause. (104)

Throughout the U.S., approximately 75 percent of houses built before 1988 contain air levels of the pesticide chlordane, a common pesticide used for termite control. Thirty-four percent contain levels over the safety limit of 5 micrograms per cubic meter of air (set by the National Academy of Sciences). (105) An estimated 10 million to 20 million U.S. residents could be breathing chlordane levels that exceed the recommended safe limit. Chlordane contamination is linked to childhood cancers and blood disorders. David Ozonoff, Ph.D., of the Boston University School of Public Health, says, "A national program for monitoring all homes treated is urgently needed to detect persistent contamination." He went on to say, "...It should also be noted that commercial chlordane formulations contain carcinogenic 'inert ingredients' and contaminants, such as propylene oxide, hexachlorobutadiene, and carbon tetrachloride, apart from some 40 other ingredients so far undisclosed by the manufacturer, formulators, and applicators of chlordane/heptachlor." (106)

In 1987, 250 adults and children were exposed to chlordane when building surfaces and soil around their apartment complex were sprayed. Subsequent testing showed many negative effects upon mental function from low levels of air chlordane in their apartments. Test scores for reaction time, balance, and memory were lower and scores were worse for depression, anger, vigor, fatigue, and mood states. Also, these chlordane-exposed people had more asthma, allergies, chronic bronchitis, wheezing, headaches, and indigestion. The researchers wrote: "Examination of subjects exposed in their homes to chlordane... showed significant, and we suggest important, impairment of both the neurophysiological and psychological functions including mood states. These impairments include probably irreversible dysfunction of the brain... chlordane use should be prohibited worldwide." (107)

Americans put about 62.7 million pounds of pesticides and 278.5 million pounds of antimicrobials (disinfectants) into their homes each year. A recent study estimated that between 78 percent and 97 percent of families (in the Midwestern U.S.) use pesticides in and around the home. A study in Jacksonville, Florida, detected pesticides in the air in 100 percent of the homes. (108)

And it's not just around the home that pesticide use is a problem. A study by Yale University researchers and Environment & Human Health Inc. found that 87 percent of schools apply pesticides on school grounds and in classrooms, often while children are on the premises. (109)

Farmers have an increased incidence of certain kinds of cancer (soft-tissue carcinomas such as non-Hodgkin's lymphomas and malignant lymphomas, the same type of cancer the dogs got when exposed to treated lawns). These cancers are on the rise in the general population as well. In fact, non-Hodgkin's lymphomas (NHL) were the second fastest-growing type of cancer in the U.S. in the 1980s and 1990s, increasing at the rate of 3.3 percent per year between 1973 and 1991. Two well-known Swedish scientists, Mikael Eriksson and Lennart Hardell, published a study in March 1999 showing that non-Hodgkin's lymphoma (NHL) is linked to pesticide exposure. One of the herbicides linked to NHL by this study is Roundup (glyphosate), a popular herbicide promoted as a safe spot-killer for weeds.

A previous study in 1998 implicated Roundup in hairy cell leukemia (cancer of the blood-forming organs). Several other animal studies have shown that

Roundup can cause gene mutations and chromosomal damage. (110,111) Jonathan D. Buckley, Ph.D., of the University of Southern California in Los Angeles conducted a study that showed that children whose mothers used pesticides in the home once or twice a week were nearly two and a half times as likely to have non-Hodgkin's lymphoma. If the pesticides were used on a daily basis, the children were seven times more likely to get this kind of cancer. Pregnant women exposed to pesticides by professional exterminators in their homes were three times more likely to have a child with that cancer and children directly exposed to pesticides were just over twice as likely to develop the disease. This from the December 2000 issue of the journal *Cancer*. (112)

A very interesting article about pesticides and aggression was published by the *Environmental Research Foundation* on April 29, 1999. It linked aggression with the use of pesticides. One study the article cited was a five-year-long investigation that looked at the possible effects of low levels of insecticides, weed killers, and artificial fertilizers on the behavior patterns in the test animals. The study concluded that:

> [The] combinations of these chemicals – at levels similar to those found in the ground water of agricultural areas of the U.S. - have measurable detrimental effects... [There were] effects on the endocrine system (thyroid hormone levels) and the immune system, and reduced body weight, from mixtures of low levels of aldicarb and nitrate, atrazine & nitrate, and atrazine, aldicarb and nitrate together... increased aggression from exposure to atrazine and nitrate, and from atrazine, aldicarb and nitrate together...

> Some, though not all, studies have shown that attention deficit and/or hyperactivity disorders in children are linked to changes in the levels of thyroid hormone in the blood. Children with multiple chemical sensitivity (MCS) have abnormal thyroid levels. Furthermore, irritability and aggressive behavior are linked to thyroid hormone levels... (113)

A recent study of four- and five-year-old children in Mexico specifically noted a decrease in mental ability and an increase in aggressive behavior among children exposed to pesticides. This study reported:

> Some valley children (exposed to pesticides) were observed hitting their siblings when they passed by, and they became easily upset or angry with a minor corrective comment by a parent. These aggressive behaviors were not noted in the pesticide-free-foothills children. The pesticide-exposed children had far less physical endurance in a test to see how long they could keep jumping up and down; they had inferior hand-eye coordination; and they could not draw a simple stick figure of a human being, which the upland children could readily do. (114)

Americans are searching for the causes of violence in their society. Some blame a decline in religious upbringing and others point to the fact that many times both parents work and no one is minding the kids. Violent movies and violence on TV, extremist Internet sites, and readily available cheap guns all contribute. But no one seems to be asking whether pesticides, fertilizers, and other toxins may be affecting our young people's mental and emotional balance and social adjustment. Former U.S. Surgeon General C. Everett Koop comments, "Regarding violence in our society as purely a sociologic matter, or one of law enforcement, has led to an unmitigated failure. It is time to test further whether violence can be amenable to medical/public health interventions." (115)

Monsanto, the company that produces Roundup, has been working on genetically engineering crops such as potatoes, corn, and soybeans to withstand the effects of Roundup. The goal is to create crops that are not affected by Roundup so that unusually large quantities of this pesticide can be applied to eradicate weeds without harming the crops. It's estimated that 20 million more pounds of toxic herbicide per year are being sprayed on American soybean fields because of this. More pesticide sales means increased profits. In 2000, Monsanto's total sales were $5.5 billion, and $2.6 billion of this was from the sale of herbicides and pesticides like Roundup. (116)

Genetic modification (GM), also called genetic engineering (GE), is where certain genes of one plant are transferred into another plant in order to have that second plant express certain traits. Some traits aren't expressed right away – they may be latent for a dozen generations. Those traits may be harmful to humans. We, then, become the experiment.

Genetic modification of crops is becoming widespread in America – more than 58 million acres are now planted with GM crops. In 1996, that figure was just six million (most all soybeans are now genetically modified). But not everyone agrees it's beneficial. Japan and most European countries are opposed to the sale of GM produce. Switzerland destroyed 500 tons of chocolate when they learned it contained GM soy lecithin. All GM foods sold in the European Union (EU) must be labeled and the entire EU and India have stopped allowing experimentation with GM foods in the field until more is known about long-term effects. Thailand and Sri Lanka have taken it a step further and banned GM foods completely. Americans are starting to speak up too. A petition with 500,000 signatures was presented in Washington D.C. in June, 1999, that demanded congress and the FDA require GM foods be labeled. So far, no response. The manufacturers of GM foods say they are safe and even beneficial. How can they say that when no long term studies have been done?

There is one bright spot in all this madness. Gerber, the nation's largest baby food manufacturer said in 1999 that it was going to stop using GM foods. (117) That's good, since we not only don't know enough about GM foods, but also so much more pesticide is used on them that they cannot be any better for your child.

Amazingly, there's more to fear in a pesticide than the "active ingredient" alone. Of the 600 million pounds of 2,4-D used in the United States each year, 60 million pounds of it are "active" ingredients (i.e., 2,4-D) and about 540 million pounds of it are "inert" ingredients. For example, an inert ingredient may be an oily substance that prevents rain from washing the poison away. A typical pesticide is 1 percent to 20 percent active ingredients and 80 percent to 99 percent inert ingredients.

The U.S. EPA Office of Pesticides and Toxic Substances lists 2,000 chemicals that have been approved for use as inert ingredients. Those so called "inert" ingredients can include such known poisons as carbon tetrachloride, chloroform, chloroethane, xylene, cadmium, and lead. Federal pesticide law does not require chemical companies to disclose what those inert ingredients really are. More shocking than that is that federal law levies a $10,000 penalty for any government employee who reveals the make-up of inert ingredients in pesticides. (118) If that's not all, a little known exemption in the RCRA (the nation's basic hazardous waste law) allows hazardous wastes to be "recycled" into pesticides as inert ingredients. Therefore, it's legal to put known carcinogens, mutagens, and teratogens into pesticides that will be sprayed all across the country.

How does the EPA account for this? EPA press officer Al Hire told a reporter that allowing recycled hazardous waste in pesticides is "a way of disposing of hazardous materials." (119)

So no one will ever know that the thing they use to get rid of their dandelions not only contains the pesticide (bad enough by itself), but has other carcinogenic ingredients as well. Considering our children's playing, getting in the dirt, touching their mouths, noses and eyes, their risk of exposure to these kinds of recognized carcinogenic compounds is increased.

Since many of you reading this are women, or perhaps the fathers of female children, and to make another point about toxic chemicals and cancer, I would like to bring to your attention the relationship of toxic chemicals to breast cancer.

Female breast cancer has increased 58 percent during the past 35 years. This is despite better diagnoses (mammography) being made. In 1940, an American woman's lifetime risk of getting breast cancer was one in 16. Today it is one in eight.

Every year more than 175,900 American women discover they have breast cancer and every year 44,500 die of it. They lose an average of 19 years of life because of it. (120)

A Japanese women living in Japan has about one quarter as much of a chance of getting breast cancer. But when Japanese women move to America, by the second generation, their risk of breast cancer has risen to "normal" American levels. We must conclude that something in the environment, not genetics, is at work here.

In Israel, deaths from breast cancer in young women less than 44 years old in the 1960s and 1970s began to sharply increase. Then, the death rate from breast cancer in women 44 or younger dropped between 1976 and 1989: but the death rate among older Israeli women continued to rise. That was an unusual pattern. Was there an explanation?

There was. In the 1970s, measurements of three carcinogenic pesticides in cow's milk and human milk in Israel found levels five to 1,000 times higher than in the U.S. These contaminants were Lindane, DDE (a chemical created when

DDT breaks down in the environment) and alpha-BHC. Cow's milk and human tissues were all found to be heavily contaminated with these. Finally, in 1978, after public protests, Israel banned these pesticides. By 1980, breast milk contamination had dropped 90 percent or more among the Israeli women. (121)

Could these pesticides have caused the unusual breast cancer pattern in Israel? Many scientists think so. A recent study in America showed women with breast cancer have significantly elevated levels of DDT, DDE, and PCBs in their fat compared to women who do not have cancer. (122) The incidence of breast cancer goes down when a woman exercises on a regular basis, and eats more green vegetables and fiber.

Food for Thought

The connection between breast milk and toxicity is not intended to discourage you to breastfeed your baby. Breast feeding gives an infant immunity against gastrointestinal diseases and respiratory infections, offers protection against food allergies, provides emotional bonding between mother and child, and is really the right food for the baby. And prepared formulas and baby foods are usually even more contaminated than mother's milk. But since not every mother produces breast milk in sufficient quantities, I will address this topic more in later chapters.

There is much evidence that links breast cancer to "xenoestrogens," chemicals strange or foreign to the human body that mimic or interfere with the body's natural estrogen, the female sex hormone. Indeed, many common industrial chemicals and pesticides mimic hormones and thus interfere with fundamental bodily processes. DDT, methoxychlor, benzene, and others can act like sex hormones and interfere with fundamental biological processes such as reproduction in wildlife and humans. It is believed that xenoestrogens stimulate the growth of cells in the breast, possibly giving rise to cancer. (123)

From epidemiological studies (studies of diseases in the human population), there's evidence that exposure of females to xenoestrogens while in the womb can increase their risk of breast cancer as adults. Not only that, but if a male is exposed to these same chemicals while in the womb, it reduces his ability to produce sperm later in life. It's estimated that the average male today produces only half as much sperm as his grandfather did, and exposure to environmental toxins may well be the cause of this decline. (If this decline were to continue at historical rates, humans in industrialized countries would have difficulty reproducing themselves by about the year 2020.) There is also evidence that prostate cancer, the second leading cause of cancer deaths in the U.S. for men, (lung cancer is No. 1), is linked to these xenoestrogens. (124)

Human breast milk can also be affected by pollution. Scientists first discovered human breast milk was contaminated with DDT in 1951. DDT, like many other chlorinated organic chemicals (pesticides), is soluble in fat but not very soluble in water. So when it enters the body, it's not easily excreted and builds up in fatty tissue. Breast milk contains about 3 percent fat and fat-soluble chemicals collect there. So, if the mother is contaminated and she breastfeeds her baby, the baby gets contaminated too.

In 1975 the U.S. EPA conducted a study of the milk of American women. Taking samples from more than one thousand women and analyzing them for only a few pesticides, they found DDT in 100 percent of the samples, PCBs in 99 percent, and dieldrin in 83 percent. All three are considered "probable carcinogens" by the EPA. (125)

Until early 1999, pesticides had never been measured in the amniotic fluid of pregnant women. (The amniotic fluid is what the fetus floats in the womb prior to birth.) But in June 1999, researchers in the United States and Canada found p,p'-DDE (a breakdown byproduct of DDT), in 30 percent of the women examined.

The concentrations of p,p'-DDE found in the amniotic fluid are a real concern. Of the various health problems associated with these chemicals, developmental abnormalities of the male reproductive tract, suppression of immune function, development of the brain, and neurobehavioral problems in children are of major concern because they are irreversible. DDE is known to interfere with male sexual development by de-activating the male sex hormone, testosterone. (126)

Several studies of laboratory animals have reported that DDE can interfere with normal sexual development of males and can cause enlarged prostate glands.) Alligators in Florida exposed to similar chemicals were reported to have much smaller than normal penises. (127,128)

In another study, test animals were exposed to different pesticides typically used in agriculture and lawn care – Lasso (containing alachlor), Basalin (containing fluchloralin), and Premiere (containing dinoseb and Maneb-80). The test animals were shown to have over 50 percent more activity (i.e., they were considered hyperactive) following a single exposure. The researchers said, "The results of this study suggest that at least some herbicides, in addition to pyrethrins, organophosphate, and carbamate pesticides, can produce behavioral manifestations following accidental exposure... The effects of the pesticides on activity also support the hypothesis that these agents may affect the central nervous system." (129)

Philip J. Landrigan, chairman of the department of community medicine at the Mount Sinai School of Medicine in New York City, says:

> Disease caused by toxic chemicals in the environment is a substantial... cause of morbidity [illness] and mortality [death] in the United States and around the world. Public health workers and the makers of public policy must recognize that toxic chemicals in the environment are important, widespread, proven causes of human disease. Each year preventable exposures to chemical toxins sicken and kill thousands of persons of all ages in the United States and around the world. These hazards must be confronted. They cannot be wished away. Reduction of exposures to chemical toxins will pre-

vent thousands of deaths and will improve the quality of hundreds of thousands of lives. (130)

Food for Thought

We are led to believe that if a product is sold to the general public, it must be safe. If we follow the label directions, we should be okay. But that is clearly not the case. There are strong political pressures from the manufacturers of these products to keep this information from getting out. Although in some instances the data are incomplete, there is sufficient proof that many chemicals do indeed contribute to cancer. It's very similar to what happened with the tobacco industry. For years the tobacco companies said no proof existed that their products caused cancer or were addictive. They kept studies that showed that they actually were to themselves and under lock and key. Now, there are all kinds of lawsuits claiming the opposite, and the courts are agreeing with the plaintiffs and awarding the victims huge settlements. I believe the same kind of scenario is being played out with pesticides. The companies manufacturing them earn millions of dollars. Are they going to come out and say "Hey, our products kill people and give dogs and children cancer!" I don't think so. It's our job, like it or not, to change our world into a safe and healthy one. Stopping the use of pesticides is a good step. Maybe some couple will be brave and take the pesticide manufacturers to court because their child got brain cancer. That will get it onto the evening news.

Household Products

We know that chemicals in the home such as pesticides are potential health hazards. However, many other products you may use around the house and yard without thinking twice can be dangerous to you and your child. And these can add up to creating a toxic living environment. How toxic? A 15-year study found that women who were homemakers had a 54 percent greater risk of developing cancer than women who worked outside the home due to continuous exposure to household cleaners, chemicals, and pesticides. (131) (Who said being a mom was easy and safe?) And the EPA rates indoor air quality among the top 5 threats to human health. (132)

The average American home has 3 to 10 gallons of hazardous materials stored in it. In 1998 there were more than one million incidents reported to poison control centers related to household chemicals – 220,000 of them specifically related to cleaning products. (133) In all, over 90 percent of all reported poisonings occur at home, and the leading cause is household cleaners. (134) Short-term acute effects such as irritation and burning can be suffered from ammonia, chlorine bleach, and other common chemicals, and ingestion of chemical products can lead to sickness and death. So make sure all chemical products are put out of reach of inquisitive toddlers and children and be sure to know what to do in case of a poisoning.

The danger of chemicals does not stop there, however. These chemicals seep into the air, making the average American home a quite toxic place to breathe. The EPA has found that indoor air contains two to five times more pollution than outdoor air. In fact, the Consumer Product Safety Commission found that in the houses they tested, the outdoor air contained less than 10 volatile organic compounds (VOCs), while the indoor air contained 150 VOCs! (135) These VOCs come from a number of sources, not just household cleaners (see below).

Many long-term chronic problems can manifest from exposure to the volatile solvents found in cleaners and other chemicals that get into your airspace. These chronic problems include:

- Neurological difficulties such as fatigue, memory problems, personality changes, headaches, sleep disorder, coordination difficulties, visual problems, and sexual dysfunction.
- Asthma. Sensitive young lungs are damaged by prolonged exposure to the chemicals in the air.
- Liver and kidney damage. These two organs are the ones most responsible for detoxification. If they are impaired, the body has difficulty eliminating toxins, which can lead to numerous health problems.
- Reproductive damage.
- Multiple Chemical Sensitivity (MCS). MCS is a recently defined condition where the person is extremely sensitive to a great number of chemicals found in air, food, water, and those that can be absorbed through the skin. It is thought to result from both acute and chronic chemical exposure.

And remember, children are especially susceptible to chemical exposure due to their developing respiratory and immune systems. So if you have any chemicals in your house, not only get them out of the reach of children, but keep them sealed up so the fumes don't escape. Better yet, put them in a separate building away from the house (not in an attached garage). This includes paint, paint thinners, strippers and other solvents, gas and kerosene cans, lubricants, cleaners, and anything else that has a chemical smell or has warnings on the label.

Speaking of attached garages, they are a potential source of significant air pollution in your house. Every time you open the door leading to the garage, the pollutants from car exhausts and any chemicals stored in the garage come into the house. If you do have an attached garage, you may consider sealing it off with tape and using the front door. This is an inconvenience, I know, but if your child is sensitive and having problems, it's really worth it.

Think twice about storing chemicals under the sink. The chlorine in that scrubbing powder not only gets through your skin as you clean the pots and pans, but also gets into the air and circulates throughout the house. It may not be noticeable, but even tiny concentrations can have effects. This goes for the automatic dishwasher soap and laundry bleach too. Oven cleaners, drain cleaners, and floor and furniture polishes are extremely toxic when ingested, and they pollute the air. Switch to more natural products (available at health food stores) without chlorine or volatile organics in them or at least put these products in airtight containers for storage.

Products such as mothballs, glass cleaners, floor and furniture polish, rug and upholstery cleaners, oven cleaners, and air fresheners are not only toxic if ingested but also pollute the air. Table 1 shows simple ways to get around using these.

Table 1
Alternatives for Toxic Household Products (136)

Product	Potential Health Effect	Suggested Alternative
Air Fresheners	Irritant, toxic to liver and kidney, affect lung function	Open window, open box of baking soda, simmer cloves, grow house plants such as spider plants which helps detoxify the air
Floor & Furniture Polish	Cancer, birth defects, fetal toxicity, lung effects, cardiovascular effects,	1 part lemon oil to 2 parts olive or vegetable oil, vegetable oil soap
Mothballs	Cancer, skin irritant, lung effects, kidney and liver damage, nerve damage	Cedar chips, lavender, aromatic herbs and spices
Glass cleaners	Skin irritant, cancer, corrosive	Use 1/4 to 1/2 cup white vinegar to 1 quart warm water, wipe with newspaper
Rug & Upholstery	Cancer, irritant, kidney damage nerve damage, corrosive, birth defects, fetal toxicity, reproductive toxicity	Baking soda or cornstarch on rug, then vacuum: replace wall-to-wall with washable area rugs.

You should be aware that wall-to-wall carpeting can be especially problematic. New carpeting emits chemicals such as formaldehyde for years. The carpeting holds in most of the dust, food, pesticide residues dragged in on shoes, and harbors dust mites. Even with vacuuming and shampooing (most carpet cleaners have toxic chemicals too), the carpeting will still be contaminated and emit toxins. This is especially bad for children who play on the carpeting. Many experts advise taking out the carpeting altogether and replacing it with nontoxic flooring and using area rugs that can be washed. And remember, your child is probably being exposed to carpet toxicity in day cares and schools. The less they're exposed to at home, the better. There are some companies that sell nontoxic carpeting and they can be found in the Resource Guide.

If you have hardwood floors, use a water-based floor finisher. If using polyurethane finishes, be sure you open all the windows and have the house well ventilated for a few days afterward.

Perchloroethylene is a chemical used in rug and upholstery cleaners and in dry-cleaning and is hazardous if inhaled. People who work in dry-cleaning stores have been shown to have a 25 percent greater chance of dying from cancer than the general public. (137) Do your best to avoid using cleaners with this chemical and to purchase clothes that don't require dry-cleaning. If you do have things dry-cleaned, let them air out outside or somewhere else so the fumes don't come into your house.

One simple way to clean up the air in your house is by having numerous houseplants. They absorb many of the pollutants that are in the air and emit oxygen. The best species to clean the air are golden pothos, nepthylis, spider plant, snake plant, aloe, and philodendron. One plant per 100 square feet is a good rule of thumb to use to determine how many you need. Getting a good air filter/purifier is not a bad idea either.

Another area of concern is the playground equipment, decks, and picnic tables that kids play on. Pressure-treated-wood is treated with chromated copper arsenate. Children playing on this kind of lumber can absorb dangerous amounts of arsenic. And these chemicals leach out into the surrounding soil, which they may get on their hands and into their mouths. Keep your child off and away from these, and replace any home equipment with nontoxic alternatives.

Other items that are a serious health risk to your baby are baby-bottle nipples and pacifiers. Many are made of polyvinyl chloride (PVC), which leach harmful chemicals such as phthalates. These have been shown to increase the risks of cancer later in life. Replace these with silicone nipples and pacifiers. They can be found at most major department-store chains.

As I state in this book several times, I recommend eating organically raised foods not just because they are more nutritious, but also because they are cleaner. But if you eat conventionally grown food, be sure to wash it well. Most health food stores sell natural cleaners designed to take the pesticides off foods. The foods shown to accumulate pesticides the most are apples, grapes, green beans, peaches, pears, spinach, and squash.

As you can see, staying home is oftentimes a hazardous proposition. Cleaning up your household environment will definitely help keep your child healthier and happier, and won't do you any harm either!

Smoking

The Centers for Disease Control and Prevention says that tobacco use is the nation's leading cause of death, accounting for about 430,700 of the more than two million annual deaths in the U.S. One in every five deaths in the U.S. is caused by tobacco use, which accounts for more than $50 billion a year in medical expenditures and another $50 billion in indirect costs. (138,139) Parental smoking contributes to 150,000 to 300,000 respiratory infections in babies causing 7,500 to 15,000 hospitalizations a year. And, as we shall see, the effects of smoking by the parents not only can affect the infant, baby, and child, but can also affect future children in the womb and even before conception.

Donna E. Shalala, Ph.D., the Secretary of the U.S. Department of Health and Human Services says, "Today, nearly 3,000 young people across our country will begin smoking regularly. Of these 3,000 people, 1,000 will lose that gamble to the diseases caused by smoking. The net effect of this is that among children living in America today, 5 million will die an early, preventable death because of a decision made as a child."

An estimated 4.5 million (20 percent) of youths age 12 to 17 years were smokers in 1995, while 48 million (24.7) percent of adults age 18 years and older currently smoke – 27.6 percent of men and 22.1 percent of women. (140) Data suggest that smoking prevalence may be increasing among young adults.

Each day, about 3,000 young people in the U.S. begin smoking. Ninety percent of smokers begin before age 20, 50 percent begin by age 14 and 25 percent begin by age 12. Since 1991, past-month smoking has increased by 35 percent among eighth graders and 43 percent among tenth graders. Smoking among high school seniors is at a 19-year-high.

Between 1988 and 1996, among adolescents 12 to 17 years old, the incidence of initiation of the first use of tobacco increased by 30 percent and of first daily use increased 50 percent. An estimated 4.1 million teenagers are smokers in this age category. (141)

Food for Thought

Many young people start smoking because of peer pressure. It takes strength of character to resist. As our children become weaker in mind, body, and spirit because of toxins in our environment and food, lack of proper nutrition and exercise and a poor family structure, they become more vulnerable to this peer pressure. Often times the strength of the biological fabric of our children determines the strength of their will and common sense. Smoking, drinking, and drug use will continue to rise as their biological strength continues to decline. Anti-smoking and drug use campaigns are great, but they will go mostly ignored by our youth until their strength of character is rekindled. That strength starts with a strong and healthy body.

The health risks of young people smoking are the same as those found in adults: death from cancer, heart and cardiovascular disease, and emphysema. There's evidence that those who begin smoking before they're 20 years old have the highest incidence and earliest onset of both coronary heart disease and high blood pressure. (142)

In fact, it's been shown that cigarette smoking by children or their exposure to smoke initiates events that lead to coronary artery disease, cancer, and chronic obstructive pulmonary disease. Smoking in children (or exposure to smoke) also changes the serum lipoproteins in the blood and increases platelet aggregation. It causes injury to the endothelial cells (the cells lining the blood vessels), which is thought to be the primary initiating event of artherosclerosis; pathological changes of the endothelial cells have even been observed in the umbilical arteries of infants born to mothers who smoke. (143)

In January 1993, the EPA officially declared environmental tobacco smoke (ETS) a known human carcinogen. It is now classified as a Group "A" carcinogen, known to cause cancer in humans – in the same category as asbestos and other hazardous substances. The EPA's report called ETS a serious and substantial health risk for nonsmokers, particularly children. (144) ETS contains more than 4,000 chemicals and at least 40 known carcinogens. Nicotine is the addictive drug in the smoke and leads to acute increases in heart rate and blood pressure. Exposure to ETS causes about 10 times as many deaths from heart and blood vessel diseases as does cancer. ETS is also associated with acute middle ear infections, tonsillectomy, cancer in childhood, slower growth, adverse neurobehavioral effects, colds and sore throats, and meningococal infections (infections of the meninges of the brain). (145)

Nine million American children under five years of age live in homes with at least one adult smoker, so they breathe secondhand smoke regularly. Children who are exposed to secondhand smoke are more likely to have upper respiratory problems, including infections, bronchitis, asthma, pneumonia, wheezing, more throat infections, and even more ear infections. Indeed, children newborn to five years old who are exposed to maternal smoking are over twice as likely to develop asthma compared to those free from exposure. A study in Italy of almost 19,000 children ages six and seven and more than 21,000 adolescents ages 13 and 14 showed parental smoking dramatically increases the incidences of asthma in children. It's estimated that 15 percent of asthma cases in children and 11 percent of wheezing cases among adolescents are attributable to parental smoking. "There is no question that a parent who smokes – especially a mother – puts her child at risk of asthma," says Norman H. Edelman, M.D., a consultant for the American Lung Association. (146) A report by the California Environmental Protection Agency estimates that parents who smoke each year cause 8,000 to 26,000 new cases of childhood asthma in the U.S. and make existing asthma worse in 20 percent of the two to five million children who already have the disease. The children of parents who smoke compared with children of nonsmoking parents have increased frequency of respiratory infections, increased respiratory symptoms, and slightly smaller rates of increase in lung function as the lung mature.

A child's lungs undergo important growth and development during the first two years of life. If an infant regularly breathes secondhand smoke, it may stunt lung growth and may cause a permanent decrease in lung function – affecting his respiratory health for the rest of his life.

If parents smoke in their home or car, their children breathe in their secondhand smoke. The nicotine from that smoke can be measured in the child's urine. Secondhand smoke contains harmful chemicals such as arsenic, cyanide, tar, formaldehyde, carbon monoxide, benzene, and nicotine. (147)

Children are especially vulnerable to respiratory hazards – their airways are smaller than adults, they breathe more rapidly and inhale more pollutant per pound of body weight than adults and they often spend more time engaged in vigorous activities.

The Centers for Disease Control gives these statistics:

- Children with parents who smoke suffer excessive and unnecessary colds, flu, bronchitis, and pneumonia.

- More than 10 million children (31.2 percent) are being exposed to cigarette smoke in their homes.

- Children exposed to smoke miss more than 28 million days of school a year, one third more than kids from smoke-free homes.

- These children have 1.7 million more colds and acute respiratory infections – 10 percent more than kids who are not exposed, and suffer over 10 million days a year of restricted activities such as missing sports practice – 21 percent more than unexposed kids. (148)

Children in homes with low income and educational levels are far more likely (48 percent) to be exposed than kids in homes with high income and educational levels (28 percent).

Smoking can cause problems even before the child is born. Smoking by the mother during pregnancy is responsible for 14 percent of premature deliveries, 30 percent of low-birth-weight babies, and 4,600 infant deaths per year. Mothers who smoke 10 or more cigarettes a day during pregnancy cause as many as 26,000 new asthma cases a year among children. Nicotine makes the mother's blood vessels smaller, so less nourishment, water, and oxygen gets to the fetus. Poisons in the smoke reach a baby through the mothers' placental bloodstream and later through breast milk. The nicotine in the smoke also raises the blood pressure and slows the heartbeat of the fetus, which can damage the baby's blood vessels and heart, even before birth. Maternal smoking increases the likelihood of SIDS (Sudden Infant Death Syndrome) by more than three times. (149) (See more on SIDS below)

A study by a team of researchers at the University of Southern California indicated that cigarette smoke damages the unborn babies' lungs at crucial points in their development leading to reduced lung capacity in later life. Passive smoking after birth had the same effect, but was not as marked as the damage done during pregnancy. The airflow was significantly impaired in the small airways of children whose mothers had smoked. Frank Gilliland, Ph.D., warned that the long-term effect for children whose mothers smoked during their bodies' development could be obstructive pulmonary disease, lung cancer, and cardiovascular disease. (150)

In fact, a study at Ohio State University suggests that the effects of environmental tobacco smoke linger long after that child has left home and is no longer exposed. It showed that children who were exposed to high levels of ETS growing up maintained higher blood pressure, mean arterial pressure, and resting heart rate, and heart rate during psychological stress compared to students who grew up with low levels of ETS. One of the researchers said, "We've learned that children who grow up in a smoking household will have small but long-lasting negative effects on their health. You don't have to be the one smoking, but you can still vicariously suffer some of the effects." (151)

Clive Bates, director of the British group Action on Smoking and Health, comments, "When babies are exposed to the chemicals in cigarette smoke while still in the womb, it is just about the nastiest form of passive smoking imaginable and it looks as though it does lasting damage. It's hard to think of a more pervasive and pernicious assault on the health of the most vulnerable infants." (152)

Smoking by the mother during pregnancy has been shown to increase the risk of miscarriages, premature birth, stillbirths, and death in the first few weeks of life. Nicotine, carbon monoxide, and polycyclic aromatic hydrocarbons are known to cross the placenta and have been identified in newborns of smokers. Carbon monoxide likes to bind with hemoglobin, which reduces the capacity of the blood to adequately transport oxygen to the fetus. The placental blood flow is reduced due to fewer fetal capillaries with smaller diameters which is believed to slow fetal growth. Studies have shown that these effects can take place even if the mother doesn't smoke, but if the father does and the mother is exposed. Pregnant smokers have a higher incidence of the placenta rupturing (called placenta previa) and premature rupture of the membranes. Anencephaly, a congenital absence of the brain and the spinal cord because the cranium does not close properly, is also higher in babies whose mothers smoked during pregnancy. (153,154)

Several studies have shown that birth weight is decreased by an average of about 200 grams in infants whose mother smoked throughout pregnancy. A low-birth weight baby is two to four times more likely to be born to a smoking mother than one who does not smoke. (155) A normal weight for a new born is considered 2,500 grams or more. Smoking increases the risk by more than 50 percent in light smokers and over 100 percent in heavy smokers that their baby's weight will be less than that. Such babies are more likely to be stillborn, to need intensive care in the hospital, or to die in infancy. (156)

In an Australian study of over 8,500 women, children of women who smoked during pregnancy were far more likely to suffer middle ear infections or ear surgery by age five than children of mothers who did not smoke while pregnant. (157) Seven percent of ear infections in children are attributed to exposure to tobacco smoke. Ear infections cause most of children's hearing loss.

Research shows that mothers who quit smoking during pregnancy may decrease the risks of potential health problems in their newborns. But even if a woman stops smoking during pregnancy and resumes later, her baby is twice as likely to die from SIDS. If a mother smokes and breastfeeds, her baby gets nicotine with every meal. Nicotine stays in the breast milk for up to five hours after smoking. Smoking can also decrease the quantity of breast milk and can change its quality and may lead to the necessity of early weaning.

Perinatal mortality (occurring at about the time of birth) is 25 percent to 56 percent greater in infants of mothers who smoke than those who do not. (158) There are also higher mortality rates in infants of fathers who smoke.

Food for Thought

Here's a risk I bet you haven't thought of: children can become sick from swallowing cigarette butts. In 1995 there were 7,917 reports of potentially toxic exposures from swallowing cigarettes among children six years of age or younger, with the greatest risk among the ages of six months to one year old. Reactions included depressed breathing, irregular heartbeat, and convulsions. (159)

SIDS is greater in infants exposed to tobacco smoke in utero (as a fetus), and postnatally (after birth) than those with only postnatal exposure. If a mother smokes during pregnancy and after birth, her child is three times more likely to die of SIDS than nonsmokers. If the mother smokes only after the child is born, the child is two times more likely to die of SIDS. Smoking by the mother during pregnancy may result in chronic fetal hypoxia (lack of oxygen), which can impair the normal development of the central nervous system. Nicotine has been shown to cause necrosis (cell death) of cells in the brain stems of fetal rats. Abnormal cell growth in the respiratory centers in the brain have been found in some cases of sudden infant death syndrome, possibly resulting from exposure to the poisons in smoke. (160)

The lead and carbon monoxide in the tobacco smoke inhaled by the mother can damage the baby's brain, leading to developmental, learning, and behavioral problems. Children of mothers who smoke during and after pregnancy are more likely to suffer from hyperactivity and impairment in school performance and intellectual achievements than children of non smokers. (161)

Sharon Milberger, M.D., of the Pediatric Psycholpharmacology Unit at Massachusetts General Hospital in Boston, says that exposure to nicotine, the most potent psychoactive component of tobacco, causes damage to the brain at critical times in the developmental process. Research has reported that 22 percent of the children with ADHD had mothers who smoked during pregnancy while maternal smoking occurred in only 8 percent of the healthy group. ADHD and behavioral and cognitive disorders from smoking causes detrimental changes in the dopamine delivery system in the brain and causes "fetal hypoxia" when the fetal brain does not get enough oxygen. The study, reported in the *American Journal of Psychiatry*, states that "it is now believed that the human fetus is actually exposed to a higher nicotine concentration than the smoking mother [and] chronic exposures during pregnancy, especially those producing hypoxia... are most associated with neuropsychiatric impairment." The study also noted that the ADHD children whose mothers had smoked during pregnancy had significantly lower IQs than those whose mothers did not smoke. (162)

The Truth About Children's Health

Children from mothers who smoked during pregnancy are more likely to commit crimes later in life. One study reported that "Our results support our hypothesis that maternal smoking during pregnancy is related to increased rates of crime in adult offspring." Although the researchers admitted that there is not enough evidence to add prenatal smoking to the list of established risk factors for adult crimes, the statistics showed that more than a quarter of the men whose mothers had the highest levels of smoking and delivery complications with their births were arrested for a violent crime as an adult. The researches did note that mothers who smoke during pregnancy are often young women who have had previous misconduct problems, so there may be an inheritability of misconduct problems. (163) (Or maybe *their* mothers smoked too!)

If you have your child in day care, you should know what the environment is like there. Children who attend licensed child-care centers are usually protected from exposure to tobacco smoke because of state and federal indoor air acts. But unlicensed centers or private-family or group day care situations are not necessarily protected by law, so it's important for you to find out if smoking occurs at the day care place.

The reasons children and adolescents start smoking have to do with being accepted by one's peers, asserting independence, feeling attractive and glamorous, and signaling maturity. Children who have a low self-image and are less academically successful have fewer skills to cope with social pressures to smoke. Girls who smoke tend to have good social skills, whereas boys do not; and girls may also believe that smoking helps them to control their weight.

Teenagers who smoke are 56 percent more likely to suffer serious sleep disturbance, and teens who smoked a little were 20 percent more likely to have mild insomnia, according to a study appearing in *Pediatrics*. The exact mechanism is not understood, but nicotine, the addictive drug in tobacco, is a stimulant that may keep them awake. (164) Lack of sleep, of course, can lead to a host of behavioral and physiological problems.

Cigarette smoking appears to be a gateway to drug and alcohol use. Twelve- to 17-year-olds who smoked cigarettes in the previous 30 days were about three times more likely to have consumed alcohol and eight times more likely to have smoked marijuana, and 22 times more likely to have used cocaine in the past 30 days. Those who use drugs rarely do so *before* smoking cigarettes. The CDC says that youths ages 12 to 17 that smoked were about eight times as likely to use illicit drugs and 11 times as likely to drink heavily as nonsmoking youths. A young person who uses tobacco daily is likely to become addicted to nicotine, and to get a young person to stop smoking is difficult. (165)

Food for Thought

It's no coincidence that the time people start smoking is one of the most tumultuous times of their lives – adolescence – when there are significant physiological, psychological, and social changes taking place. Young people are in a most vulnerable position and are attempting to come to

---

grips with their own bodies and lives. Those who feel most secure emotionally will be less likely to start smoking to fit in with the crowd, to show their independence or to rebel against authority. A loving environment in the home is important to establish this attitude. And a loving environment begins with a healthy environment. It's been shown that children from lower income families are more likely to start smoking. It's also known that lower-income families often-times do not get proper nutrition. When a child is not fed adequately, numerous aberrations may result. Could the need for stimulation from cigarettes or the development of an inadequate self-image be a result of having an undernourished and underdeveloped brain? Does a really healthy, happy child feel the need to inflict damage upon himself or to get a "rush" from some harmful substance? On second thought, does a healthy, happy adult feel the need to do the same?

Protecting your child from smoking isn't easy. Besides the peer pressure to start, the tobacco industry spends $6 billion a year advertising and promoting their products in the U.S. One study found that 30 percent of three-year-olds and 91 percent of six-year-olds could identify "Joe Camel" as a symbol of smoking. (This kind of advertising – blatantly targeting youngsters with cartoon characters – has since been banned.) (166) The tobacco industry must recruit 5,000 new young smokers every day to maintain the total number of smokers, and advertising is an effective way to do this. They have also targeted women more in recent years, introducing different brands that appeal to their sense of independence and sexuality. They have been successful as evidence in the increase in women smoking. Lung cancer has become the leading cause of cancer death among women, having increased by nearly 400 percent in the past 20 years. More than 145,000 women die every year from smoking-related diseases. As former U.S. Surgeon General Antonia Novello said, "The Virginia Slims Woman is catching up to the Marlboro Man." (167)

On the bright side, those who quit smoking decrease their risk of heart disease by half after one year off cigarettes. After 15 years, the risk of heart disease is similar to that of people who've never smoked. The body can regenerate itself. In five to 15 years off cigarettes, the risk of stroke returns to the level of those who've never smoked. (168)

Parents, to raise as healthy and bright a child as possible, try to make it as easy for them as possible. Don't smoke, find a day care where the attendants don't smoke, and educate your teens about smoking. You can even give your kids a reward – like a college fund or a car when they turn 16 – if they don't smoke.

Smoking and pregnancy, along with the hazards of alcohol are further discussed in Chapter IX.

Food for Thought

The human mind is an amazing and sometimes puzzling thing. How can we be so intelligent and so stupid at the same time? How can we be convinced to spend our hard-earned money on things that make us feel bad and continue using them until we're addicted, sick, and dead? Are we really that insecure that we believe these little white tubes filled with a carcinogen can make us more popular, independent, and cool? Advertising and peer pressure can make us do incredible things. There's also the attraction of cheating death. We feel powerful when we do things that are dangerous and thrilling – as long as we come out seemingly unharmed. Smoking, drinking, taking drugs, extreme sports, and other dangerous activities are obstacles we place in front of ourselves to remind us that yes, we are powerful. We met the enemy and overcame it. That's part of the nature of man. Hopefully, some of us can tame these compulsions and overcome our need to prove ourselves – to ourselves and anyone else. This healthy attitude manifests as self-esteem.

There was a kid in my high school class, Frank, who was a pretty good baseball pitcher. He had a wicked fast ball and could "smoke" it by just about anyone. I remember going to parties my senior year and seeing all the "cool" kids – many of whom smoked and drank. And although Frank was part of the crowd and very much liked, he didn't do either. I thought it kind of strange to see this kid seemingly defy the peer pressure and still fit in. It didn't seem to matter to anyone that he didn't smoke or drink. He was cool enough just being Frank. A few years later I turned on the TV to watch a ball game, and guess who was on mound pitching? Frank had made it all the way to the major leagues, and was a relief pitcher for more than 10 years. I wonder if he would have made it if he succumbed to the peer pressure and had started those nasty habits. The message? If a child has self-esteem, he or she will fit in anywhere without the need of "props." And if you raise a healthy kid, they will naturally have self-esteem.

Obesity

The Centers for Disease Control's (CDC) 2000 report on Nutrition and Physical Activity found that the percentage of children and adolescents who are overweight has more than doubled in the past 30 years. And most of the increase has occurred since the late 1970s. (169) Roughly 25 percent of U.S. children are considered overweight or obese. (170)

Between 1991 and 1999, obesity (defined as being over 30 percent above ideal body weight) for the total U.S. population increased 57 percent, from 12 percent in 1991 to 17.9 percent in 1998. Obesity increased in every state, in both sexes and across all age groups, all races all educational levels and among smokers and non-smokers alike. By region, the largest increases were seen in the South, with a 67 percent increase in the number of obese people. Georgia had the largest increase: 101 percent.

Food for Thought

It's interesting to note that of the occurrences of childhood violence sited in the previous chapter, five of the 10 were in Southern States. I don't know if these children were overweight, but I would venture to say the increased number of people overweight in a region has to reflect their lifestyle and state of overall health.

As the weight of our children has increased, physical activity has gone down. Nearly half of young people ages 12 to 21 are not vigorously active on a regular basis. Participation in all types of physical activity declines as children and adolescents get older. The percentage of high school students who participate in daily physical education classes has declined in recent years from 42 percent in 1991 to 25 percent in 1995: 40 percent of high school students are not enrolled in any type of physical education class.

The ever-present television and the explosion of the Internet have not helped matters when it comes to exercise. Our children are much more likely to sit in front of the tube or computer than go out and play. Many schools have done away with or cut back on physical education.

It's obvious that our young are simply not getting enough exercise. And that fact no doubt contributes to their discontent. Remember the old saying "a sound body, a sound mind?" Science bears that out. One of the recommendations for people with clinical depression is physical exercise. It's a stress reliever and a self-esteem builder. It causes the release of endorphins, the body's natural "feel-good" chemicals. Exercise simply makes you feel better. And by the way, have you ever known a happy person to get violent?

CDC Director Jeffrey P. Koplan says that the American lifestyle of convenience and inactivity has had a devastating toll on every segment of society, particularly on children. Research shows that 60 percent of overweight five- to 10-year-old children already have at least one risk factor for heart disease, including hyperlipidemia (increased levels of fat in the blood) and elevated blood pressure or insulin levels. Koplan says, "Overweight and physical inactivity account for more than 300,000 premature deaths each year in the United States, second only to tobacco-related deaths. Obesity is an epidemic and should be taken as seriously as any infectious disease epidemic. Obesity and overweight are linked to the nation's No. 1 killer – heart disease – as well as diabetes and other chronic conditions."

Obese children and adolescents are more likely to become obese adults. This extra weight carries with it increased risks for heart disease, high blood pressure, stroke, diabetes, some types of cancer, gallbladder disease, and osteoporosis. And even the health of the parents has a tremendous effect on whether a child will be obese or not: Children with two obese parents stand an 80 percent chance

The Truth About Children's Health

of being obese themselves and a 40 percent chance if one parent is obese. And sadly, "once you're fat, you're fat:" Eighty percent of obese teenagers will become obese adults. (171)

The CDC is taking steps to help children get healthier. In 1996 they started the PAN Program – Improving Child and Adolescent Health Through Physical Activity and Nutrition. It's a multifaceted approach to helping young people develop healthy behaviors and lifestyles through prevention and interventions strategies. (172)

This program "seeks to understand the multiple influences on the lives of children: families, peers, schools, communities, health care, and media. While any one of these influences may be sufficient to encourage healthy behaviors, it is more likely that a synergistic effect will be required."

The key words here are "healthy behaviors." Sitting in front of the television for three hours a day (average time for youngsters), spending even more time in front of the computer, not even taking gym class in school, eating a large percentage of fast food, do not contribute to "healthy behavior." There are just some natural laws we must abide by to remain healthy, happy, and nonaggressive. And achieving and maintaining good physical condition is one of them.

Koplan also states that "schools must offer more physical education that encourages lifelong physical activity; urban policy makers must provide more sidewalks, bike paths, and other alternatives to cars; and parents need to reduce their children's TV and computer time and encourage outdoor play. In general, restoring physical activity to our daily routines is critical."

Being obese and overweight is clearly a problem for our children, and a new problem at that. Mary Horlick, a pediatric endocrinologist at St. Luke's Roosevelt Hospital, sums up the increase in childhood obesity this way: "But today we have an unprecedented epidemic of childhood obesity, and kids are growing up in a 'obesogenic' environment, which did not used to be the case." She noted that today's grandmothers were more physically active and better nourished as children than today's youngsters. They didn't grow up eating fast foods, drinking soda instead of milk and spending hours sitting in front of a television or computer. (173)

William Dietz, M.D., head of clinical nutrition at New England Medical Center Hospital in Boston says that television viewing is the second most important predictor of adolescent obesity behind childhood obesity. A child who watches four or more hours of television a day has twice the risk of obesity than the child who watcher less (see Figure 1). Dietz attributes this to a decrease in physical activity and an increase in eating while watching TV. (174)

Figure 1

Television and Obesity: A child who watches four or more hours of TV a day has twice the risk of being obese.

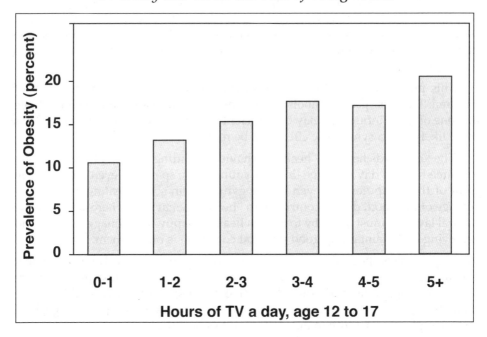

Television

Perhaps more than any other factor, television is to blame for our children's weight gain. Satellite dishes and cable make literally hundreds of shows available at the click of a button. Street play – which is sometimes not an option given today's legitimate safety concerns – can scarcely compete with the hypnotic lure of the tube. The prevalence of day care, after school care, and even latchkey kid situations make television an all too convenient "activity."

Unfortunately, there's nothing "active" about it. The American Academy of Pediatrics confirms that "Increased television use is documented to be a significant factor leading to obesity." (175) What's more, the *Journal of American Medical Association* showed that children lost weight, and lost inches around the midriff, if they simply watched less television. (176)

To better realize the overall impact television has on the lives of our children, consider these sobering statistics:

- The national average for all children is more than three hours of TV per day – about 21 to 28 hours a week. This translates into 20 percent of their waking hours glued to the tube. That doesn't include time watching video movies, surfing the Internet, playing video games or watching music videos. By age 70, today's typical American child will have spent seven to 10 years watching television.

- The average American child views 20,000 television ads per year (2,000 of them for beer and wine).

- Children as young as three are influenced by pressure from ads.

- Young children are not able to distinguish between commercials and television programs. They don't recognize that commercials are attempting to sell then something.

- In one year's time of average viewing, the child will be exposed to more than 14,000 sexual references. So 21 hours a week of viewing will show them one sexual reference every five minutes. (177)

In 1999 the American Academy of Pediatrics (AAP) made the recommendation that children younger than two years old should not be allowed to watch television at all, stating that it may stunt the development of their brains. The emotional and intellectual development of young children depends upon interaction with adults, and when children watch TV, that is lacking. (178)

The academy explains, "Pediatricians should urge parents to avoid television viewing for children under the age of two years. Although certain television programs may be promoted to this age group, research on early brain development shows that babies and toddlers have a critical need for direct interactions with parents and other significant caregivers for healthy brain growth and development of appropriate social, emotional and cognitive skills. Therefore, exposing such young children to television programs should be discouraged."

The academy goes on to advise parents to limit all children's TV viewing to one to two hours of "quality programming" per day: "Time spent with media often displaces involvement in creative, active or social pursuits."

The academy also blames TV for some of the violence exhibited by some children. "More than 1,000 scientific studies and reviews conclude that significant exposure to media violence increases the risk of aggressive behavior in certain children and adolescents, desensitizes them to violence, and makes them believe that the world is a 'meaner and scarier' place than it is." In 1995, the academy said that "by age 18 the average American child has viewed an estimated 200,000 acts of violence on TV alone. Video games increase that number... Although media violence is not the only cause of violence in American society, it is the single most easily remediable contributing factor."

Food for Thought

My drama professor in college said that theater is a reflection of life – a reflection, not a cause. I have to agree that exposing children to violence can do nothing but harm them, as the studies show, and I would endorse any legislation to limit violence and sex on TV. I would like to point out, however, that the reason there is so much violence on TV today is because it sells. And it sells because it's what people want to watch. And it's what people want to watch because it's what they identify with. And they identify with it because they are in fact becoming more violent themselves. As we

---

are seeing, there are many reasons for this tendency toward violence (including "The Ancestry Factor" explained in Chapter XII). And these reasons are not just psychological and sociological, but biochemical and physiological as well. Mainstream theater, movies, and TV are reflecting what our society is becoming – one of decreased morals, sick and aggressive minds, and sick bodies.

An American child has viewed about 360,000 advertisements before graduating from high school. The AAP states, "In 1750 BC, the Code of Hammurabi made it a crime, punishable by death, to sell anything to a child without first obtaining a power of attorney. In the 1990s, selling products to American children has become a standard business practice." The AAP "...believes advertising directed toward children is inherently deceptive and exploits children under eight years of age" because children who are developmentally younger than eight "are unable to understand the intent of advertisements and, in fact, accept advertising claims as true." (179)

Children age 12 and younger spent or influenced the spending of around $500 billion in 1997. More and more commercials are geared to children to try and get their share of that money.

The American Psychological Association (APA) says in its brochure titled *Violence on Television*, "Violent programs on television lead to aggressive behavior by children and teenagers who watch those programs." This was from a report by the National Institute of Mental Health, a report that confirmed and extended an earlier study done by the Surgeon General. (180)

Other psychological research has shown three major effects of seeing violence on television:

- Children may become less sensitive to the pain and suffering of others.
- Children may be more fearful of the world around them.
- Children may be more likely to behave in aggressive or harmful ways toward others.
- Children who watch a lot of TV are less aroused by violent scenes than those who watch a little. They are bothered less by violence in general and less likely to see anything wrong with it.

In several studies, children who watched a violent program instead of a non-violent one were slower to intervene or call for help when, a short time later, they saw younger children fighting or playing destructively.

George Gerbner, Ph.D., of the University of Pennsylvania, has reported that children's TV shows contain about 20 violent acts each hour. (Imagine how many in an adult program!) He also reported that children who watch a great deal of television are more likely to view the world as a mean and dangerous place.

Gerbner's ground-breaking research was done in the early 1980s. Back then there were an estimated 22 acts of violence per hour on TV. Since then the numbers have increased: In 1992 one prime-time show ("Young Indiana Jones") registered 60 acts of violence per hour; "Cookie's Cartoon Club" averaged 100; "Tom and Jerry" averaged 88; and "Looney Tunes" averaged 80. (181)

In a study at the Pennsylvania State University, close to 100 preschool children were observed both before and after watching television. One group watched cartoons containing much violence, the other group shows that had no kind of violence. Significant differences in behavior were observed in the two groups: "Children who watch violent shows, even 'just funny' cartoons, were more likely to hit out at their playmates, argue, disobey class rules, leave tasks unfinished, and were less willing to wait for things than those who watched the nonviolent programs," Aletha Huston, Ph.D., reported. (182)

A report in *The Christian Science Monitor* reinforces the fact that young children are very impressionable when it comes to watching TV. When a class of two- to five-year-olds watched "Barney", they sang along, marched along, held one another's hands, and laughed together. The next day the same class watched the aggressive "Power Ranger." Within minutes they were karate-chopping and high-kicking the air – and one another. (183)

Leonard Eron, Ph.D., at the University of Illinois, found that children who watched a lot of TV violence when in elementary school tended to show a higher level of aggressive behavior when they became teenagers. He and his team of researchers observed a group of youngsters until they were 30. They found that the ones who had watched a lot of TV when they were eight were more likely to be arrested and prosecuted for criminal acts as adults. (184)

Even though some broadcasters do not believe there is enough evidence to prove that TV violence is harmful, scientists do. The 1992 American Psychological Association's Task Force on Television and Society confirms this view in a report entitled "Big World, Small Screen: The Role of Television in American Society." They say that just by limiting the number of hours children watch television will probably reduce the amount of aggression they see. And this will help keep the child in a more peaceful, less agitated state - not just at the time, but later on in life. (185)

Parents should also watch at least one episode of the programs their kids are watching. That way they'll know what their children are being exposed to and can talk to them about it. Or, parents can outright ban any programming they deem too offensive and limit viewing to shows that have less or no violence.

Food for Thought

Here's a totally radical recommendation: Sell your TV! Or box it up and put it in the basement. Or put it away somewhere and take it out only for special occasions or emergencies. Can you imagine? Life without TV? My goodness, how will you survive? How did the human species make it without "Seinfeld," "Days of Our Lives," "60 Minutes," "Sesame Street,"

Hazards Our Children Face

"Barney," and "Blue's Clues?" They must have been strong individuals back then to be able to function and not get bored out of their skulls. No TV! Aaaauuuuugggggghhhhhh!!

I have an interesting personal story to tell you. I've had a number of children's books published, and I go to elementary schools to read the books, do a show and give writing workshops. Invariably, one of the students will ask me how I got started writing. This is what I tell them, and it's absolutely true: After I finished graduate school (in Environmental Sciences and Engineering), I loaded up my hatchback with just about everything I owned to go off and look for a real job. You know, be a responsible adult and do something with my degree. I crammed that little Plymouth Horizon to the ceiling (books, clothes, toaster oven, bed, food). And just when it was totally full with just the driver's seat clear to sit in, I looked down on the sidewalk and saw my little 13-inch black-and-white TV sitting there. I was tired of packing and didn't want to open a door because everything would have fallen out, so I left it with a friend. I got down to Florida (yes, I wanted a job, but you can't forget golf!) and rented an apartment. Those first few days, coming home after job hunting, I found my hand reach out for the TV's "on" button. Problem was, it was still in Virginia. You see, I had become conditioned, kind of like a Pavlovian dog, to turn on the TV the moment I entered my living room. (I don't think I started salivating, but I can't say for sure.) Well, poverty is good for some things, because I could barely feed myself, so I surely couldn't afford a new TV.

As a kid, I hadn't watched much TV – I was always out playing ball. I was more interested in doing something than watching something. But from what I've learned from researching this book, if I had watched more TV as a kid, maybe I wouldn't care so much about sports. Anyway, to keep myself from climbing the walls, I started to read. Yes, read. I read *Moby Dick, War & Peace, Crime & Punishment, The Castle*. And then, one night, I picked up a pen, I put it on the paper and out came a paragraph! It was sorrowful and depressing. It was bad writing. Really bad writing. But, I kept doing it anyway. And one thing lead to another, and I started writing a novel. And then a couple years later, a book for kids. The moral of the story is that I became a writer because I didn't have a TV to pass the time. It's amazing what you can do when you don't have one. It's amazing what you *want* to do when you don't have one.

When I go to schools now and tell this story, I ask the kids what they think it would be like to not have a TV. I get groans of agony in reply. So, I dare you. I double dare you. Turn off the TV. Put it away. Find out what life can be like. It won't just be good for you, but more so for your kids. Just remember, you'll go through a withdrawal period, so brace yourself.

The Truth About Children's Health

I remember reading about a study once years ago where researchers wanted to see what effect TV was having on us. So they had a small community go off TV cold-turkey for about a month. What happened was very interesting. The first several days after taking away all the TVs, crime went up. That was not what they expected. But after a short period of time, the community settled down to become much more peaceful and harmonious than when they had TV. The researchers likened it to coming off drugs. There is an initial "withdrawal" period, followed by better health. You can't go wrong watching less TV.

In recent years, professional wrestling has become quite popular on TV. Although adults readily recognize that it's all a big show and not real, children, oftentimes, do not. It's estimated that 15 percent of the wrestling audience (more than one million viewers) is 11 years old or younger; 25 percent are children and teenagers age two to 17. Not only is there violence in professional wrestling (kicks to the groin, chairs, tables and brooms used as weapons, head butting, urination, etc.), there is also quite a bit of sexual references (crotch-grabbing, pointing at the crotch, simulated sexual activity, obscene finger gesturing, and scantily clad women). Not only are the shows themselves bad for children, but they run tons of commercials. One two-hour segment contained 103 commercials. These commercials are geared toward violence, sex, junk food – the kind of things people who like wrestling will buy.

Professional wrestling is big business. Sales in 2000 were estimated at $340 million, up from $250 million in 1999. (186) I believe it's a reflection of our times, our bodies, minds and morality. Wrestling reminds me of the gladiators in the Coliseum in Rome, before the Roman Empire fell – barbaric entertainment. A healthy society is not barbaric. It is compassionate and kind because the people in it are compassionate and kind because these people are healthy and happy. America, my dear reader, is not. Not these days. Barbaric, crude, mindless, sensational and violent entertainment is popular because the people demand it. And they demand it because it's a reflection of the violence occurring within their bodies and minds.

Yes, it's probably good to keep your kids away from watching television. But you should ask yourself the question as to why they want to watch it in the first place. A healthy, happy child is a lot less likely to watch raunchy things simply because they will not identify with those kind of shows. A child is more likely to watch the nature channel, history channel, or read a book. If your child likes professional wrestling, you may want to examine more closely his or her overall health, their diet, exercise pattern. The healthier your child is, the more likely he or she will explore more wholesome things. And as the health of your child improves, so will his or her viewing preference.

Of course, there's always the alternative of not having a TV in your house at all. It's best to remove it before your child is born, and keep it out until they are at lease six or seven. By that time, most of their psyche is already developed and it's a lot less likely they will be overly influenced by TV shows and commercials.

Of course, if you put your child in day care, that may well be impossible. If you take the TV out of your house after the child has become accustomed to it, you may be in for a tough time. You could always say it's broken and you don't have the money to fix it! (Just a little white lie.) Or, you could hide it, put it away except for special occasions, or simply put a blanket over it so you and your children forget it's there.

It's not just the content on TV that is the problem, it's the very nature of the TV itself. TV puts the viewer in an altered state of consciousness similar to a hypnotic state It has been scientifically shown that as little as 30 seconds induces a semi-hypnotic, sleepiness or inattentive state of mind. (187) (That's why violence on TV works so well – those kinds of images keep the watcher awake!) Humans are more open to suggestion in this state - which the advertisers love.

Since the image on the screen is ready-made, our minds do not have to create it's own as is done in reading. This has lead psychologist Bruno Bettelheim to say "TV traps the fantasy, it doesn't free it. A good book motivates thinking and simultaneously frees it." Valdemar W. Setzer, Ph.D., a professor of Computer Science, has studied and published on the problems of the influence of TV, video games, and computers on children for almost 30 years. He says, "If you wish to develop your thinking, do reading. If you wish to impair your thinking, dampening it more and more, watch TV." (188)

Not only that, but the TV gives off low levels of radiation. Some researchers believe that prolonged exposure can cause a host of problems including insomnia, lack of attentiveness, hyperactivity and discipline problems, lack of ability to concentrate, and possible cancer risks.

The pioneer of time-lapse photography and photo biology, John Ott, performed some interesting tests on the effects of exposure to television radiation and biological functioning. He used white laboratory rats in his experiment. Two rats were placed in each of two cages, directly in front of a color TV. The set was turned on for six hours a day and 10 hours on Saturday and Sunday. One cage was shielded from the TV tube with black photographic paper, and the other cage was shielded with one-eighth inch of lead shielding. The sound was turned off and the rats couldn't see the picture (so they weren't influenced by violent scenes – just kidding).

What Ott observed was that the rats protected with only the black paper became increasingly hyperactive and aggressive within three to 10 days. After that, they became progressively lethargic. At 30 days they were extremely lazy and it was necessary to push them to make them move.

The rats shielded with lead showed some similar patterns of behavior, but they took longer to manifest and were not as severe. Dr. Ott noted that there was another TV (black-and-white) in the area – approximately six feet away, which at the time was considered a safe distance – that was unshielded. He concluded that the lethargic behavior of the shielded rats was probably due to the exposure from the second set. His experiment was repeated three times with different rats, and the results were the same in each experiment.

The Truth About Children's Health

The unshielded rats, when exposed to both the color and black-and-white TVs, were even more severely impacted. All the young rats in one of the cages died within 10 to 12 days. Autopsies were performed, and microscopic investigations indicated brain tissue damage in several instances.

Also of note is what happened in a room nearby – about 15 feet away from the color set. That room had been used for animal breeding purposes successfully for more than two years. But immediately after the color TV was placed in the adjacent room, the breeding program was completely disrupted. Litters of rats that had been averaging eight to 12 young dropped to one or two, and many of those did not survive. It took approximately six months for the breeding program to return to normal after the color TV was removed. (189)

These experiments were performed around 1965. And you may be thinking that since then, we've gotten wiser and have made televisions cleaner. After all, we have regulatory agencies to protect us. At the time of Dr. Ott's experiments, the National Committee on Radiation Protection and the International Commission on Radiation Protection set a limit of 0.5 mr/hr* measured at 5 centimeters from the surface of the set. Sadly but not surprisingly, this standard has not changed. (190) That's more than 35 years with the same standard, despite evidence that it causes harm!

Consumer advocate Ralph Nader spoke up in the '70s to the Senate Commerce Committee: "The standards are too low. Millions of people are being exposed to the risk of physical, genetic, and eye damage." I guess no one was listening.

*5 millirems per hour, a standard way to measure radiation

Video Games

Although there has not been any conclusive research done on the effects of video games on children, it's safe to say that playing them is not the healthiest activity a child could undertake. These games often present extremely violent, bloody, and sometimes sexually explicit scenarios that, considering the research done on TV shows, may carry over into life and encourage violent and uncaring behavior. Indeed, John Naisbitt, in his book *High Tech, High Touch: Technology and our Search for Meaning*, tells us that the youngsters who committed the crimes at Littleton, Colorado and West Paducah, Kentucky, actually trained and practiced their acts on video games! (191)

Dr. Setzer says that "…the prolong use of these games can cause, mainly upon children, a number of physical and psychological problems which may include the following: obsessive, addictive behavior; dehumanization of the player; desensitizing of feelings; personality changes; hyperactivity; learning disorder; premature maturing of children; psychomotor disorders; health problems due to lack or exercise and tendonitis; development of anti-social behavior; loss of free thinking and will." (192)

Only time and further research will tell just how harmful these games can be on our children. But since so many companies are making so much money selling them and the demand for them is so high, there has been no push to find out if or to what degree they may be harmful.

But while we're waiting for research to catch up with life, use your own common sense. Do you really think your child's blowing things and people up on a screen is helping him become a mentally healthy and well-balanced adult? Instead of letting your child go off to play a video game alone, why not break out the good old Monopoly, Scrabble or other board game and have some fun with them. (You can find the time to do this by not watching TV!)

Light and Health

Phillip Hughes, Ph.D., a specialist in neurological sciences, physiology and psychology, says:

> Along with food, air and water, sunlight is a most important survival factor in human life. Solar radiation activates other important biochemical events in our bodies involved in endocrine control, timing of our biological clocks, entrainment of 24-hour circadian rhythms, immunological responsiveness, sexual growth and development, regulation of stress and fatigue, control for viral and cold infections, and dampening of functional disorder of the nervous system. (193)

It's only logical, then, that under natural light or an artificial source that duplicates natural light, there is less human fatigue and stress and better visual acuity and production. Yet, our children are indoors most of the day at school, where they are not only being deprived of natural sunlight, but are also being subjected to regular fluorescent lighting, with its very distorted spectrum that contributes to health and behavioral problems. Not to mention that many children go home and sit in front of the TV or play video games now instead of going out to play after school. Again, a double whammy. They are not getting the natural light they need and instead come home to be bombarded with low level radiation and artificial light.

Dr. John Ott started researching light back in the 1950s when Disney hired him to produce the first time-lapse photographs of flowers growing. During the course of making the plants grow, he discovered that they would only flower and grow normally under certain lighting conditions.

As he learned more, he expanded his investigations on the effects light and certain kinds of light have on animals and humans. It can indeed be dramatic. The most important findings of Ott's research is that the quality of light can effect our health, and the health and behavior of our children.

In experiments on first grade students in Sarasota, Florida, researchers found that children in a classroom with cool-white fluorescent lighting were more hyperactive than students in another classroom with full-spectrum fluorescent tubes that duplicated natural sunlight. "Under the standard, cool-white fluorescent lighting, some first graders showed nervous fatigue, irritability, lapses of attention and hyperactive behavior." says Ott. "Within a week after the new lights were installed, the children settled down and paid more attention to their teachers." (194)

The Fort Worth, Texas, school system was one of the first to install fluorescent lighting years ago in a dozen schools. But they soon removed them because of all the complaints of eyestrain, headaches, and other health related problems. Ott demonstrated that radiation from regular fluorescent lights can grossly weaken muscle strength and affect both academic achievement and behavior. Fluorescent lights can cause eyestrain, headaches, insomnia, irritability, hyperactivity, fatigue, and increase dental caries. Dr. Fritz Hollowich showed that exposure to cool-white fluorescent lights resulted in the release of the stress hormones ACTH and cortisol. Under full-spectrum lights, this did not occur. (195) Is it any wonder that our children, forced to sit in school all day under fluorescent lights, have difficulty staying calm?

The Greek athletes used to sunbathe naked before competitions because they believed it increased their strength. In many ways, they were right. Without natural light, our whole endocrine system suffers since light directly influences both the pituitary gland and the pineal gland. The pituitary gland is often referred to as the "master gland" since it is the prime regulator of the whole endocrine system.

The pineal gland is instrumental in setting and controlling sleep cycles and our body's internal clock. It also produces a hormone called melatonin that helps us to fall asleep at night, and helps regulate estrogen production. Not enough melatonin, and estrogen levels rise. The over-abundance of estrogen in the system has been correlated with a high incidence of female type cancers such as breast and uterine cancers. Not enough sunlight means too much melatonin is produced which causes too much estrogen. So women, be sure to get some pure, unfiltered sunlight!

Sunlight has gotten bad press in recent years, as evidence has suggested over-exposure leads to skin cancer and eye problems. The media has made people afraid of going out in the sun without sunblock or low UV eyewear. However, without question, adequate exposure to ultraviolet light is required for maximum health. It's needed to convert nutritional precursors to active forms of vitamin D, which the body needs to perform many healthy functions including and especially the development and maintenance of strong and healthy bones. Consider one study by British researchers that demonstrates the importance of adequate sunlight (replete with UV rays), in children's bone development. The study was performed in two areas of India: downtown Delhi, where there was significantly more haze and less sunlight; and Gurgoan, which had less haze with more sunlight. The researchers measured serum levels of calcium, vitamin D, and other markers of bone growth in 56 children. Children who lived in hazier downtown Delhi with less exposure to sunlight had a lower mean level of vitamin D, which would impact bone growth and development. The researchers concluded that children living in more polluted and high-haze areas should be offered vitamin D supplements. (196)

Vitamin D deficiency is not only a problem of developing or "Third World" nations. Rickets, a bone-softening condition in children that was common years ago, was becoming so rare in the United States that the government stopped keeping statistics on it. It's been making a comeback in recent years however, and is now affecting more and more youngsters. Government officials contribute the comeback to three things: the popularity of milk substitutes such as soy that lack certain nutrients; the failure to supplement breast milk with vitamin D; and a lack of sufficient childhood exposure to sunlight. Vitamin D deficiency has also been linked to increased risk for colon carcinoma. (197) If a child often stays inside or otherwise does not get enough exposure to pure, unfiltered sunlight – without the UV block – he or she may not get adequate vitamin D production and bone development could suffer.

Sunlight is not just important for a growing child, but the amount of it the mother is exposed to during pregnancy has been found to affect the baby's height later on in life: the more sunlight the mother receives, the taller the person will grow. (198)

Although there has been an increase in the incidences of skin cancers in recent years, there have also been increases in many other kinds of cancer. As you already witnessed, our present cancer epidemic is new and unique to the highly technological and polluted society we live in. Lack of adequate sunlight could be partly to blame. Zane Kime, M.D., tells us of a rabbit study, which showed that the animals kept in dim light were more susceptible to cancer. An increase in the light, however, resulted in a decrease in cancer. Another study in Russia was undertaken to prove that UV rays induced cancer. However, much to the researchers' surprise, the lab animals living under lights with UV rays, as compared with those living under fluorescent lights, developed significantly *less* cancer! (199)

I'm not saying a lot of sun cannot cause problems; too much of it can. Overexposure to UV rays can cause tissue damage. But overexposure to *anything* can be hazardous. Consider that people of generations ago working the land under the hot sun to provide for themselves did not have sunblock or sun glasses. And cancer was rare. Ott tells an interesting story about some members of a Congolese tribe that had suddenly developed cancer when the disease had been previously unknown to them. The natives, who wore nothing but loin cloths, had recently taken to wearing sunglasses as a symbol of status. Dr. Ott speculates that the lack of full-spectrum light entering the eye was the cause of their cancer. (200)

Food for Thought

Instead of exposure to sun or UV rays, could it be that other factors are making us generally more sensitive and skin cancer is manifesting due to different reasons? In a 1965 research study, Dr. Frederic Urbach et al., concluded that, "more than one-third of all basal cell carcinomas occurred on areas receiving less than 20 percent of the maximum possible ultraviolet dose. This suggests that some factor in addition to ultraviolet radiation

---

plays a significant role in the genesis of basal cell carcinoma." (201) It is my contention that our overall health and vitality, or lack thereof, plays a significant role in whether we get cancer – skin or any other kind.

Speaking of overdoing it, one study that has contributed to our fear of UV rays was titled "Phototherapy Exposure Tied to Retinal Damage." (202) In that experiment, newborn piglets were exposed to a bank of 10 high intensity 20-watt fluorescent lights filtered to deliver only UV light (this is the equivalent of 300 foot candles of light). One eye was held open and dilated for 72 hours straight and the other covered with a patch. It's not surprising that the eyes not protected showed retinal damage! The general conclusion was that light with UV rays is bad and causes damage. That's like holding a mouse under water for 10 minutes and saying water is dangerous.

In his classic book Health and Light, John Ott shares a couple stories about how ultraviolet light can affect health. The manager of a certain restaurant that used black lights (UV rays) to set the desired mood said that he had essentially the same group of men working for him as he had when they had opened the restaurant 18 years before. He said that the ultraviolet lights had been in use continually during that time, and that the health record of his men had been so consistently excellent that the manager of the hotel had checked into the situation, with medical supervision, to try to determine why this particular group of men was always on the job, even during flu epidemics, when other departments in the hotel would be short-handed because of employees' illness... "These men working in the restaurant seemed to be a particularly happy group – courteous and efficient, and all seemed to get along well together... Not one of them wore glasses... and none had ever complained of any eye problems or discomfort as a result of the ultraviolet light."

At the Seaquarium in Miami, Dr. Ott noticed a similar black light ultraviolet light over some of the fish aquariums.... "I learned that these lights had originally been placed over some of the aquariums for decorative purposes, to give the fish an eerie but attractive appearance... [The curator] told me that the added black light seemed to solve one of their main problems in keeping fish. This was a condition of exophthalmus, or pop-eye, recently identified as due to a virus. I was told that it is rare that any aquarium fish are troubled with exophthalmus when kept in an outdoor aquarium under natural daylight and nighttime conditions. Another problem of fin-nipping also disappeared under natural conditions..." (203)

The "fin-nipping" is obviously an aggressive behavior. Could some of the aggression children (and adults alike) exhibit be due to a lack of a vital nutrient – that being full-spectrum light with the UV included.

As children spend more and more time indoors, are commonly wearing glasses, sunglasses, and contact lenses (all of which block the UV light from entering the eye), and are slathered with sunblock because mom and dad have been brainwashed into believing all sunlight is hazardous to our health, they are getting less and less healthy and more and more emotionally disturbed. Sun is a vital nutrient necessary for the health of your child. Sensible exposure to it (and full-spectrum indoor lighting) will do much to improve it.

CHAPTER III
Cancer

To assess the present-day health of our children and determine if it is improving or declining, let's examine the occurrences and severity of chronic, long-term illnesses in our young, starting with cancer. Acute diseases, are transient and less indicative of an overall, systemic breakdown; I think of them as a snapshot of health that may not tell the whole story. They're more difficult to get reliable long-term tracking information on simply because many acute illnesses never need hospital care and are otherwise seldom reported.

Although some may argue that many chronic, degenerative diseases are a result of genetic factors, many health care professionals believe that even if an individual may have an inherent predisposition towards a specific illness (for example, a weakness in the pancreas in the case of diabetes), the disease will not manifest from this tendency alone.

Food for Thought

I believe we create in our bodies (and minds) the soil for diseases to take root and grow. We are responsible for our health, or lack there of – even if we have a predisposition towards a certain illness. The human body is incredible and, if properly maintained, can overcome and reverse most infirmities. Avoiding a genetic predisposition to disease is something I've done in my own personal life. My grandmother had diabetes, as did others in my family. I, however, have normal blood sugars, and my doctor assures me that I am in no danger of developing diabetes. That is in large part due to my having changed my diet 15 years ago. I have a much stronger system now than when I was in my twenties and thirties and eating pizza five nights a week and hamburgers from fast-food restaurants for lunch every day. If I had continued abusing my body in that way, I feel confident that I would now be in need of daily insulin injections. Again, even if you have a genetic tendency, if you stay healthy and take care of yourself within the laws of nature and biology, you won't get sick. In fact, you'd probably regenerate and get biologically younger.

Dorland's Medical Dictionary, defines cancer as: "any malignant, cellular tumor..." A tumor is defined as "1. swelling, one of the cardinal signs of inflammation; morbid enlargement. 2. neoplasm; a new growth of tissue in which cell multiplication is uncontrolled and progressive." A malignant tumor is "one having the properties of invasion and metastasis and showing a high degree of anaplasia." A benign tumor is "one lacking the properties of invasion and metastasis and showing a lesser degree of anaplasia than do malignant tumors."

(anaplasia – loss of differentiation of cells and of their orientation to one another and to the axial framework and blood vessels, a characteristic of tumor tissue.) (1)

In a nutshell, cancer is a cell or cluster of cells that is out of control. A cancer cell replicates without the cellular mechanisms intact so it can differentiate into the correct kind of cell (i.e., if healthy, a liver cell replicates to form new liver cells, a skin cell will replicate to form new skin cells, etc.). What's worse, it doesn't know when to stop replicating. A cancer cell is a cell that has gone haywire. It's totally confused. It's the ultimate expression of a cell that has lost its integrity and health. Essentially, cancer is evidence of a system that has broken down completely. The cancer not only starts and spreads, but is unchecked by other healthy cells because those cells are too weak to overcome the aberrant ones.

A cancer cell is close to extinction. That's why it replicates so voraciously. When an organism is stressed, it reproduces faster and more often, attempting to ensure its own kind does not perish. (Interestingly, that same principle relates to humans overall; as our species has become stressed, we are seeing changes in fertility characteristics such as women menstruating sooner, multiple births, and so on. More on that later.)

In fact, "cancer cells" are in us all the time. But, if the body is healthy and strong, these aberrant cells are eaten up (by phagocytes – the "garbage men"), rendered harmless and disposed of easily. Only when the total body system is in such a state of internal degeneration will normal cellular processes be overcome by uncontrolled cellular processes. Notice the word "internal." Someone may look healthy, but inside, his or her cells are scrambled and weak.

Food for Thought

There has been so much study and research into the causes of cancer, that it is without doubt the traditional medical community's biggest and longest-running enigma. Billions and billions of dollars have been poured into research over the years, and the situation is only getting worse. The medical community looks to new drugs and more technology to solve the puzzle. But considering their track record, maybe they're looking in the wrong direction for answers. It is my contention that we must look backwards to nature, not forward to drugs and technology if we are to find the solutions.

In 1900, there were reported 64.0 deaths from "cancer and other malignant tumors" per 100,000 people of all ages and races in the U.S. In 1948, that number had risen to 134.9, and by 1989, the figure was 199.99. (2) Between 1950 and 1988, for U.S. whites, incidences of all forms of cancer rose by 43.5 percent and age-adjusted cancer mortality (deaths) increased by 2.9 percent. (3)

In 1998, approximately 12,400 children younger than 20 years of age (which make up nearly 30 percent of the U.S. population), were diagnosed with cancer; and 2,300 died. (4) Cancer overall, is the second leading cause of death among children after accidents. (5) The probability of developing cancer prior to age 20 varies slightly by sex. A newborn male has 0.32 percent probability of developing cancer by age 20, (i.e., a one in 300 chance). Similarly a newborn female has a 0.3 percent probability of developing cancer by age 20 (i.e., a one in 333 chance). (6)

Table 2 shows the incidence rates and the 20-year trends from the period 1973 - 1992. (7) As you can see, in 1973-1974, the incidence of cancer in ages 0 to 14 years old was 12.9 per 100,000 children, and in the 0 to 19 age group, the incidence was 13.8 per 100,000.

Table 2

Age-Adjusted Cancer SEER Incidence Rates* and 20-Year Trends, 1973-92
by Primary Cancer Site
All Races, Males and Females

Site	Ages 0-14 Average Rate‡ 1973-74	Ages 0-14 Average Rate‡ 1991-92	Ages 0-14 % Change 73-92	Ages 0-19 Average Rate‡ 1973-74	Ages 0-19 Average Rate‡ 1991-92	Ages 0-19 % Change 73-92
All Sites						
All Races	12.9	13.9	8.4	13.8	15.9	15.0
Whites	13.3	14.4	8.7	14.2	16.5	16.1
Blacks	10.3	12.1	17.4	11.1	12.7	14.7
Bone & Joint	0.7	0.7	3.6	0.8	0.9	10.8
Brain & Other Nervous	2.4	3.3	35.4	2.2	3.1	39.8
Hodgkin's Disease	0.7	0.5	-25.8	1.3	1.4	11.6
Kidney & Renal Pelvis	0.7	0.8	13.3	0.6	0.6	12.8
Leukemias	4.3	4.1	-4.2	3.8	3.7	-2.7
Acute Lymphocytic	2.7	3.2	14.7	2.3	2.7	15.1
Non-Hodgkin's Lymphomas	0.8	0.9	12.1	0.8	1.0	32.4
Soft Tissue	0.7	0.9	24.9	0.8	0.9	14.5

* SEER Program. Rates are per 100,000 and are age-adjusted to the 1970 U.S. standard standard population. Each rate has been age-adjusted by 5-year age groups.

‡ The Average Rate is the Average Annual Rate over the specified two-year period.

By 1991-1992, the incidence had increased to 13.9 in the 0 to 14 age group and 15.9 in the 0 to 19 age group. Therefore, there was an 8.4 percent increase in the younger age group and a 15.0 percent increase in the age group through 19 years old. That is most definitely a significant rise in both age groups, and is not due to just statistical variability or probability.

The National Cancer Institute (NCI) reports that the incidence (per 100,000 children) of many childhood cancers has increased steadily during the period 1973-1990. All childhood cancers combined have increased at the rate of 0.9 percent per year. Brain cancer and central nervous system cancers have increased at 1.8 percent per year. Leukemias have increased at 1.8 percent per year. Non-Hodgkin's lymphomas have increased at 1.4 percent per year. Kidney cancer has increased at 1 percent per year. (8) The data from another survey by the National Cancer Institute are similar. Figures 2 and 3 show the overview of childhood cancer patterns from this study. (9)

Figure 2

Trends in the age-adjusted* SEER incidence and U.S. mortality rates for all childhood cancers age <20, all races, both sexes, 1975-1995

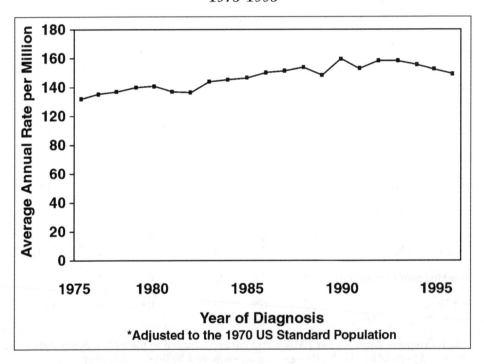

The Truth About Children's Health

Figure 3

Trends in age-specific incidence rates for all childhood cancers by age, all races, both sexes, SEER, 1975-1995

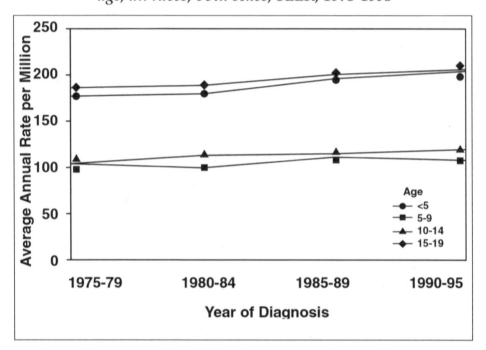

Again, it is apparent that childhood cancer is on the rise. Of course, part of the "increase" results from better diagnosis and better recording of cases by state and federal agencies, but the SEER report recognizes that "taken together [changes in record keeping] cannot explain the magnitude of the increases that have been observed over the last several decades." (10)

In adults, cancers occur after a delay of seven to 20 years (or more) between the time of exposure to cancer-causing agents and the manifestation of a cancer. However, in the case of childhood cancers, these delays are often much shorter. That makes it seem as if many childhood cancers occur in children who are somehow predisposed to getting the disease. If they are exposed to a carcinogen before or shortly after birth, their disease manifests quickly. Perhaps the predisposition is inherited, or it may be caused by something in the environment. (11) Whatever the reasons, our children are breaking down sooner. Cancer is becoming an "epidemic" not just for the population at large, but for our children too. Clearly, their overall health is impaired, allowing cancer cells to flourish and take over.

Two questions arise: Why is cancer increasing at all, among adults and children alike? And why is it affecting people at younger and younger ages?

The second question will be discussed later – in Chapter XII. The answer to the first question may not be obvious to the traditional medical and scientific community, but is readily apparent when you just look at our history, society and environment.

Causes of Cancer

There are a myriad of reasons people get cancer – from alterations in the foods we eat and nutritional problems to the chemicals and impurities in our environment. The list of causative agents seems almost endless, and many have already been discussed.

Sometimes it may appear as if there's no way to avoid cancer. Many people are beginning to believe that getting cancer is inevitable and just a fact of life. But we are not predisposed to cancer. Many of the causes can be eliminated or lessened simply by changing your lifestyle. In fact, a recent study reported in the *New England Journal of Medicine* examined 44,788 pairs of twins and found that environmental factors such as diet and lifestyle are a much better indicator of cancer risk than genetics. (12) You can do much to protect yourself from cancer (and any other disease for that matter) if you live properly and take precautionary measures. You have the power to save yourself and your child from the miseries and expense of ill health. The first step to doing so is to know the enemy.

Chemicals

Since the 1940s, thousands of new chemicals have been introduced into our lives – roughly 300 each year. The production of synthetic materials has increased from 1.3 million pounds in 1940 to 320 billion pounds in 1980. The health effects on children for a majority of those compounds is unknown. And fewer than 10 percent of these chemicals have been tested for their effects on the central nervous system. (13)

But don't hold your breath if you expect testing these chemicals for adverse health effects, as important as you may believe it to be, will happen soon. John Wargo, Ph.D., of Yale University comments, "Thousands of synthetic chemicals need to be tested to understand their toxicity. By the time the federal government completes these tests, my children will have children." (14) Wargo, one of the country's top experts on toxic chemicals, goes on to give us some sage advice, "It is just common sense to reduce exposure to toxic substances. Eat low on the food chain, test your water, buy organic food when possible, renovate [your house] with special care, and don't allow smoking around children."

But is there *proof* that these chemicals cause problems in humans? Many people think that modern synthetic chemicals pose little or no risk. But in a 1969 study, the causes of death among 3,637 members of the American Chemical Society (ACS) revealed that chemists die at unusually high rates from cancer of the pancreas and lymph system and female chemists had an elevated risk of breast cancer. The study also revealed that chemists tend to commit suicide more than other people do. (15) In another study 347 white female members of ACS who died between 1925 and 1979, there were increases in breast cancer, ovary, stomach, pancreas, lymphatic, and hematopoietic (blood-forming) cancers. Suicide among those women was five times higher than other U.S. white females. (16)

In a study reported in the *Journal of Occupational Medicine*, employees of a large pharmaceutical company revealed an increase in the occurrence of several kinds of cancer – lung, skin, and brain – among males and an increase in leukemia, breast, and large-intestine cancers in females. [17] Another study, of Exxon employees, revealed an increase in leukemia and lymphatic cancers among scientists, engineers, and research technicians, as compared with managerial employees who had less potential for chemical exposure. [18]

Apparently, chemicals affect adults in adverse ways if they are overly or consistently exposed. The risk of these kinds of exposures to children is probably less, but they are still exposed to chemicals during day-to-day activities. The evidence shows that minimizing exposures to any unnatural chemicals may help reduce the chances of cancers later in life.

As the use of chemicals in our society increases, so do the occurrences of brain cancer. Table 3 shows the increase over a 35-year period. The steady increase in brain cancer is true for all industrialized countries (who use various chemicals consistently). In addition, there are similar increases occurring in children, so the increases are not just an effect of aging.

Table 3
Number of Brain Cancers [19]

Year	Per 100,000 Population
1940	1.95
1945	2.25
1950	2.90
1955	3.40
1960	3.70
1970	4.10
1975	4.25

Clearly there is a correlation between chemical exposure and disease. To protect our children from harm, we need to clean up our environment.

Our Food Supply

Can the foods we eat contribute to cancer? Most experts now think so. But is it just the *kinds* of foods we choose to eat, or could it be the very *nature* of the food itself?

Since the early part of the 20th century, our society has changed from a small-farm, mostly rural one to a big-city, industrial one. In the early 1900s most people lived in the country on small, largely self-sufficient farms. (Remember that cancer rates were very low in the early part of the 20th century.) People ate food grown locally, raised without chemicals, pesticides, and herbicides because they did not exist. Essentially, everything was raised organically. Also, there was very little processing of the food, and there was little transportation of food.

As more people moved to the city for jobs, the small farms slowly gave way to large agribusiness. Food had to be transported from the country to the city, so the shelf life of the food needed to be extended.

Enter processing and chemical additives to accomplish this. Case in point: white flour. The outer "germ" of wheat is rich in oils and fats that are needed by the human body. The problem is, those fats and oils turn rancid easily and quickly once the wheat is milled. The shelf life of whole-grain bread is therefore short. When bread goes bad, the manufacturers lose money. But, if the germ is removed, and only the white pulp is used to make bread (or pasta, bagels, pastry, etc.) then the shelf life is prolonged. Bread doesn't spoil as easily, transportation and storage are no longer such a problem, and less bread goes "bad" before it reaches the consumer. It makes *economic* sense.

The same is true for milk. The reason milk is pasteurized is not so much to kill bacteria (as health officials insist) as to prolong shelf life. If you drink fresh milk within a few days of collecting it – like they did down on the farm long ago – you need not worry about bacteria which develops only after a period of storage. To get milk to market sometimes thousands of miles away, the bacteria that could develop in transit needs to be kept in check to prolong the shelf life. Pasteurization does nothing to increase the nutrition of milk. In fact, vital minerals, vitamins, and fatty acids are altered and made less bio-available when they are heated as in the pasteurization process.

The end result of this overprocessing of our food is that it is less nutritious and more contaminated. This leads to weaker bodies, minds, and emotions. Weaker bodies are more susceptible to diseases – including cancer. In addition, the food additives themselves must be handled by the body (a food additive is not a "food," but an impurity), and energy must be expended to do this. Often the additives may be poisonous themselves and contributors to the formation of cancer.

Food Additives

The regulation of food additives in the U.S. began in 1938 under the Federal Food, Drug, and Cosmetic (FD&C) Act, which created the FDA and gives it authority over food and food ingredients and defined requirements for truthful labeling of ingredients. The Food Additives Amendment to the FD&C Act, passed in 1958, requires FDA approval for the use of an additive prior to its inclusion in food. It also requires the manufacturer to prove an additive's safety for the ways it will be used. Unfortunately, all substances that the FDA or the U.S. Department of Agriculture (USDA) had determined were safe for use in specific food prior to the 1958 amendment were designated as prior-sanctioned substances and "grandfathered in" as acceptable no matter what future research found. The problem here, of course, is that these "prior-sanctioned" substances may not, indeed, be safe. Examples of prior-sanctioned substances are sodium nitrite and potassium nitrite (used to preserve luncheon meats), substances that have come into question many times over the years. (20)

The FDA estimates that there are more than 3,000 different additives, mostly synthetic chemicals, used in our foods – only 2,000 of which the FDA has chemical and toxicological information on. The other 1,000 the FDA has only administrative and chemical information on. (21)

Here is a very partial list of some food additives (dyes) and their potential health effects. These additives do not increase shelf life. They do not make the food more nutritious. They don't even make it taste better! You may remember when FD & C Red No. 2 dye was removed from general use because it caused cancer in lab animals. But there are many other questionable coloring agents still widely in use. These are dyes used to color our foods so they look pretty:

Table 4
Food additives and their health effects (22)

Additive	Health Effects
FD&C Red No. 2	Angioedema (swelling of the heart), cancer
FD&C Red No. 3	Thyroid tumors, chromosomal damage
Citrus Red No. 2	Cancer in animals
Allura Red AC	Tumors/lymphomas
FD&C Yellow No. 5	Allergies, thyroid tumors, lymphocytic lymphomas, chromosomal damage, trigger for asthma, hives, hyperactivity
FD&C Yellow No. 6 (Sunset Yellow)	Allergies, kidney tumors, chromosomal damage, abdominal pain, vomiting, indigestion
FD&C Green No. 3 (Fast Green)	Bladder tumors

It's quite unrealistic to think that all the additives used in foods are 100 percent safe and do no harm. Food additives are chemicals not natural to our body. They're not used as fuel and are not needed for any cellular processes. They just get in the way. Many studies indicate that many additives may be cancer causing or cause behavioral or other problems. Even if the additive is not outright poisonous or cancer-causing, it's not a food and therefore only a burden the body must get rid of or store – often times in fat cells. And you know how hard it is to get rid of fat cells (with their accumulated poisons)!

It's interesting to consider how the FDA approves a food additive for use. The following is a section of text taken straight out of the January 1992 FDA/IFIC Brochure titled "Food Additives." I've added emphasis to those phrases I find most alarming:

How Are Additives Approved for Use in Foods?

To market a new food or color additive, a manufacturer must first petition FDA for its approve. Approximately 100 new food and color additives petitions are submitted to FDA annually...

A food or color additive petition must provide convincing evidence that the proposed additive performs as it is intended. Animal studies using large doses of the additive for long periods *are often necessary* to show that the substance would not cause harmful effects at *expected levels of human consumption*. Studies of the additive in humans also *may be* submitted to FDA.

In deciding whether an additive should be approved, the agency considers the composition and properties of the substance, the amount likely to be consumed, its probable long-term effects and various safety factors. *Absolute safety of any substance can never be proven.* Therefore, FDA must determine if the additive is safe under the proposed conditions of use, based on the best scientific knowledge available.

If an additive is approved, FDA issues regulations that may include the types of foods in which it can be used, the maximum amounts to be used, and how it should be identified on food labels...

Federal officials then *carefully monitor the extent of Americans' consumption* of the new additive and results of any new research on its safety to assure its use continues to be within safe limits.

In addition, FDA operates an Adverse Reaction Monitoring System (ARMS) to help serve as an ongoing safety check of all additives. The system monitors and investigates all complaints by individuals or their physicians that are believed to be related to specific foods; food and color additives; or vitamin and mineral supplements. The ARMS computerized database helps officials *decide whether reported adverse reactions represent a real public health hazard associated with food*, so that appropriate action can be taken. (23)

I would like to discuss each italicized section to help you realize just what we're dealing with here:

"Animal studies *are often* necessary to show no adverse effects." That really means that they are not always necessary, and a food additive may be approved with no toxicological or epidemiological studies (i.e., animal testing).

"...the substance would not cause harmful effects at *expected levels of human consumption.*" So if someone consumes more than the expected level, they may get sick? Well, yes. As an example, let's look at sulfites, a common food additive. The above-referenced brochure comments on sulfites as follows: "Sulfites added to baked goods, condiments, snack foods and other products are safe for most people. A small segment of the population, however, has been found to develop hives, nausea, diarrhea, shortness of breath or even fatal shock after consuming sulfites. For that reason, in 1986 FDA banned the use of sulfites on fresh fruits and vegetables intended to be sold or served raw to consumers. Sulfites added as preservative in all other packaged and processed foods must be listed on the product label." In the case of sulfites, it took people dying to change the regulation, and since they're still in some foods, the possibility exists others may still have severe reactions.

"Studies of the additive in humans also *may be* submitted to FDA." "May be" means "a manufacturer has permission to." So it's not required to have any information on the effects of a proposed additive on humans to get FDA approval, but the FDA is giving permission for someone to submit the information if they so choose!

"Absolute safety of any substance can never be proven." So what the FDA does is look at "relative" safety. Then, it all becomes a matter of opinion as to what is safe.

"Federal officials then *carefully monitor the extent of Americans' consumption* of the new additive..." I would believe that it's pretty much impossible to track the consumption of FD&C Red No. 3 among our population and see who is consuming it and what effects, acute (short-term) or chronic (long-term), it may be having. The "monitoring" is really a case of disaster regulation. When a disaster occurs, like when people start dying from ingesting too many sulfites, then and only then is the regulation changed. Essentially, what is occurring is that the U.S. population has become the lab test animals.

But back to the FDA's words: "The ARMS computerized database helps officials *decide whether reported adverse reactions represent a real public health hazard* associated with food, so that appropriate action can be taken." In many cases, adverse reactions may not be recognized as coming from a food additive. How many people would attribute their allergies or asthma to FD&C Yellow No. 5? Then, there's the subjectivity of the officials to determine if reported reactions represent a real public health hazard.

Food for Thought

There are two major points I'd like to make using food additives as the example. First, it's virtually impossible to effectively regulate substances used as food additives. Any additive may have adverse effects – either acute or chronic – on certain people. The FDA or any regulatory agency simply cannot ensure that anything used in food is safe. It then becomes the responsibility of the consumer to determine if a certain food is safe for his or her own consumption. And the regulations are based on "the population at

---

large." If someone is overly sensitive, he or she may have an adverse reaction, where most people do not. Too bad for the sensitive individual. Second, you must understand the human body and how it works to fully appreciate why any additive is really deleterious. If the body cannot use a substance as a nutrient, it sees it as a waste. The more polluted a body becomes, the more likely it will fail to function to its optimum or will function incorrectly. Considering that, it's not a mystery at all why the body breaks down, gets cancer or some other "disease," or becomes ill whether physically, mentally, or emotionally. A clean and well-fed body and mind will perform the way nature intended it to – without disease and without aggression.

The FDA, like most individuals, views the human body in shades of gray, where really the body operates more as black or white. The FDA believes that if a substance does not cause "apparent and obvious" negative effects, then it is having no negative effect. That is simply not true. Even if a substance does not cause an obvious health problem or risk, if the body is not using it as a nutrient, then it is really a pollutant that will rob the body of energy and cause long-term problems, premature aging, and disease. And as we saw earlier, children and fetuses are often times more sensitive to adverse effects than adults are.

It's all a matter of energy dynamics. Your body takes in fuel, nutrients, air, water, and sunlight and converts them into usable energy. That energy is used to operate the muscles, nerves, brain, and so on. There is not an endless supply of energy. It is limited. We eat food and get a certain amount of energy from it. That energy is either used for movement, regeneration and repair, or waste disposal. The more used for waste disposal (i.e., getting rid of unusable dyes and other additives, not to mention other pollutants we must expel), the less is available for movement (daily living) and regeneration and repair of our body. The less available for regeneration and repair, the less regeneration and repair occur – and the more susceptible we become to lack of energy, diseases, and systemic breakdowns. It's not unlike the operation of a car engine or other mechanical devises. If the engine oil gets dirty, if the spark plugs are fouled, if the gas and air filters are clogged, is the car going to operate at peak efficiency? Or is it more likely to sputter and break down?

If waste cannot be eliminated, the body tucks it away somewhere – usually in soft tissue or fat. Over time, those accumulations build up and can cause problems. For example, the intake of the wrong kind of calcium - one being dicalcium phosphate which is used in many health supplements as a binding agent – can not only interfere with nutrient absorption, but also contribute to deposits of inert calcium in joints and arteries, contributing to arthritis and arteriolosclerosis.

We do not live in some magic never-never land. With all the science that we use to determine health effects, we are assuming that dyes, additives, preservatives, and other toxins are somehow magically removed or rendered harmless by the human body. Have there been any radioisotope studies to determine where that molecule of "Sunset Yellow" goes once it's been ingested? It would be interesting to find out. A computer operates digitally: Every switch in the computer is just an on/off switch; either yes or no. The human body is the same. Every substance is either good or bad. Good if it gives energy. Bad if it robs us of energy. That's it. Keep this in mind when making decisions on what you put into it.

Aspartame - The Worst Food Additive

Aspartame is an artificial sweetener (more than 200 times sweeter than sugar) used in diet sodas, "lite" yogurt and ice cream, sugarless gelatin desserts, and a number of other products. It's the technical name for the brand names NutraSweet, Equal, Spoonful, Indulge, Canderel, Benevia, and Equal-Measure. It is now the most popular artificial sweetener on the market, with sales of more than $100 million a year. In 1987, the last year that NutraSweet publicized its records, Americans consumed around 17,100,000 pounds of aspartame. Now our estimated consumption is over 25 million pounds per year. (24)

Aspartame was discovered by accident in 1965 and approved for use in dry goods in 1981 and carbonated beverages in 1983. It had been approved for use as early as 1974, but objections from neuroscientist John W. Olney, Ph.D., and consumer groups made the FDA revoke its approval, which was later reinstated. (25)

Aspartame has been called "by far, the most dangerous substance on the market that is added to foods." (26) In all, there have been more than 90 different documented symptoms. Many of these reactions are minor, but some are quite serious. A February 1994 Department of Health and Human Services report lists many reactions to aspartame, two of which are seizures and death.

Mary Nash Stoddard is the founder of the Aspartame Consumer Safety Network and author of a book about aspartame (*Deadly Deception*). She's a recognized expert on aspartame and is a board member of the National Natural Foods Association and a former judge on the State of Texas Board of Adjustments. Way back in 1995 she spoke out against aspartame. She said that at that time, about 78 percent of all "Adverse Reaction" complaints to the FDA concerned aspartame, and at one time, the figure was 85 percent! She called this "a well-hidden secret."

She went on to say:

> Aspartame not only causes individual symptoms, it can mimic entire syndromes! For example... it can mimic the symptoms of CFIDS [chronic fatigue and immune deficiency syndrome]. It can also cause grand mal seizures. According to H.J. Roberts, M.D., it

can cause decreased vision, pain in the eyes, decreased tears, ringing in the ears, hearing impairment, headache, dizziness, and unsteadiness, confusion, memory loss, drowsiness, sleepiness, slurring of speech, numbness and tingling, tremors, depression, irritability, aggression, anxiety, insomnia, phobias, heart palpitations, shortness of breath, high blood pressure, nausea, diarrhea, abdominal pain, itching, hives, menstrual changes, weight gain, hair thinning and hair loss, urinary burning and frequency, excessive thirst, fluid retention, bloating, increased infections, and even death.... Five deaths were reported prior to 1987. We don't know the number since then.... (27)

Stoddard sees big money behind the approval of the artificial sweetener. After removal from the market, she says aspartame was finally approved again, but not without supposed payoffs and other questionable political occurrences. Even though the FDA approves a substance, it *may not* be as safe as it sounds. There's big money involved here, and big money has a tendency to sway some people into twisting the truth. One example is how Dr. Arthur Hull Hayes Jr., as the commissioner of the FDA, approved NutraSweet for soft drinks. Two months later, he took a position with a subsidiary of the company that manufacturers aspartame (Monsanto) as the senior medical advisor in their public relations firm to the tune of $1,000 a day. This is in the public record. Just one isolated incident? Stoddard had this to say:

> Watch out, diabetics! The NutraSweet Company has given money, money, money to the American Diabetes Association. And remember when you hear a registered dietitian say aspartame is safe for pregnant women, children, and everyone else, the registered dietitian's professional association has been given $75,000 to expound on the virtues of aspartame. The American Dietetic Association has even stated that the NutraSweet Company writes their "Fact Sheets." Aspartame approval and persistence on the market has everything to do with money and politics, and almost nothing to do with science and reason. Even the FDA's own reviewers were against aspartame until those political [and] financial events I've mentioned. There are reports that many research reports to justify aspartame's use were poorly conducted and outright fraud. Senator Edward Kennedy said that "the extensive nature of the almost unbelievable range of abuses discovered by the FDA on several major Searle products is profoundly disturbing." [Searle Pharmaceuticals manufactures NutraSweet.] (28)

Aspartame is made up of three chemicals: aspartic acid (40 percent), phenylalanine (50 percent), and methanol (10 percent). It's considered by many to be a "chemical poison." Russell L. Blaylock, M.D., a professor of Neurosurgery at the University of Mississippi medical school and author of the book *Excitotoxins: The Taste That Kills*, cites almost 500 scientific references which show how excess excitatory amino acids (of which aspartic acid is one - and also the glutamic acid found in the popular flavor-enhancer monosodium glutamate commonly known as MSG) are causing serious chronic neurological disorders and other acute symptoms. The effects of aspartic acid together with glutamic acid (from MSG) are cumulative – meaning that when both are taken together, their individual adverse effects are multiplied. (29) So don't drink a diet soda when you're having Chinese food.

Blaylock says that too much aspartate (or glutamate from MSG) in the brain kills certain brain cells because it "excites" or stimulates the neural cells to death. The blood-brain barrier (BBB) normally protects the brain from toxins, but it cannot always do so. During childhood, the BBB is not fully developed, and aspartate (and glutamate) can get into the brain. Therefore, children and fetuses are especially vulnerable. Even in adulthood, excess aspartate (and glutamate) can seep through the BBB causing damage. And there are some parts of the brain that the BBB does not fully protect. The areas of the brain most affected are the hypothalamus, medulla oblongata, and corpus striatum – each intricately involved in regulating various processes in the body. (30)

Blaylock goes on to say that excessive buildup of phenylalanine in the brain can cause seizures or even schizophrenia. When aspartate (and glutamate) are in the brain, they slowly destroy neurons. And they are silent killers: the majority (more than 75 percent) of the brain cells in a particular area are killed before any clinical symptoms of a chronic illness are evident. Long-term exposure to these excitatory amino acids can contribute to multiple sclerosis, ALS, memory loss, epilepsy, Alzheimer's disease, Parkinson's disease, hypoglycemia, AIDS, dementia, brain lesions, neuroendocrine disorders, brain tumors, mental retardation, lymphoma, birth defects, fibromyalgia, and diabetes.

Ingesting aspartame can lead to excess levels of phenylalanine, an amino acid that's normally found in the brain. People with a genetic disorder called phenylketonuria (PKU) are especially susceptible to this (sometimes causing death), but people without PKU can also be vulnerable. Also, excessive levels of phenylalanine in the brain can cause serotonin levels to decrease, which can lead to depression.

In testimony before the U.S. Congress, Dr. Louis J. Elsas, M.D., professor of pediatrics at Emory University for 25 years, showed that a high blood level of phenylalanine can indeed be concentrated in parts of the brain, and is especially dangerous for infants and fetuses. (31) Even a single dose of aspartame can raise the blood level of phenylalanine. He said:

> First of all, in the developing fetus... the mother is supplying that fetus with nutrients. And if she were dieting, let's say, and increasing her blood phenylalanine uniquely by taking Crystal Lite or Kool-Aid, or any of the various diet foods now, to maintain her weight, and increased her blood phenylalanine from its normal 50 to 150 umoles/liter [micromoles per liter] by chronic ingestion at 35 milligrams of aspartame per kilo per day – which everyone agrees could be reached – the placenta will concentrate her blood phenylalanine twofold. So the fetal blood circulation to her baby in utero is now 300 umole [of phenylalanine per liter]. The fetal brain then

Cancer

will increase further that concentration into the brain cells of that baby two to fourfold. Those are neurotoxic levels in tissue culture and in many other circumstances. (32)

Dr. William M. Pardridge, M.D., a Professor of Medicine, says that increases in phenylalanine concentrations in the blood of the pregnant mother can cause a drop in the IQ of the child born of that mother and a lowering of the higher cognitive function (the ability to make key decisions). Another study by Elsas showed that "there are quantitative changes in the human electroencephalogram when the blood phenylalanine is raised threefold – something that clearly will happen in children who consume nearly five servings per 50-pound body weight." (An electroencephalogram, or EEG, is a devise to measure the electrical activity of the brain. Variations from a normal reading indicate the brain has unbalanced and unhealthy electrical activity.)

One account of harmful aspartame use is noteworthy here. A man by the name of John Cook was drinking six to eight diet drinks every day. He started experiencing memory loss and frequent headaches. Then came wide mood swings and violent rages. Even though he did not have PKU, a blood test revealed a phenylalanine blood level that was extremely high. Cook showed abnormal brain function and brain damage. When he went off aspartame, his symptoms improved. (33)

Food for Thought

Since a large percentage of our youngsters are now overweight, I wonder how many of them are consuming diet sodas, maybe on advice of their parents. Which leads one to wonder if some of the violent acts by our youth may be partially due to the neurological effects of aspartame.

Ten percent of aspartame is wood alcohol or methanol. That's a known deadly poison. It's caused "skid row" alcoholics to end up blind or dead. Methanol is released in the small intestine when aspartame is digested. Absorption is sped up when aspartame is heated because free methanol is then created. That's what happens when you make sugar-free Jell-O (or when aspartame-containing products are stored above 86 degrees F). Yet, in 1993, the FDA approved aspartame as an ingredient in numerous foods that are typically heated above 86 degrees F. Mary Nash Stoddard has this to say about aspartame and methanol:

> Among other things, [aspartame is] about 10 percent methanol (wood alcohol), famous for causing blindness in alcoholics. In the body, methanol metabolizes into formaldehyde, a neurotoxin; formic acid, a venom in ant stings; and diketopiperazine, which causes brain tumors in animals. It's so bad that in July of 1983, the National Soft Drink Association presented official objections to putting aspartame in beverages. I'll read you one of their objections: "It is well established under Section 402(a)(3) that a food which contains a decomposed substance... is subject to seizure by FDA." It's thoroughly

established that after a number of weeks and at temperatures over 86 degrees F, there's no aspartame left in a soft drink, only breakdown products. So, why isn't FDA seizing it under Section 402 (a) (3)?... Aspartame was originally approved in 1974, but when the brain-tumor issue arose, the approval was withdrawn.... Many of the test animals fed aspartame developed large tumors. These were actually cut out, and the animals returned to the study. In some cases, the tumors weren't even examined for malignancy, and the tumors weren't reported to FDA. In several cases, animals were reported as dead and later reported as alive again. (34)

Food for Thought

Ah... the FDA. Just knowing they're there makes you feel all warm and fuzzy and safe, doesn't it? In 90 non-industry-sponsored studies of aspartame, 83 identified one or more problems with it. Of the seven studies that did not find a problem, the FDA conducted six of them. (Soon after the FDA approval of aspartame, numerous FDA officials went to work for the aspartame industry.) Of the 74 industry-sponsored-studies of aspartame, 100 percent of them claimed there were no problems with it. (35) Some of these experiments lasted a grand total of one day. (36) Monsanto (makers of aspartame) funded a study on the possible birth defects caused by aspartame. When preliminary data showed "damaging information" in the study, funding was stopped. (37) By the way, there are currently class action lawsuits being filed against Monsanto concerning aspartame. (Go to www.holisticmed.com for more information.)

You hear that regular table sugar is bad for you, and it is. But aspartame goes beyond the hazards of sugar, in some cases causing severe changes in the brain's activity. In an independent double-blind study in children with generalized absence epilepsy, a single dose of aspartame worsened the EEG spike wave discharges that indicate a seizure's severity. The authors concluded, "Aspartame appears to significantly increase the duration of time that children with absence epilepsy have spike wave on their EEG. In this study, the children spent 40 percent more time in spike wave after aspartame than after sucrose." Simply put, children with epileptic tendencies will be more likely to have a seizure if they ingest aspartame. (38) Of course, the proponents of aspartame will cite different research. However, those studies are hopelessly flawed. For example, one study reported aspartame didn't increase the likelihood of seizures. But 16 of the 18 subjects were on antiseizure medication during the study! And the study consisted of only a single dose of aspartame! (39) Don't these researchers have any shame? Again, methanol is a poison. An EPA assessment of methanol says it "is considered a cumulative poison due to the low rate of excretion once it is absorbed. In the body, methanol [breaks down] to formaldehyde and formic acid; both of these metabolites are toxic." They recommended a limit of 7.8 mg/day of methanol. A 1-liter (about 1-quart) bottle of an aspartame-sweetened beverage has about *56 mg* of methanol in it. Someone who drinks four 1-liter bottles a day consumes as much as 250 mg of methanol daily, or 32 times the EPA limit. (40) Concerning formaldehyde, "...formaldehyde formation from aspartame ingestion is very common and does indeed accumulate within the cell, reacting with cellular proteins (mostly enzymes) and DNA (both mitochondrial and nuclear). The fact that it accumulates with each dose, indicates grave consequences among those who consume diet drinks and foodstuffs on a daily basis." Formaldehyde also causes retinal damage, is a known carcinogen, interferes with DNA replication, and causes birth defects. (41)

The best known results of methanol poisoning are eyesight problems, which may include misty or blurry vision, progressive contraction of visual fields, retinal damage, and blindness. Other symptoms include headaches, ear buzzing, dizziness, nausea, gastrointestinal disturbances, weakness, vertigo, chills, memory lapses, numbness and shooting pains in the extremities, behavioral disturbances, and neuritis.

Some fruit juices and alcoholic beverages contain small amounts of methanol. However, in these cases ethanol (another alcohol) is also present. Ethanol is an antidote for methanol toxicity so it's presence essentially cancels out the methanol.

Diketopiperazine (DKP) is another byproduct of aspartame metabolism. It's been implicated in the occurrences of brain tumors and uterine polyps. In 1981, an FDA statistician named Satya Dubey stated that the brain tumor data on aspartame indicated it was so bad that he could not recommend its approval. Aspartame has caused large brain tumors in animal experiments at a dose that could be considered within the "Acceptable Daily Intake" of humans (after adjusting for differences in metabolism between humans and the test animals).

The late Adrian Gross, Ph.D., a former FDA toxicologist, testified before Congress that aspartame was capable of producing brain tumors:

> In view of all these indications that the cancer-causing potential of aspartame is a matter that had been established way beyond any reasonable doubt, one can ask: what is the reason for the apparent refusal by the FDA to invoke for this food additive the so-called Delaney Amendment to the Food, Drug, and Cosmetic Act? Is it not clear beyond any shadow of a doubt that aspartame had caused brain tumors or brain cancer in animals, and is this not sufficient to satisfy the provisions of that particular section of the law? Given that this is so (and I cannot see any kind of tenable argument opposing the view that aspartame causes cancer) how would the FDA justify its position that it views a certain amount of aspartame (50 mg/mg body-weight) as constituting an ADI [Allowable Daily Intake] or "safe" level for it? Is that position in effect not equivalent to setting a "tolerance" for this food additive and thus a violation of that law? And if the FDA itself elects to violate the law, who is left to protect the health of the public? (42)

The Truth About Children's Health

Between the years 1973 and 1990, the incidences of brain tumors in people over 65 years of age has increased 67 percent. Brian tumors in all age groups have jumped by 10 percent. (43) The researchers of study on the carcinogenicity of aspartame reported in the *Journal of Neuropathology & Experimental Neurology* concluded:

> ...the artificial sweetener aspartame is a promising candidate to explain the recent increase in incidence and degree of malignancy of brain tumors... An early animal study revealing an exceedingly high incidence of brain tumors in aspartame-fed rats compared to no brain tumors in concurrent controls, the recent finding that the aspartame molecule has mutagenic potential, and the close temporal association. (44)

Aspartame was introduced into U.S. foods and beverage markets several years prior to the sharp increase in brain tumor incidence and malignancy. Aspartame was approved for use in 1974, revoked, and then approved again in 1981. Our "watchdog" government on patrol again. They say it's safe, but what do you think? Are those few calories you save by using aspartame products really worth a brain tumor?

The American Diabetes Association (ADA) is recommending aspartame to people with diabetes. But according to research conducted by H.J. Roberts, M.D., a diabetes specialist who is also a member of the ADA and an authority on artificial sweeteners, aspartame can lead to clinical diabetes, causes poorer diabetic control for those on insulin or oral drugs, leads to the aggravation of diabetic complications such as retinopathy, cataracts, neuropathy, gastroparesis, and causes convulsions. (45) When patients avoided aspartame Roberts saw "Dramatic improvement... and the prompt predictable reoccurrence of these problems when the patient resumed aspartame products..."

Roberts states: "I regret the failure of other physicians and the American Diabetes Association to sound appropriate warnings to patients and consumers based on these repeated findings which have been described in my corporate-neutral studies and publications." (46)

Ralph G. Walton, Ph.D., conducted a study to see what the effects of aspartame are on people with mood disorders. Symptoms got so bad that the Institutional Review Board forced him to stop the study. Walton said, "Individuals with mood disorders are particularly sensitive to this artificial sweetener; its use in this population should be discouraged." (47) Walton later stated, "I know it causes seizures, I'm convinced also that it definitely causes behavioral changes. I'm very angry that this substance is on the market. I personally question the reliability and validity of any studies funded by the NutraSweet Company." (By the way, when Walton tried to buy aspartame from NutraSweet for his study, they would not sell it to him! He had to get certified product somewhere else.) (48)

The ADA is not the only organization approving aspartame. The Epilepsy Foundation is also promoting it as safe. Yet at the Massachusetts Institute of Technology, 80 people who had suffered seizures after ingesting aspartame were studied. It was concluded that "These 80 cases meet the FDA's own definition of an imminent hazard to the public health, which requires the FDA to expeditious-ly remove a product from the market." (49) One of the first studies performed on aspartame was in 1969 by Harry Waisman, Ph.D., who studied its effects on infant primates. Out of the seven infant monkeys, one died after 300 days and five others had grand mal seizures. (50)

The U.S. Air Force magazine *Flying Safety* has published articles warning about the many dangers of aspartame, cautioning that its ingestion can make pilots more susceptible to seizures and vertigo. Other magazines echo that warn-ing, among them, *National Business Aircraft Association Digest* (NBAA Digest, 1993), *Aviation Medical Bulletin* (1988), *The Aviation Consumer* (1988), *Canadian General Aviation News* (1990), *Pacific Flyer* (1988), *General Aviation News* (1989), *Aviation Safety Digest* (1989), and *Plane and Pilot* (1990). More than 600 pilots have reported symptoms from aspartame including grand mal seizures in the cockpit. (51)

Aspartame is everywhere: breath mints, cereals, sugar-free chewing gum, cocoa mixes, coffee beverages, frozen desserts, gelatin desserts, juice beverages, laxatives, *multivitamins*, milk drinks, pharmaceuticals and supplements, shake mixes, soft drinks, tabletop sweeteners, tea beverages, instant teas and coffees, topping mixes, wine coolers, puddings, chewing gum, candy cough syrups, yogurt, and others. And this is just the tip of the iceberg. You may wonder why aspartame is used in all these products. Do you think the reason could be because it's cheaper than sugar? In closing this section, I quote an adult victim of aspar-tame poisoning:

> I know that the average consumer has a devil-may-care, some-
> thing-is-gonna-kill-me attitude... but they don't realize that before

this stuff kills they are going to have a miserable declining existence with *lots* of pain and other problems (not to mention cancer, tumors, and maybe even Alzheimers or similar things) before death solves the problem. (52)

Parents, whatever you do, don't feed your child products with aspartame - such as diet sodas. You're looking at trouble. Play it safe – always. Feed them something natural.

Food for Thought

In some cases children that have already suffered from aspartame toxicity have had similar toxic reactions to aspartame and some people suspect products that contain aspartame are not labeled as such. If that is happening, it is clearly against the law. To be safe, you may want to purchase products from a health food store, since it is less likely that those products contain aspartame. Some health food stores refuse to even sell any product containing aspartame. Many health food companies are quite vigilant since they were born out of a concern for health and the environment.

CHAPTER IV
Diabetes

D iabetes mellitus (Greek for "honey that passes through") is a group of diseases characterized by high levels of blood glucose resulting from defects in insulin secretion, insulin action, or both. Diabetes can be associated with serious complications and premature death. (1)

Diabetes is a disease of the endocrine system, specifically, a disorder of the pancreas. The pancreas produces hormones that help digest your food, but the pancreas has another important function: it creates hormones that regulate your body's use of glucose, a form of sugar that fuels most of the daily activities of all your body's cells.

The pancreas produces three hormones: insulin, glucagon, and somatostatin. When the concentration of sugar rises in your blood (i.e., after a meal), insulin stimulates muscle and fat cells to recover glucose from the blood and store it. Insulin also stimulates storage of excess glucose in the liver in the form of a starch called glycogen.

When more sugar is needed in the blood, the pancreas produces the hormone glucagon to break down glycogen in the liver and turn it back into glucose (blood sugar), which is then released into the blood stream. The third pancreatic hormone, somatostatin, is not so well understood as the other two, but is thought to also help regulate sugar levels in the blood.

When the pancreatic system fails to control glucose properly, the blood can end up containing too much sugar, a condition called hyperglycemia. Eventually, this sugar gets dumped in the urine, so a diabetics urine sugar will be higher – thus the Greek "honey that passes through."

Nearly 16 million people in the United States have some form of diabetes. That's roughly 5.9 percent of the population. Of these 16 million people, it is estimated that 5.4 million of them are undiagnosed cases. Many people suffering from diabetes symptoms do not realize they have the disease. There are 800,000 new cases of diabetes diagnosed each year. In 1996, diabetes was considered a major contributing cause of death in 192,140 people, and was ranked as the sixth leading cause of death. (2)

Diabetes may be underreported on death certificates, both as a condition and as a cause of death. However "I expect diabetes to be one of the major killers of the world in the year 2010," says Jak Jervell, president of the International Diabetes Federation. "What is bothering me is that the developing world will bear the brunt of this increase," referring to people adopting an American lifestyle of fatty fast food with little or no physical exercise. (3)

In 1947 there were about 600,000 cases of diabetes in the U.S. (4) And although the U.S. population has approximately doubled since the 1940s, the number of diabetics has risen more than 20 times. (5) Between 1990 and 1998 diabetes in the adult population as increased 33 percent. The CDC is predicting an alarming and steady rise in diabetes in the near future. The highest increase is in young adults between 20 and 30 years of age, which has gone up 70 percent from 1990 to 1998. The American Diabetes Association projects that at a conservative 3.5 percent growth rate, 50 million Americans will have diabetes by the year 2025 – that's one in every five or six citizens. (6)

Diabetes and obesity go hand in hand. According to Dr. Ali Mokdad, a senior epidemiologist at the CDC, the main reason behind the rise of diabetes is a concurrent rise in obesity and the association of obesity and diabetes is as strong as the association of cigarette smoking and lung cancer. Many researchers have noted a relationship between obesity and diabetes in both adults and children – and considered it one of the major contributing causes of diabetes. With roughly 25 percent of U.S. children being overweight or obese, diabetes is concomitantly a major problem. In fact, a study of adolescents in Cincinnati found 92 percent of 1,027 children with diabetes were obese. (7)

Food for Thought

Parents, if your child is overweight, that's not just a problem in itself or something he or she will just grow out of. There's a very good chance he or she will develop diabetes later in life. It's vital that you change your child's (and your own) dietary habits now before it's too late (see Chapter XIV for recommendations). As more and more people are getting diabetes at a younger age, in the not to distant future, we will see more and more children getting diabetes too (along with other degenerative and emotional disorders). This is due to what I call "The Ancestry Factor," which is fully explained in Chapter XII.

In both human and economic terms, diabetes is one of our nation's most costly diseases. It's the leading cause of kidney failure, blindness in adults, gangrene, and amputations. It's a major risk factor for heart disease, stroke, and birth defects, it shortens average life expectancy by up to 15 years, and it costs the nation in excess of $105 billion annually in health-related expenditures. At present, more than one of every ten health-care dollars and about one of every four Medicare dollars are spent on people with diabetes. (8)

It's expected that over the next decade, these numbers will grow as the number of people afflicted by diabetes continues to increase at an alarming rate. Since 1981, the death rate due to diabetes has increased by 30 percent.

Diabetes is not just a single disease, but occurs in several forms. The most common forms are Type I (insulin-dependent or IDDM) diabetes, which usually starts in childhood or adolescence (this is also called juvenile-onset diabetes), and Type II (non-insulin dependent or NIDDM) diabetes, which typically affects adults and increased dramatically with age and obesity. As the name implies, IDDM requires a person to take insulin, usually by daily injections. About 10 percent of all diabetics have IDDM. NIDDM usually appears after age 40 and the people who get it are usually obese. These people do not need to take insulin because the insulin levels in the blood are about normal, but their body seems to be unable to make good use of the insulin. They must control their blood sugar by controlling their diet – not an easy task for someone who already has a weight problem. About 90 percent of diabetics have NIDDM. The main effect of diabetes (any kind) is to cause changes in the body's small and large blood vessels. These changes in turn effect nearly every system in the body:

- Diabetic eye disease (retinopathy) is the most common cause of blindness in working age adults.

- Diabetic kidney disease (nephropathy) accounts for 42 percent of new cases of end-stage renal disease, and is the fastest growing cause of kidney dialysis and transplantation (over 100,000 cases per year).

- Nervous system damage (neuropathy) affects over 60 percent of diabetics, causing impaired sensation or pain in the feet or hands, slowed digestion of food in the stomach, impotence, and other problems.

- More than half of lower limb amputations in the U.S. occur among people with diabetes.

- About 80,000 amputations are performed each year on people with diabetes.

- Heart disease death rates in adults with diabetes are about two to four times those people without diabetes. Premenopausal women lose their protection from heart disease and have even more markedly increased risk.

- High blood pressure affects over 60 percent of people with diabetes. As a result of the combination of hypertension and diabetes the risk of stroke is increased two to four times.

- The rate of major congenital malformations and death of the fetus and newborn are increased three to four times when the mother is diabetic.

- Higher rates of infection, periodontal disease, and many other problems occur in people with diabetes. (9)

I bring the above details to your attention because there are so many people who do not even know they have diabetes. We will go into the symptoms a little later. If, after you read this chapter, you believe you may have diabetes or have many of the symptoms, I suggest you consult a trained health care professional.

It's estimated that one out of every 600 children in the U.S. has diabetes, which is about 125,000 children under the age of 20.

Most of these cases are Type I, IDDM diabetes. It is one of the most frequent chronic diseases in children in the United States. The incidence of IDDM is higher than all other chronic diseases of youth. Much has been written about the frequency of childhood AIDS, which is certainly a major health concern. However, the number of children who develop IDDM each year is about 13,000, more than 14 times that seen for cases of childhood AIDS. The economic impact of IDDM is large, with a cost to age 40 years of almost $40,000 per case. (10)

There are 13,171 new cases of IDDM a year in people less than 20 years old and 16,542 cases of IDDM in people 20 years old or older. If we compare the 13,171 new cases of IDDM for young people with rates of other diseases, onset diabetes is clearly a major problem: There are an estimated 796 cases of muscular dystrophy a year, 8,829 cases of cancer a year and 2,822 cases of leukemia a year for the same age group. "In the United States... rapid rises during certain years and in certain areas ...may be suggestive of epidemics." (11)

IDDM is largely a disease of children, while NIDDM is largely a disease of adults. However, in recent years more and more children are getting NIDDM. Prior to 1992, only 2 percent to 3 percent of pediatric patients had NIDDM and 97 percent to 98 percent had IDDM. But in a study of youngsters in Cincinnati, Ohio, in 1994, NIDDM accounted for 16 percent of all new diabetes cases. Among diabetes patients 10 to 19 years of age in this study, NIDDM accounted for 33 percent of diagnoses of diabetes that year. This represents a staggering tenfold increase in NIDDM among children in recent years. (12)

The most accepted theory about how diabetes develops is that the repeated and heavy intake of sugar causes the body's energy system to become defective. When sugar enters the bloodstream, the beta cells of the pancreas are signaled to secrete more insulin and they continue to do so until the blood sugar level drops to normal. Repeated intakes of large amounts of sugar forces the pancreas to work overtime to produce more and more insulin. Eventually, the pancreas becomes exhausted and production of insulin slumps. So when children consume too much sugar too often, they will be more likely to wear out the pancreas and the chances of developing diabetes increases. (13) A more detailed discussion about sugar and its effects is presented later in this chapter.

Another contributing factor to the development of diabetes was brought to light by Walter Mertz, Ph.D., former chief of the U.S. Department of Agriculture's Vitamin and Mineral Research Division. His experiments showed that a shortage of chromium in the diet can bring on diabetes. This is because insulin needs small amounts of chromium to help get glucose through cell walls. Mertz thinks that most adult-onset diabetes results from a diet of chromium-poor, overprocessed foods. He recommends including chromium-rich foods such as brewer's yeast, beef liver, chicken and various meats, and whole grains in the diet to avoid this problem.

Since epinephrine, a hormone released by the adrenal gland, increases free fatty acids in the blood and turns off the release of insulin, it is thought that continued stress can upset the balance of pancreas hormones and bring on diabetes (epinephrine is released when we're under stress or in "fight-or-flight" situations). (14)

Although excess fat is a contributing cause of diabetes, the traditional medical establishment knows of no biological mechanism to explain just how the presence of this excess body fat might cause diabetes. However, one researcher has a plausible explanation:

W. John H. Butterfield, M.D., Professor of Medicine at Guys Hospital in London, has done experiments to determine why overweight individuals are more prone to developing diabetes. His research showed a striking similarity in how the body handles carbohydrates in overweight individuals and those with diabetes. In the book *Solved: The Riddle of Illness*, authors Stephen E. Langer, M.D., and James F. Scheer write:

> Obese subjects handled carbohydrates almost like diabetics... As obesity progresses, less and less insulin reaches the insulin-respon-sive muscles, so less and less glucose uptake occurs there, making it necessary for more and more insulin to be formed. When obesity increases to certain proportions, the pancreas can't keep up produc-tion of insulin to meet demand, and hyperglycemia results. Reversible-obesity diabetes, then, adds up to a breakdown of the body's insulin-glucose economy. Another significant insight of Dr. Butterfield's about the propensity of diabetes in obese people is that body fat competes with muscle for insulin, and fat wins. Then car-bohydrates are changed into more fat. (15)

James Anderson, M.D., of the University of Kentucky, says that both obese and lean diabetics are helped with a diet high in fiber. This usually reduces blood fats and the need for insulin. Diets containing large amounts of raw foods, fruits, vegetables, whole grain breads, nuts, and seeds all contain a lot of fiber. Specific foods that have been shown to help are prunes, corn, spinach, fresh peas, sweet potatoes, apples, blackberries, whole wheat bread, broccoli, almonds, raisins, potatoes, zucchini, plums, and kidney beans.

Professor Somasundaram Addanki, Ph.D., of the Ohio State University College of Medicine, says that a high-fiber diet is good not only for managing dia-betes, but also for preventing it. Ninety percent of people prone to diabetes can avoid the disorder by not eating the typical American diet high in fat and sugar and low in fiber. Drawing from his own personal experience, he said that he and his wife did not develop diabetes until they came to America from their native India and started eating American foods. He thinks that only about 8 percent of diabetic cases can be strictly attributed to heredity, based on research in Africa and Japan. That theory is backed by the findings that many Japanese living in Japan did not develop diabetes; however, when they moved to Hawaii and started eat-ing American food, they developed diabetes in great numbers. (16)

Although many people believe that heredity plays a major role in diabetes, many researchers now rule this out:

> There is a definite genetic component to the development of Type I diabetes and some of these genes are known... But genetic predis-position to diabetes is far from the whole story. For one thing there is a high prevalence of these so-called susceptibility genes in the general population, yet this is not reflected in the incidence of the disease. Even in identical twins, one of which may develop dia-betes, in about half the cases the other twin, who carries the same genes, does not develop diabetes. Furthermore, in recent years the disease has been increasing in the general population at about 2.5 percent a year. (17)

Do any environmental factors contribute to the development of diabetes? In a study of Vietnam veterans, the level of dioxin levels in the blood correlated with the development of diabetes. The study compared 989 veterans who had participated in Operation Ranch Hand (which sprayed roughly 12 million gallons of Agent Orange over 10 percent of South Vietnam between 1962 and 1971) with 1,276 Air Force veterans who served in Southeast Asia during the same period but did not participate in the herbicide-spraying program. Dioxin was at about 3 parts per million in the Agent Orange.

Blood dioxin levels were significantly higher in the Ranch Hand group, and these men were about 50 percent more likely to get diabetes compared with the control group. And the severity of diabetes increased in the Ranch Hand group as the level of dioxin in the blood increased. Also, the time-to-onset of diabetes was shorter among those with more dioxin in their blood. The study found consistent increases in the likelihood of glucose (blood sugar) abnormalities with increasing dioxin levels. (18)

This finding linking diabetes to a chemical like dioxin, which is a known endocrine-disrupting chemical, offers another explanation as to why obesity contributes to diabetes. It's well recognized that human fat accumulates toxic chemicals. For any particular chemical, our fat often has a concentration 100 times as high as the concentration found in our blood. It's also known that chemicals can be released from fat to recirculate in the blood stream during times of pregnancy, stress, illness, or fasting. Many fat-stored chemicals are known to interfere with our endocrine systems by mimicking or blocking natural hormones. (19)

So it may not just be the fat that's contributing to more diabetes. It could be that the unnatural, harmful chemicals stored in the fat are causing endocrine problems which leads to diabetes. It would be interesting to find out if years ago, before all these chemicals were introduced, there was the same kind of correlation between obesity and diabetes. If there wasn't, then it very well could be that the chemicals stored in the fat, and subsequently recirculating in the blood, could be responsible for disrupting the endocrine system.

There are also theories that vaccines could cause diabetes in children. This will be explored in more detail in Chapter XI.

For now, suffice it to say that the "epidemic" of diabetes may not just be from our lifestyle of bad food and no exercise, but also from exposure to water, food, and air that has been contaminated with a myriad of chemicals, many of which mimic or interfere with our hormones. Problems, such as diabetes, can arise from this.

Dealing with Diabetes

The telltale signs of diabetes are excessive thirst, frequent and copious urination, a highly acid system, rapid weight loss, constant hunger, severe itching, weakness, fatigue, and high sugar levels in the blood and urine.

If you've been determined to need insulin, it's best to take it. However, by adopting a better, cleaner and more natural lifestyle, the symptoms and severity of your disease can be handled and alleviated. I have heard of many people who have changed their diet and exercise patterns and decreased their need for insulin. In rare cases, some have even been able to go off it completely.

A most important thing to do is to change your diet and the diet of your child – whether you are diabetic or not. The typical American diet of fast food hamburgers, pizza, coke, and chips is certainly not conducive to the health of your pancreas! In fact, if you keep eating like that, diabetes is probably just around the corner. Fresh fruits, vegetables, whole grains, good organically grown meats, nuts, seeds, greens, fresh vegetable juices, raw milk, and spring water are what the pancreas and the body need to function correctly. Remember, it's the repeated spike of sugar in the blood that causes the pancreas to work too hard. Over time, it wears out, and blood sugar problems arise.

Killing Our Children Softly

What do you think this substance is?

It removes rust spots from chrome car bumpers.

It cleans corrosion from car battery terminals.

It removes grease from clothes. Just put some into your washer and run through a regular cycle.

It's great to clean a stained toilet. Put some in and let it sit for one hour, then flush clean.

It has a pH of 3.4, which is very acidic. (Car battery acid is around 2.0. The pH of human blood is normally 7.4. And if the pH of your blood dips below 7.2, you die.)

It will dissolve a tooth or human bone. Put a tooth in this stuff and in ten days it will be gone.

It will also dissolve a common metal nail.

It will loosen a rusted bolt in minutes because it is extremely corrosive.

Did you guess a household cleaner, disinfectant or maybe even a industrial chemical? Sorry. The "substance" I'm referring to is the All-American cola drink. That's right. Soda pop. And in 1998, children between the ages of six and 11 drank an average of 15 ounces of this substance a day. (20)

We feed this to our children? One fifth of one- and two-year-old children consume soft drinks, averaging seven ounces (almost a cup) per day.

The biggest consumers are 12- to 19-year-old males, drinking an average of almost 2.5 12 ounce sodas (28.5 ounces) per day. That's 868 cans of soda pop a year. Teenage girls drink about 1.7 12-ounce sodas per day. Twenty years ago, the average consumption for boys was just three quarters a can per day.

Back in 1942, the average consumption of soft drinks per person per year was just sixty 12-ounce cans. Now children drink almost 900 cans a year. Between 1942 and 1998, production of soft drinks increased ninefold.

One reason for the increase in consumption, aside from the ubiquitous advertising, is that over the past 40 years, bottles and cans have grown in size from 6 1/2 ounces to 12-ounces to the present 20-ounce bottles. The larger the container, the more beverage people are likely to drink, especially when they assume they are buying single-serving containers.

In 1998, Americans spent over $54 billion to buy 14 billion gallons of soft drinks. That's an average of 576 12-ounce sodas per year for the average consumer – or 1.6 12 ounce cans per day for every man, woman and child in America. In 2000, sales were even higher, topping $57 million. (21)

Although soft drinks are now commonplace, they are a very recent addition to the human diet. We survived and thrived for millions of years without them. Now they are connected to a host of health problems: obesity; diabetes and other blood sugar disorders; heart disease; osteoporosis and bone fractures; nutritional deficiencies; eating disorders and food addictions; neurotransmitter dysfunction; and neurological and adrenal disorders. (22) To say, as a National Soft Drink Association's poster (intended for teachers) proclaims, that soft drinks are a "positive addition to a well-balanced diet" is positively untrue. The poster goes on to say: "As refreshing sources of needed liquids and energy, soft drinks represent a positive addition to a well-balanced diet... These same three sugars also occur naturally, for example in fruits... In your body it makes no difference whether the sugar is from a soft drink or a peach." (23)

First, it's true that the body needs liquids. Specifically, it needs water. Although a soft drink does contain about 90 percent water, it also generally contains caffeine (six of the seven top-selling soft drinks contain caffeine). Caffeine is a known diuretic, a substance that causes increased urine and water excretion. It's estimated that for every can of soda a person consumes, the body requires about two glasses of water to replenish what was lost due to the caffeine's diuretic action. That holds true for any caffeinated beverage, coffee and tea included. You may think you're replenishing water in your body when you drink that soda, but in reality, you're actually contributing to dehydration.

Second, the sugars in the soft drink may, on paper, look like the sugars found in fruits, but they are not. A manufactured, synthetic or processed sugar does *not* have the same effect on the human body as a sugar found in its natural state.

Many soft drinks now contain artificial sweeteners to cut down on calories from sugar. Two of the major ones used are saccharin and aspartame, and both have been linked to urinary-bladder cancer. Now Congress has required products made with saccharin to have a warning label – but this has done little to curtail consumption. Acesulfame-K, another artificial sweetener approved in 1998, is considered suspect by some cancer experts. (24)

Soft drinks are Americans' single biggest source of refined sugar (we'll go into the problems with refined sugars more below) Twelve- to 19-year-old boys get about 44 percent of their 34 teaspoons of sugar a day from soft drinks. Girls get a little less – only 40 percent. That translates to about 15 teaspoons of sugar a day for boys and 10 teaspoons a day for girls.

One thing to keep in mind here is that these are averages for all children. Considering that some kids don't drink any pop at all, the children who do drink it are really taking in more than that average.

As teens have doubled or tripled their consumption of soft drinks, they now drink 40 percent less milk. Twenty years ago, boys consumed twice as much milk as soda and girls consumed 50 percent more milk than soda. Now, boys and girls consume twice as much soda pop as milk. Michael Jacobson, executive director of the nonprofit Center for Science in the Public Interest (CSPI) says, "Many teens are drowning in soda pop. It's become their main beverage, providing many with 15 percent to 20 percent of all their calories and squeezing out more nutritious foods and beverages from their diets. It's time that parents limited their children's soft-drink consumption and demanded that local schools get rid of their soft-drink vending machines, just as they have banished smoking." (25)

Marianne Manilov, the executive director of the Center for Commercialism-Free Public Education (in Oakland, California), castigated schools "for sacrificing their students' health by selling out to Coca-Cola. The marketing agreements virtually ensure that more kids will be drinking more soda – while their health classes are discouraging consumption. Taxpayers must provide schools systems with adequate funds so schools don't become reliant on junk-food companies." (26) Since the adult market is essentially stagnant, the soft-drink companies are going after the young and the innocent. An article in *Beverage* magazine stated: "Influencing elementary school students is very important to soft-drink marketers." (27) So important they spend billions of dollars each year on advertising aimed at children. They run ads on Channel One – the classroom TV network seen by eight million junior and high school students every day. Coca-Cola paid one Colorado school district $11 million over more than 10 years to advertise in the hallways and sides of busses. Amazingly, the schools have quotas, so consumption, even in the classroom, is encouraged by the administration. (28)

If that's not bad enough, get this: At a press conference, CSPI displayed baby bottles with Pepsi, Seven-Up, and Dr Pepper logos. Those companies have licensed their logos to a major maker of bottles, Munchkin Bottling, Inc. One study found that parents are four times more likely to feed their children soda pop when their children use those logo bottles than when they don't. (29)

Let's look more closely at the documented health impacts of soft drinks. When you consider soft drinks in the context of obesity and overweight, it's interesting to note that obesity rates have risen in tandem with soft-drink consumption. Heavy consumers of soda pop have been shown to have higher calorie intakes. Michael F. Jacobsen, Ph.D., writes, "While those observations do not prove that sugary soft drinks cause obesity... Heavy consumption is likely to contribute to weight gain in many consumers." (30)

The National Institutes of Health recommends that people wanting to lose weight cut back on consuming soft drinks and drink water instead. Nutritionists and weight-loss experts routinely advise overweight people to consume fewer calories, especially "empty-caloric foods" such as soft drinks. Soft drinks now account for about 25 percent of sugar consumption and sugar is an empty-calorie food.

They are called "empty-calorie foods" because they have no nutritional value besides calories. A soft drink contains no vitamins, minerals, enzymes, or fiber that give a food its nutritional value. All you get when you drink a can of soda is calories (and caffeine, artificial flavoring, and acid) which can be used for energy production or stored as fat. Since we're exercising less, guess where most of it goes?

Several additives used in soft drinks can cause occasional allergic reactions. Yellow No. 5 dye causes runny noses, hives, and asthma as well as lymphoma, thyroid tumors, and chormosomal damage. (31) Cochineal, a red coloring agent, can cause life-threatening allergic reactions, and other dyes have been shown to cause hyperactivity in sensitive children. (32)

Osteoporosis

It's a well-recognized fact that low calcium intake contributes to osteoporosis, a disease that leads to fragile and broken bones. Currently, 10 million Americans have osteoporosis, with another 18 million having low bone mass. (33) It's estimated that teenage girls in the United States are getting only 60 percent of the recommended amount of calcium, with soft-drink drinkers consuming almost one fifth less than non soft-drink drinkers. (34) This means these girls are replacing healthier beverages such as milk (although super-market milk is not so healthy these days – see Chapter VI).

Not only that, but the very nature of soft drinks is that they deplete calcium in the body. It's all a matter of simple chemistry. The pH of most soft drinks is around 3.4. That's highly acidic. Neutral pH is 7. The pH of healthy blood is slightly alkaline, being 7.4. It's fatal if your blood pH drops to 7.2. When you ingest acidic food or drinks (such as a soft drink), the body must neutralize the acid. It does so by drawing on its stores of calcium from the bones, teeth, and muscles.

I'm sure you've heard of the calcium in heartburn medicine; some antacid brands even go so far as to promote their product as "bone-building" (which they are not). It's there to neutralize the acid in your stomach that causes gas and heartburn. Not unlike a farmer liming his field. Lime is calcium carbonate, which he spreads on the field to raise the pH to a more neutral condition, which promotes better plant life. That's what our bodies do naturally when we consume a substance so high in acid (low pH). We have to neutralize it (by robbing calcium out of our bones, muscles, and teeth). The end result? Osteoporosis and weak and brittle bones.

Do soft drinks cause this? In a study published in *Pediatrics & Adolescent Medicine* in June 2000, the researchers concluded that cola beverages were "highly associated with bone fractures." They expressed "...concern and alarm about the health impact of carbonated beverage consumption on teenaged girls..." (38) Another study reported in the *Journal of Adolescent Health* also found a "Strong association between cola beverage consumption and bone fractures in girls... The high consumption of carbonated beverages and the declining consumption of milk are of great public health significance for girls and women because of their proneness to osteoporosis in later life." (36)

To drive this important point home one more time, Dr. Bess Dawson-Hughes, a bone-disease expert at the Jean Mayer USDA Human Nutrition Research Center on Aging at Tufts University in Boston, says, "I'm particularly concerned about teenage girls. Most girls have inadequate calcium intakes, which makes them candidates for osteoporosis when they're older and may increase their risk for broken bones today. High soda consumption is a concern because it may displace milk from the diet in this vulnerable population." (37)

Caffeine is one of the ingredients in soft drinks that contribute to calcium loss. Linda Massey, Ph.D., a bone researcher at Washington State University in Spokane, says that caffeine can indeed be hard on your bones. "The more regular coffee a woman drinks, the more calcium is excreted in her urine," she says. Janet Barger-Lux of Crieghton University's Osteoporosis Research Unit in Omaha, Nebraska, goes further: "This loss amounts to about 5 milligrams of calcium for every 6 ounces of coffee or two cans of cola." (38) Yes, soft drinks also increase the excretion of calcium the urine. Drinking 12 ounces of a caffeine-containing soft drink can cause the loss of about 120 milligrams of calcium (roughly 2 percent of the U.S. Recommended Daily Allowance). (39)

It's a simple equation: Soft Drinks + Human = Soft Bones (and Rotting Teeth, as we shall see). If things keep going the way they have been, it may not be long before you start seeing hip replacement surgery on teenagers!

Tooth Decay

Drinking soft drinks regularly bathes the teeth in and acidic sugar-water for long periods of time. Refined sugars promote tooth decay. So it's not a surprise that a study between 1971 and 1974 found a strong correlation between the frequency of between-meal consumption of soda pop and cavities. (40)

The phosphoric acid in soft drinks also plays havoc on teeth. As this acid lingers in the mouth after a sip of soda, the body must pull calcium ions from the teeth in an attempt to normalize the saliva's pH (which should be around 7.4). As the calcium is stripped away, so is the enamel. This explains why dentists are noticing a condition in teenagers that was previously found only in the elderly – a complete loss of enamel on the teeth, resulting in yellow teeth. (41)

Food for Thought

When dentists do cosmetic bonding, they first roughen up the enamel by removing some of it with a chemical compound. That chemical is none other than phosphoric acid - the same found in soft drinks!

Upset Stomach

There's another risk from phosphoric acid (and other acids in sodas such as acetic, fumaric, gluconic) and caffeine: stomach aches. These acids and caffeine upset the fragile acid-alkaline balance of the stomach, creating a continuous acid environment that leads to inflammation. (42) Oftentimes the lament of "Mommy, I have a tummy ache" can be prevented by keeping the child away from sodas or other acidic and caffeinated beverages.

Heart Disease

In some people, a diet high in sugar may promote heart disease, some researchers contend. An estimated one quarter of adults have high levels of triglycerides and low levels of HDL cholesterol (the "good" cholesterol – HDL stands for High-Density Lipoprotein) in their blood. When these people eat a diet high in carbohydrates (sugar is a refined carbohydrate), their triglyceride and insulin levels rise. It's been shown that sugar has a greater effect than other carbohydrates in producing this result. No wonder excessive sugar intake also contributes to developing diabetes.

A study in Louisiana determined that overweight children were at increased risk for developing heart disease. Fifty-eight percent of the overweight kids ages five to 10 had one additional risk factor such as elevated cholesterol or high blood pressure. Twenty percent were found to have two or more additional risk factors for heart disease. (43) Since so many kids are overweight these days, there's a significant number that are close to or already have heart problems. Part of the reason is that they are getting less exercise. Another is that they are consuming more sugar, thus leading to heart problems similar to what happens in adults.

One of the most painful disorders, kidney stones affected more than one million people in 1985. (44) It's estimated by the National Institute of Diabetes and Digestive and Kidney Diseases (NIDDK) that 10 percent of all Americans will have a kidney stone during their lifetime – more in men than women. Men, incidentally, are the heaviest consumers of soft drinks.

One study linked soft drink consumption with kidney stones. (45) More research is needed, but the NIDDK does include cola beverages on a list of food that patients with kidney stones should avoid.

Caffeine

Caffeine is a mildly addictive stimulant drug found in most cola and other soft drinks of all colors and tastes. An average soda pop drinker, drinking Mountain Dew, would have ingested 92 mg of caffeine. That's equivalent to one six-ounce cup of coffee.

Caffeine causes nervousness, irritability, sleeplessness, and rapid heartbeat. It's been documented that children who normally do not consume much caffeine become restless and fidgety, develop headaches, and have difficulty going to sleep when they do consume it. When children age six to 12 stop consuming caffeine, they suffer withdrawal symptoms that impair their attention span and performance. (46)

Roland Griffiths, professor in the department of psychiatry and behavioral sciences at the Johns Hopkins University School of Medicine, says, "Caffeine is a mildly addictive drug, and parents might wish to limit their children's consumption of it." He goes on to say, "Americans should be mindful about their caffeine consumption. Drinking the caffeine equivalent of several cups of coffee a day can lead to insomnia, anxiety, and difficulty concentrating. Ceasing the consumption of caffeine often leads to withdrawal symptoms, such as headache and fatigue." (47) And again, these symptoms have been reported in children as well as in adults.

Yes, caffeine is a drug. According to more than 40 scientific studies, it may cause miscarriages, insomnia, and other problems. Dr. Michael Jacobson, executive director of CSPI, says, "Caffeine is the only drug that is widely added to the food supply and consumers have a right to know how much caffeine various foods contain. Knowing the caffeine content is important to many people – especially women who are or might become pregnant – who might want to limit or avoid caffeine." (48) The Food and Drug Administration advises pregnant women to "avoid caffeine-containing foods and drugs, if possible, or consume them only sparingly." Why? Because they have been implicated in causing birth defects and underweight babies. In laboratory animals, very large amounts of caffeine seem to cause females to bear young that are malformed. (49) As far as humans are concerned, the jury on whether they in deed do cause birth defects is still out. But one report stated, "The risk for any kind of congenital abnormalities is 3.5% in individuals who consume caffeine and 1.7% in those who do not. The difference is statistically significant." (50)

Caffeine has been more strongly implicated in low-birth weight babies. Among nearly 4,000 women who gave birth in New Haven, Connecticut, in the early 1980s, those who consumed between 150 and 300 milligrams of caffeine a day during their pregnancies, had more than twice the risk of delivering underweight babies (less than about five pounds) than those who consumed less. The risk was almost five times greater for women who consumed more than 300 milligrams a day, just three cups a day! Unfortunately, researchers haven't been able to tell if it's the caffeine, the coffee, or something else about women who consume these substances that's causing the low-birth-weight babies. And, a 1996 study showed more than double the risk of miscarriage in women who were consuming more than 300 mg a day of caffeine. (51)

There are also studies that show that caffeine consumption by pregnant mothers may cause decreased placental circulation, smaller brain size in offspring, and decreased learning capacities. (52) Potential mothers, why take the chance? Just don't drink coffee and don't drink soft drinks while you're pregnant. Period. You're more likely to have a normal, healthy baby.

Food for Thought

"You know," you might say. "I understand all these things about soft drinks and coffee. But really, how bad can they be? I mean, everybody drinks them. And wouldn't the FDA or some other government agency say they were harmful if they really were? You're just being a worrywart." And people smoked for decades thinking there was nothing wrong with it. Now, there's so much scientific evidence to the contrary, I doubt you'll find many people not admitting that it's bad for your health. It's just a matter of time before people wake up to the fact that these drinks are harming not just ourselves, but our children, who do not get adequate nutrition or are fed harmful substances. As a child's health is impaired, so is his or her enjoyment of life. That child is then more likely to get depressed or despondent or even violent. I'm not saying soda pop necessarily causes violent behavior. What I am saying once again is that the healthier a person is, the less likely he or she will have mental or emotional problems. And the more a child consumes harmful substances, the less likely that child will be healthy. All these things add up. Soda pop here, food additives there, pesticides over there, TV over there. They're all straws added to the backs of someone growing up – straws that can eventually break that child's back and make that child snap. It's estimated that one in five kids may have some sort of mental problem. They're three times as likely to have an emotional or behavioral disorder today as they were 20 years ago. That means that psychological disorders in kids almost tripled in the last 20 years. (53)

Personally, I have not had a soda in close to 20 years. I stopped in graduate school when I figured that just by not buying a cola at lunch, I would save over $100 a semester. ($100 was a lot of money back then!) I didn't realize the health risks associated with drinking the stuff back then; I quit because I needed the money. Now, when I see people who may be struggling to make ends meet drinking soda, I have to shake my head. Considering the average male teenager drinks 868 cans of this stuff a year, they're spending over $500 a year for something that will undermine their health.

One other thing: When I worked as an environmental engineer for the State of South Carolina, we would inspect industrial plants to make sure all the waste and hazardous wastes were disposed of properly. It was somewhat of a joke among us inspectors that if we found a drum of cola on the site, it would, according to EPA regulations, be required to be disposed of at a hazardous waste disposal facility. Recently I checked with the EPA to see if that is really the case. I found that if a substance has a pH of less than 2.0, it is considered hazardous. So soft drinks don't meet this criterion because they have an average pH of 3.4. But, if a substance corrodes steel at a rate greater than 6.35 millimeters a year – roughly 1/4 inch (at a temperature of 65 degrees centigrade), it is considered hazardous. (54) I do not know if soft drinks will corrode steel at that rate, but I did discover some comments on this subject in the book *Sugar Blues* which quotes Dr. McCay, who had been in charge of nutritional research during World War II. Besides reporting to a Congressional committee that cola beverages typically contained about 10 percent sugar, he also commented that they were very corrosive. An excerpt of the committee records is interesting:

Dr. McCay: "I was amazed to learn that the beverage contained substantial amounts of phosphoric acid. At the Naval Medical Research Institute, we put human teeth in a cola beverage and found they softened and started to dissolve within a short period. The acidity of cola beverages... is about the same as vinegar. The sugar content masks the acidity, and children little realize they are drinking this strange mixture of phosphoric acid, sugar, caffeine, coloring, and flavoring matter."

A congressman asked the doctor what government bureau was in charge of passing on the contents of soft drinks.

Dr. McCay: "As far as I know, no one passes upon it or pays any attention to it."

Congressman: "No one passes on the contents of soft drinks?"

Dr. McCay: "So far as I know, no one."

Another congressman asked if the doctor had made any tests of the effect of cola beverages on metal and iron. When the doctor said he hadn't the congressman volunteered: "A friend of mine told me once that he dropped three ten-penny nails into one of the cola bottles, and in forty-eight hours the nails had completely dissolved.

Dr. McCay: "Sure. Phosphoric acid there would dissolve iron or limestone. You might drop it on the steps, and it would erode the steps coming up here... Since soft drinks are playing an increasingly important part of the American diet and tend to displace foods such as milk, they deserve very careful consideration." (55)

According to this anecdotal information about corrosion then, cola drinks and probably most other soft drinks would indeed be classified as a hazardous waste according to EPA guidelines.

Sugar

In 1975, the book *Sugar Blues* by journalist William Dufty was published. It is a shocking exposé of sugar, its history and the health problems that arise from its continued use. Before going into its possible health effects, a brief discussion about just what sugar is and how it evolved is in order so that you will better understand just what we're dealing with here.

Sugar is refined sucrose, often called simple sugar. It's produced by a number of chemical processing steps from the juice of the sugar cane or sugar beet. In processing, all fiber, protein, and minerals (which comprise about 90 percent of the plant itself) are removed.

Simple sugars (monosaccharides and disaccharides) are sometimes called "rapid sugars" because they don't need digestion and are rapidly absorbed into our bloodstream. Most sweeteners, natural or otherwise, are composed of simple sugars. When they are absorbed into the bloodstream, they cause a rise in blood glucose levels that are unnaturally high. Glucose is a single sugar molecule. It results from the breakdown of disaccharides and is the only sugar used by the cells in the body. In fact, it is the only thing the body ever uses as fuel. When the blood glucose level in the blood rises, it results in a condition called hyperglycemia, and is one of the symptoms of diabetes. When the pancreas functions as it should, it will produce and release enough insulin to remove the excess glucose from the bloodstream. If the pancreas is impaired, it cannot keep up and hyperglycemia results.

As the body senses the increased glucose in the blood, insulin production increases, but when the intake of sugar is stopped, the pancreas does not recognize this right away. There is a time lag. So as the insulin keeps pouring into the bloodstream, there's less and less sugar to go around. The result is that the glucose level in the blood falls too much. Low blood sugar, or hypoglycemia is the result. Symptoms of hypoglycemia include depression, dizziness, crying spells, aggression, insomnia, weakness, and in extreme cases loss of consciousness.

When the blood glucose level falls too low, the adrenal glands kick in to mobilize the body's stores of glycogen (a carbohydrate found in the liver and muscles – the "storage" form of glucose) to bring the sugar level up to normal. Glucose is also synthesized from proteins, and other substances when the blood level of glucose falls too low.

So, when too much sugar is ingested, there's a seesaw effect of the metabolism. The pancreas reacts to produce insulin. This results in hypoglycemia. Then the adrenals react and glycogen is released from the liver to bring the blood sugar up to normal. Not only is the sugar level of the blood going up and down in extremes, but also the pancreas, adrenals, and liver are being overworked.

When the pancreas wears out, diabetes manifests. But there are other effects. As the sugars are absorbed, the body turns them into saturated fatty acids and cholesterol. If these are not burned off through activity, they accumulate under the skin, in our liver, kidneys, arteries, and other organs. That's why so many diabetics have weight problems and cardiovascular complications. If they don't exercise (and they are less likely to not to want to since their blood sugar levels are so inconsistent), they get fat.

Since sugars increase our body's production of adrenaline by fourfold, two major things happen. One is that the body goes into a state of stress – the "fight or flight" response. This stress reaction increases the production of cholesterol and cortisone. Cortisone is known to inhibit the immune system – so allergies and infections are more likely. Also, as insulin levels rise, the release of growth hormone is decreased. Growth hormone is known to activate the immune system. So, the more sugar, the more insulin, the less growth hormone, the weaker the immune system.

The second thing is that along with the pancreas, the adrenals simply get tired and wear out. Eventually they cannot produce the necessary hormones for proper cellular function. Stress cannot be handled as well.

Another reason that sugar is so bad is that it does not contain the vitamins, minerals, and cofactors necessary for its own metabolism in the body. So the body must draw on its stores of these nutrients in order to metabolize it. Sugar leaches out vitamins B, C, and D, and minerals like calcium, iron, zinc, chromium, and phosphorous. The more sugar you eat, the more minerals and vitamins you need, and the less minerals remain in your body.

Sugar not only robs the teeth, bones, muscles, and blood of a great percentage of their minerals, but also causes irritation and weakens mucous membranes. This irritation and inflammation can result in breathing problems (i.e., asthma and emphysema) and digestive problems such as heartburn.

As vitamins and mineral stores in our body decrease, the body is less able to carry out other functions that require them. It cannot metabolize fats and cholesterol as efficiently or convert cholesterol into bile acids. So cholesterol levels rise, the metabolic rate goes down, fats burn more slowly and gall stones are formed. As all this is happening, the person certainly feels less and less like exercising, so body weight increases even more. A vicious cycle.

William Coda Martin, Ph.D., believes that sugar is a poison because it depletes the body of its life forces, vitamins, and minerals. He says,

> What is left consists of pure, refined carbohydrates. The body cannot utilize this refined starch and carbohydrate unless the depleted proteins, vitamins and minerals are present. Nature supplies these elements in each plant in quantities sufficient to metabolize the carbohydrate in that particular plant. There is no excess for other added carbohydrates. Incomplete carbohydrate metabolism results in the formation of toxic metabolites such as pyruvic acid and abnormal sugars containing five carbon atoms. Pyruvic acid accumulates in the brain and nervous system and the abnormal sugars in the red blood cells. These toxic metabolites interfere with the respiration of the cells. They cannot get sufficient oxygen to survive and function normally. In time, some of the cells die. This interferes with the function of a part of the body and is the beginning of degenerative disease. (56)

Essentially, eating sugar is worse than eating nothing at all since it robs the body of minerals and vitamins, along with the energy demands of detoxification and elimination from the body. You can survive for quite some time on nothing but water, but eating sugar and water can kill you sooner. In fact, in 1816 the French physiologist F. Magendie published his results of a series of experiments with dogs in which he fed them nothing but sugar or olive oil and water. All the animals died in a shorter time than if they consumed nothing but water. (57)

Diabetes

If you eat sugar every day, a continuously over-acid condition results and more and more minerals are required from deep in the body in the attempt to rectify the imbalance. Finally, in order to protect the blood and keep it in a slightly alkaline condition (since sugar creates an acid condition), so much calcium is taken from the bones and teeth that osteoporosis and decay, respectively, result.

Excess sugar eventually affects every organ in the body. Initially, it is stored in the liver, as already mentioned, in the form of glycogen. Since the liver's capacity is limited, it will soon expand like a balloon. When the liver is filled to its maximum, the excess glycogen is returned to the blood in the form of fatty acids. These are taken to every part of the body and stored in the most inactive areas – the belly, buttocks, breasts, and thighs.

When these places are filled, the fatty acids are then distributed to the active organs such as the heart and kidneys. This causes their activities to slow down and tissues to degenerate and turn to fat. The whole body is affected by their reduced ability, and abnormal blood pressure is created. The circulatory and lymphatic systems are taxed, the red corpuscles change, an overabundance of white blood cells are created, and tissue regeneration and repair are slowed. The parasympathetic nervous system is affected and the organs governed by it (such as parts of the brain) become inactive and paralyzed.

As you can see, it's not just the body that suffers, but the mind also. Dr. E. M. Abrahamson and A.W. Pezet, in Body, Mind, and Sugar, says that "since the cells of the brain are those that depend wholly upon the moment-to-moment blood sugar level for nourishment, they are perhaps the most susceptible to damage. The disturbingly large and ever-increasing number of neurotics in our population makes this clearly evident." [58]

The late endocrinologist John W. Tintera said, "It is quite possible to improve your disposition, increase your efficiency, and change your personality for the better. The way to do it is to avoid cane and beet sugar in all forms and guises." [59]

Nobel Prize winner Linus Pauling, M.D., and other prominent doctors believe that mental illness is a myth and that emotional disturbances are the first symptom of a person's inability to handle sugar. In Orthomolecular Psychiatry, Dr. Pauling writes, "A deficiency of [vitamin B-12] whatever its cause, leads to mental illness, often even more pronounced than the physical consequences... Other investigators have also reported a higher incidence of low B-12 concentrations in the serums of mental patients than in the population as a whole and have suggested that B-12 deficiency, whatever its origin, may lead to mental illness." [60]

Remember that sugar is stripped of its vitamins when it is processed. The B vitamins are leached from the body to help metabolize the sugar when we eat it. Thus, this could lead to a vitamin B-12 deficiency. The B vitamins play a major role in brain function, so their presence in our body is of utmost importance. They are not only supplied to us from the food we eat (provided it's unprocessed!), but also a significant amount of them are normally produced in our intestines by "friendly" bacteria. However, refined sugar actually kills these bacteria, and in so doing our stock of B vitamins can get depleted.

In *Megavitamin B3 Therapy for Schizophrenia*, A. Hoffner, M.D., advised patients to follow a good nutritional program with the restriction of sucrose and sucrose-rich foods (i.e. sugar). An inquiry into the dietary history of patients diagnosed as schizophrenic showed that their choice of foods was rich in sweets, candy, cakes, coffee, caffeinated beverages, and foods prepared with sugar. These foods stimulate the adrenals as noted earlier and can cause adrenal exhaustion. (61)

In the 1940s, John Tintera, Ph.D., found that the symptoms of hypoadreno-corticism (the lack of adequate adrenal cortical hormone caused by adrenal exhaustion) were similar to those found in people whose systems were unable to handle sugar. These symptoms were fatigue, nervousness, depression, apprehension, craving for sweets, inability to handle alcohol, inability to concentrate, allergies, and low blood pressure. He started using a simple glucose tolerance test (GTT) to find out if a person could handle sugar. He said:

> A glucose tolerance test... could alert parents and physicians and could save innumerable hours and small fortunes spent in looking into the child's psyche and home environment for maladjustments of questionable significance in the emotional development of the average child. The negativism, hyperactivity, and obstinate resentment of discipline are absolute indications for at least the minimum laboratory tests: urinalysis, complete blood count, and the five-hour glucose tolerance test... (62)

Dr. Tintera stressed that improvement was "dependent upon the restoration of the total organism... the importance of diet cannot be overemphasized."

Obviously, if a child is consuming large amounts of sugar his or her metabolism and brain function is being compromised. This not only affects his or her resistance to diseases like diabetes, but also impacts their mental health as well. Sugar can undermine just about every area of the body. Dr. Joseph Mercola, director of the Optimal Wellness Center, has listed 78 ways sugar can destroy your health. He compiled this list in conjunction with Nancy Appleton, Ph.D. (You can see the list at his website www.mercola.com/sugar.) Along with the list are 78 different scientific references concerning the hazards of sugar from a number of doctors and researchers. Evidence enough of the hazardous nature of this white powder.

Patricia Hardman, Ph.D., Director of Woodland Hall Academy, a school for children with hyperactivity and learning disabilities in Maitland, Florida, says,

> We can change a child's behavior dramatically by lowering his or her intake of sugar. If a child comes to school extremely depressed or complains that nothing is going right, or if he flies off the handle and can't be controlled, we ask him what he's been eating. It's almost always the case that the night before he had ice cream or soda or some other food with a lot of sugar. We had one child who was tested for his IQ and scored 140. Three days later he was tested and scored 100! It turned out that grandma had come for a visit and, that morning had made the child pancakes for breakfast. Of course, they were smothered in store-bought sugary syrup. We waited another

three days without sugar and tested him again. Sure enough, he scored 140. There's no doubt about it. Sugar makes children poor learners. At Woodland Hall, sugar is eliminated from the diet of every child." (63)

It's not just disposition and intelligence that is affected by sugar. The very survival of your child may depend on avoiding it. In his book, *Type A Type B Weight Loss Book*, H.L. Newbold writes:

The teenage suicide rate has doubled since 1968, largely because mothers demonstrate their love by keeping the refrigerators stocked with sugary soda drinks and feed them cereals for breakfast and spaghetti for dinner. [Author's note: Remember, white flour products quickly turn into sugar in the stomach and have essentially the same effect on metabolism as sugar does.] Why do we insist upon rotting the brains of a whole generation of children, turning them into scholastic failures, delinquents, dropouts and welfare recipients? Why do we drive more and more of them to suicide by feeding them ever more processed foods? I'll tell you why: Many people are getting rich at their expense. We look askance at African tribes when they cut faces and rub dyes into the wounds and when they circumcise women. That's child's play compared to what we do to our children. In our society, it's perfectly all right to maim and kill – so long as we do it in a socially acceptable way." (64)

Food for Thought

I have also gone to "pro-sugar" web sites to see if there was any documentation on the benefits of sugar consumption. Although I found comments like "sugar represents a positive addition to the diet" and "sugar is a good, pure food that supplies much needed energy," I found nothing to the effect that there has been any research done to prove it. On the other hand, *Time* magazine reported back in 1958 that a Harvard biochemist and his assistants had worked with mice for more than 10 years – bankrolled by the Sugar Research Foundation Inc. – to find out how sugar causes dental cavities and how to prevent this. In the 10 years of research, they discovered that there was simply no way to prevent sugar from causing dental decay. When the researchers reported their findings in the *Dental Association Journal*, the Sugar Research Foundation Inc. withdrew their support. (65)

I like to think of myself as an open-minded person. I try to look at both sides of the story and then come to a decision on what the truth is. But try as I might, I cannot find one good or even harmless reason to eat sugar or sugar products (like high fructose corn syrup – which actually cheaper than sugar which explains it's presence in more and more products. By the way, high fructose corn syrup is even worse than table sugar for the body). And little do people realize that sugar is so bad for their health and well-being.

William Dufty quoted one author as saying, "It is a rule of thumb. The more you see a product advertised, the more of a rip-off it is." I would add, "and bad for your health." Do you ever see fruit and vegetables advertised? But they have to brainwash you into drinking sodas and eating junk food. I remember the first cola I drank when I was about four years old. I threw it up all over the refrigerator door. (It's one of my first memories!) My body naturally rejected it – literally – because as we now know, it's a toxic waste. My body knew better, but my mind kept forcing it on me until I built up a tolerance, and then a craving. Just like alcohol, cigarettes, and drugs. You first reject these poisons, then grow to need them. That's the way addictions are. And I don't mean to be a hardnose, but if you need that coke, pastry, candy bar, or coffee, you've got a little food addiction going. Want proof? Just try going without them for a day or two. Spare your child the same fate. Keep them away from all that junk food as long as possible and as best you can.

History of Sugar

If you want to learn about how sugar has become such a staple in our diet, I suggest you read the book I've already cited a number of times, *Sugar Blues* by William Dufty. It's an incredible exposé about how and why sugar is so popular and ubiquitous in our society.

Briefly, much of the colonization of the Western world has resulted because of the sugar trade and the fight to control it. From the early settlers of the West Indies to the American Revolution to the slave trade, sugar has played a major role. At first it was a very expensive commodity, used only by kings, royalty, and the very rich. They used to snort it like cocaine, and it was taken precisely because it gave people a "high." (People now are so used to this "high" that it's a normal state of being. Kind of like a drug addict needing more and more drugs to feel an effect and not being able to feel normal without at least some in his system.) Certain diseases were associated only with the rich, and the poor, sugarless farmers seemed to be immune. But as the industry grew and processing methods improved, the price came down more and more people could afford this high. The diseases started to spread to the common folks. Natural healers were seen as witches, burned at the stake, and hanged, because they admonished people to abstain from sugar. "The great confinement of the insane," as one historian called it, began in the late 17th century, after sugar consumption in Britain had escalated for 200 years from a pinch or two in a barrel of beer, here and there, to more than two million pounds per year. Sailors suffered when sugar was introduced as rations, and scurvy became rampant. Sir Frederick Banting, the codiscoverer of insulin, noticed in 1929 in Panama that among sugar plantation owners who ate large amounts of their refined stuff, diabetes was common. Among the native cane-cutters, who only got to chew the raw cane (replete with vitamins and minerals), he saw no diabetes.

Some researchers believe that sugar was the cause of or instrumental in causing the bubonic plague. "By 1662, sugar consumption in England had zoomed from 0 to some 16 million pounds a year... Then, in 1665, London was swept by a plague. More than 30,000 people died that September... People who lived in the country virtually without sugar seemed to escape the plague. Had anyone called it the sugar plague, they might have been denounced as menaces to commerce and crown and strung to a gibbet." (66)

Could it be the cause of tuberculosis too? "In relation to consumption, now called tuberculosis and blamed on a bacillus, evidence suggests that a sugar-rich diet may create the necessary conditions in our bodies [for the disease to take hold]... Three hundred years ago, in the 1700s, deaths from tuberculosis... increased dramatically. The highest incidence occurred among workers in sugar factories and refineries... In 1910, when Japan acquired a source of cheap and abundant sugar in Formosa, the incidence of tuberculosis rose dramatically." (67)

Dr. Weston Price traveled the world examining the dietary habits of primitive tribes and cultures. He noticed without exception that when these peoples were exposed to the white-man's food (white flour and white sugar), they invariably contracted tuberculosis and the amount of dental caries (cavities) increased dramatically.

Why don't we see tuberculosis now? When the human body is first exposed to a harmful substance, it is very sensitive to it, and the reactions can be very severe. Over time and through the generations, the body builds up resistance and adapts to some degree to overcome the toxicity. This is not to say that it is no longer toxic, but the manifestations of symptoms may take longer and change characteristics. Instead of tuberculosis, we may see diabetes or cancer instead. But a poison is still a poison that eventually takes its toll on the body.

Now sugar is in just about everything. And it's not required to be listed on food labels if it's used in certain ways in the product. In addition, the labeling is often misleading or difficult to understand. "Made from Natural Ingredients" on the label means nothing these days. Heck, plastic is made from petroleum, which is a natural product. And the label may call sugar corn syrup, dextrose, or a carbohydrate. Oftentimes people don't realize they are still buying a product with sugar in it. You'll be hard-pressed to find things with absolutely no sugar added. Finding a product with a label that specifically states "No Sugar Added" is the safest bet.

A press release from the Center for Science in the Public Interest titled, "America: Drowning in Sugar," states that a petition was made to the Food and Drug Administration to require food labels to declare how much sugar is added to soft drinks, ice cream, and other foods. The petition was filed in 1999 by 72 health experts and organizations and spearheaded by the Center for Science in the Public Interest (CSPI). Michael Jacobson, executive director of CSPI, says, "Sugar consumption has been going through the roof. It has increased by 28 percent since 1983, fueling soaring obesity rates and other health problems. It's vital that the

FDA require labels that would enable consumers to monitor - and reduce - their sugar intake." As of the date of the publication of this book, the change to the "Nutrition Facts" label has yet to occur. (68)

"Listing added sugars on labels would alert consumers as to how much added sugars are in a serving of food," Jacobson says, "It's vital that food labels give consumers the information they need to reduce their consumption of added sugars."

Another press release from CSPI in June 2000 said:

> The USDA advises people who eat a 2,000-calorie healthful diet to limit themselves to about 10 teaspoons of added sugars. However, USDA surveys find that the average American consumes 20 teaspoons a day, twice the recommendation... Just one month ago, the federal government's new edition of *Dietary Guidelines for Americans* recognized that many consumers are eating too many sugar-rich foods. The document urges consumers to "Choose sensibly to limit your intake of beverages and foods that are high in added sugars." (69)

However, if the "added sugars" are not listed on the label, there is no way consumers can know just how much sugar they are consuming. Many typical American foods provide a large fraction of the USDA's recommended 10-teaspoon-a-day sugar limit in just one serving! A typical cup of flavored yogurt provides 70 percent of a day's worth of added sugar (i.e., seven teaspoons). A cup of regular ice cream has six teaspoons, a 12-ounce Pepsi has just over 10 teaspoons, as does a quarter-cup of pancake syrup.

As you can see, if you eat like a typical American, you're going to get your dose of sugar because it's hidden in many products. The best way to go is to shop at a health food store, buy mostly unprocessed, fresh food, and maybe even grow a garden. If you do go off sugar, or at least eat less of it, you may experience withdrawal symptoms. So be prepared. (Remember, it was treated as a drug when it was first used centuries ago.) The same holds true for your kids. They may temporarily complain. But the long-term benefits greatly outweigh the inconvenience - for both you and your children.

CHAPTER V
Asthma

Throughout the United States, asthma is on the rise and becoming a serious health risk, especially to our children. "Asthma is a chronic inflammatory disorder of the airways characterized by variable airflow obstruction and airway hyperresponsiveness in which prominent clinical manifestations include wheezing and shortness of breath." (1)

The underlying causes of asthma are not understood but doctors know some of the things that trigger it in susceptible individuals. A U.S. Public Health Service pamphlet says, "There are irritants in the environment such as cigarette smoke, cooking odors, and aerosol sprays that can adversely affect a person with asthma. These should be avoided as much as possible. An asthmatic should not smoke nor be active outdoors for prolonged periods of time during air pollution alerts." (2)

Asthma expert Dr. R. Michael Sly says, "Air pollution is an established cause of increased morbidity (illness) from asthma, and intense air pollution has caused increased mortality (death)." (3)

The prevalence rate for asthma increased 75 percent from 1980 to 1994. By 1993-1994, an estimated 13.7 million people reported asthma during the preceding 12 months. This increasing trend in rates was evident among all races, both sexes, and all age groups.

The most substantial increase occurred among children ages 0 to four years (160 percent from 22.2 per 1,000 to 57.8 per 1,000), and children aged five to 14 years (up 74 percent from 42.8 per 1,000 to 74.4 per 1,000).

During the 1993-1994 period, the prevalence rate for asthma was slightly higher among children 14 years old or less than among people 15 years old or greater. The increasing trend in asthma rates during 1980-1994 was evident and significant in every region of the U.S. (See Figure 4 below)

From 1975 to 1993-1995, the estimated annual number of office visits for asthma more than doubled from 4.6 million to 10.4 million. Between 1979 and 1994, the estimated national number of asthma-related hospitalizations increased from 386,000 to 466,000. (4)

Figure 4.

Estimated average annual number of people with self-reported asthma during the preceding 12 months, 1980-1994

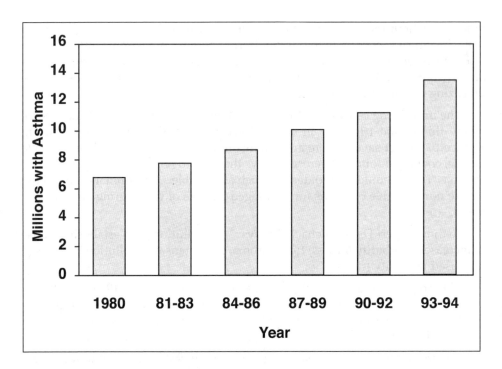

According to the report "Action against Asthma" from the Department of Health and Human Services:

> We are facing an asthma epidemic. Through newspaper stories and personal experiences, we hear more about asthma every day... The statistics support these impressions. From 1980 to 1996, the number of Americans with asthma more than doubled, to almost 15 million, with children under five years old experiencing the highest rate of increase. Reasons for these increasing rates are unclear. Yet even if rates were to stop increasing, asthma would remain an enormous public health problem. Not only does it keep children in fear and pain - it keeps them out of school. In every classroom with 30 children, there are likely to be at least two with asthma. That adds up to over 10 million school days lost to asthma each year. And the problem is not limited to children. Asthma is the leading work-related lung disease. Moreover, the disease kills over 5,000 Americans and results in half a million hospitalizations every year. As serious as asthma is, it doesn't strike evenly. Minorities and the poor are hit especially hard.

The report continues:

The steady rise in the prevalence of asthma constitutes an epidemic, which by all indications is continuing. Even if rates were to stabilize, asthma would continue to be a profound public health problem, responsible for 9 million visits to health care providers per year, over 1.8 million emergency room visits per year, and over 460,000 hospitalizations per year... Asthma is a common chronic disease of childhood, affecting an estimated 4.4 million children... Taking care of asthma is expensive and imposes financial burdens on patients and their families, including lost workdays and income, as well as lost job opportunity. In 1990, the annual cost of asthma to the U.S. economy was estimated to be $6.2 billion, with the majority of the expense attributed to medical care. A 1998 analysis... estimated the cost of asthma in 1996 to be over $11 billion per year. (5)

The traditional medical community says the causes of asthma are not known and sites an interaction between environmental and genetic factors as the most likely culprits. Some studies suggest that indoor allergen exposure is a risk factor of the initial onset of asthma.

There is also widespread agreement among physicians that one outdoor air pollutant – sulfur dioxide (SO2) – causes asthma attacks in susceptible individuals. The 24-hour atmospheric legal limit for SO2 is not to exceed 0.14 parts per million (ppm). One article about asthma (published in 1991) made note that during the Reagan administration the limit was 0.4 ppm and that the "EPA opposed the tighter regulation, saying that asthma is a 'transient and reversible' condition (even though it kills more than 5,000 Americans each year) and it's simply not worth it to force reductions in SO2 to benefit asthmatics. The electric power industry applauded." (6)

Sulfites added to food to prevent discoloration can also trigger asthma attacks. Manufacturers put sulfites in all sorts of foods without having to clear it with the U.S. Food and Drug Administration (FDA), which regulates most food additives. Sulfites are one of the food additives that have been around for so long that they were placed on the list known as "Generally Recognized As Safe" (the GRAS list) in 1958 when food additive regulations began.

In 1986, the FDA banned the use of sulfites on fresh fruits and vegetables, largely because of the hazard to asthmatics. Health advocates wanted the FDA to ban all uses of sulfites on food, period. The FDA said in a memo (which was leaked to the press in 1988) that they knew that a million asthmatics were endangered by sulfites in other food, but that the FDA had decided, after much thought, not to do anything about the problem. This time, the food industry applauded.

The official position of the U.S. EPA is that either asthma isn't related to pollution or that asthmatics are such a small fraction of the population that setting pollution standards to protect them isn't worth the effort. Considering the fact that now many believe that asthma is an "epidemic," it's hard to believe it isn't worth the trouble.

In a recent review of the current scientific literature, the Institute of Medicine (IOM) drew several conclusions about the role of numerous indoor air exposures and the initial development of asthma. The IOM found that exposure to house dust mite allergen can cause the development of asthma in susceptible children. They also determined that exposure to environmental tobacco smoke is associated with the development of asthma in younger children. Maternal smoking during pregnancy was suggested to have a stronger adverse affect than exposure after birth. (7)

Reducing exposure to certain allergens has been shown not only to reduce asthma symptoms and the need for medication, but also, in some studies, to improve lung function. The IOM committee found that exposure to allergens produced by cats, cockroaches, house dust mites, and environmental tobacco smoke causes exacerbations of asthma in sensitized individuals. Common air pollutants such as ozone, sulfur dioxide, and particulate matter are known to be respiratory irritants and can also worsen asthma symptoms. Any of these pollutants or irritants can combine synergistically, thus exacerbating the problem.

The report from the Department of Health and Human Service concludes: "In summary, we have made progress but we are not yet close to understanding the causes of the asthma epidemic nor to providing optimal care..."

Food for Thought

It's my opinion that the increase in asthma in the U.S. is no real mystery. As we saw with cancer, obesity, and diabetes, and as we shall see with other degenerative diseases and fertility, the increases can be correlated with the degeneration and pollution of our environment and food supply. While the medical community tries to point the finger at genetics and luck as the "evil spirits," the truth of the matter is that as our environment (internal as well as external) degenerates, so do we.

The goal of medical research is to find the cause of asthma. (All they need to do is read this book. But then, all those researchers would be out of jobs, the pesticide industry and other industries would be forced out of business, money would be spent on cleaning things up instead of scratching our fannies wondering what the heck is going on.) Throwing another drug at it is not the answer, as has been proven so often in the past. Drugs do not solve any medical problem – they just delay the inevitable and suppress symptoms.

This is what drugs – the kind from the drug store or the kind on the streets – do to the body: Drugs interrupt, interfere with, delay, or stop the normal transmission of nerve impulses or communication between nerves in the central nervous system (brain and spinal cord) or peripheral nervous system (everything else). That's it. They do nothing to build up or repair the body. They simply alter the transmission of nerve impulses. Sometimes this will change the expression of a disease – the acne, cancer, herpes, or whatever, may go away, but the underlying source of the problem is still

---

there and then manifests in another part of the body with different symptoms. People with one disease usually have multiple problems. If someone gets "cured" of cancer with radiation, chemotherapy, or drugs, you can bet that there's something else still wrong with them.

Medical research – as performed in medical schools and universities all around the world – focuses on how a disease or illness can be ameliorated (lessened) by administering a substance into or onto the human body. I spent a year in medical school studying for a Ph.D. in anatomy and physiology and saw what goes on there first-hand. The professors were concerned with two things: teaching the medical students and doing research. The research was *always* aimed at finding a way to alter the biological system by administrating a new drug or combination of drugs or performing a destructive procedure such as radiation. I repeat – these do nothing to nourish the body. They simply stop the symptoms from appearing.

The best analogy is that of the oil gauge on your car. If the oil gets low, the oil gauge light will go on. It's a warning signal that something is wrong. The sensor in the engine detects the absence of oil, transmits its message through a wire to the light on the dashboard which alerts you of the problem. You may not like to see the light go on, and it may be an inconvenience or even discomfort to have to stop and add oil – but you'd better stop and do it or your engine will burn up.

But what if when you saw the light go on, you simply cut the wire to the gauge and kept on driving? Would this be smart? Would you be able to drive very long? That's what drugs do. They stop you from sensing something is wrong, or they alter the transmission of the nerves so the problem may seem to be gone, but is just rerouted to another part of the body.

In some instances, a drug will actually increase the activity of nerves. The best example of this is to watch how pesticides work. If you've ever watched a bug after you sprayed it with a pesticide, you probably noticed how it twitches violently until it dies. The pesticide gets inside the bug and floods the synapses of the nerves (the gap between the nerve cells – kind of like the gap on a spark plug) with the appropriate neurochemical (the spark that jumps the gap). The nerve cells fire and fire like crazy until the bug's little body is totally exhausted and depleted and then it dies.

If you have a pain or other aberration in your body, it's a signal that something is wrong. The receptors in your body have detected something is out of whack and send messages to your brain, where the problem is recognized and you sense this as pain in that area. But what if you just cut the nerves between the problem and your head? The pain stops, and you think everything is back to normal. This is exactly what aspirin and all other pain relievers, alcohol, and recreational drugs do. The nervous transmission is interrupted, and you "feel no pain."

In the case of heart medication, often times the intricate actions of the cells in the heart are altered to affect a change that is perceived as beneficial. I distinctly remember my physiology professor saying in reference to one heart medicine: "You see, in this case we had to effectively poison the heart cells to modulate the contractions."

Yes, I agree that in some extreme emergency cases this may be necessary. But even so, the underlying cause of the problem is not corrected at all. And as the heart is poisoned over a long period, other problems will manifest. Any drug – from the innocent-looking aspirin to chemotherapy drugs, from caffeine to illegal street drugs such as cocaine and heroin, and from something as seemingly harmless as sugar to the overprescribed Ritalin – *any* drug injures some part of the body in order to make another part function differently.

And it's not just manmade drugs that can do this. Many pharmaceuticals were derived originally from plants. The classic case is Valium. Its active substance is valerium, which comes from the valerian plant. This has been known for centuries to decrease pain and put a person in a calmer state. But does that justify its use? Not everything natural is suited for the human body. Cocaine is from coca leaves of the South American shrub *Erythroxylon coca*. Eating some plants may actually kill you. So just because something grows and is not processed in a chemical plant does not necessarily make it good. The way to overcome, and I mean truly conquer a disease is to get the body back to functioning correctly. This is done by: 1. Supplying the body the proper building blocks for repair, regeneration, and maintenance; and 2. Eliminating and/or removing any interfering substances like pollutants or normal cellular waste products. That's all you have to do. The basic fundamentals to health are really not that complicated, although specific problems may require specific remedial solutions that may be more complex. But the underlying solutions to any health problem is to treat the body in accordance with natural law and in harmony with our biology and physiology.

CHAPTER VI
Attention-Deficit and Hyperactivity Disorders

Attention disorders have been known by several names over the years. They were first documented in children in 1902 by George Still, who described 43 children with aggression, defiance, emotionality, limited sustained attention, and deficient rule-governed behavior. (1) Since then, the disorder has been given numerous names including minimal brain dysfunction, hyperkinetic reaction of childhood, attention deficit disorder (ADD), and the most current, as defined by the *Diagnostic and Statistical Manual, 4th Edition*, of "Attention-Deficit/Hyperactivity Disorder" (AD/HD). This current name reflects the importance of the inattention/distraction aspect of the disorder as well as the hyperactivity/impulsivity aspect. (2)

Symptoms of AD/HD usually arise in early childhood around the age of three unless there is some type of brain injury later in life. It is marked by behaviors that are evident for at least six months with their onset before the age of seven.

There are three basic subtypes of AD/HD:

I. AD/HD - Primarily inattentive type (AD/HD-I). A person with this disorder:

- Fails to give close attention to details or makes careless mistakes.
- Has difficulty sustaining attention.
- Does not appear to listen.
- Struggles to follow through on instructions.
- Has difficulty with organization.
- Avoids or dislikes talks requiring sustained mental effort.
- Is easily distracted.
- Is forgetful in daily activities.

II. AD/HD - Primarily hyperactive/impulsive type (AD/HD-HI). Someone with this dosorder:

- Fidgets with hands or feet or squirms in chair.
- Has difficulty remaining seated.
- Runs about or climbs excessively.
- Has difficulty engaging in activities quietly.
- Acts as if driven by a motor.
- Talks excessively.
- Blurts out answers before questions have been completed.

- Has difficulty waiting or taking turns.

- Interrupts or intrudes upon others.

III. AD/HD - Combined type (AD/HD-C). These individuals exhibit both sets of attention and hyperactive/impulsive criteria above. (3)

For purposes of this discussion, we will be talking about the AD/HD combined type. It will be referred to as ADHD. To determine if a child has ADHD, the symptoms must be more frequent or severe than other children the same age. In adults, the symptoms must affect the ability to function in daily life and persist from childhood. And, the behaviors must create significant difficulty in at least two areas of life, such as in the home, at school, at work, in social settings, and so on

Since there is no single test to diagnose ADHD, a comprehensive evaluation is needed. This requires time and effort and is largely a subjective process. A history of the child should be taken from the parents, teachers, and child and the child's academic, social, and emotional characteristics all need to be evaluated. Often a clinician will use nothing more than a checklist for rating ADHD symptoms. It's shocking to find out that a diagnosis of such a serious problem can be made by a nonphysician by simply checking eight of 14 items on a behavior checklist. (4)

Some behaviors that are prevalent in children with an attention and/or hyperactivity disorder can manifest at any time – even when the child is still in the womb! Some mothers have described their children as "punching their way out of the uterus." As infants, children may do excessive head banging or crib rocking, have long bouts of crying and screaming, be overly restless, have great thirst and large amounts of saliva and dribbling, or have fitful sleep or little need for sleep. As toddlers, these children can be easily excited, cry easily or burst into tantrums if their demands are not instantly met. They run and climb on everything and can't sit still or concentrate for more than a few seconds. Often they will bump into furniture and walls so often that it looks as if the parents are battering them.

By the first grade, symptoms can get worse. ADHD children are easily distracted, make careless errors, don't follow-through on requests, forget to write down school assignments, or can't play games for the same amount of time as other children their age. They are not able to listen to an entire story or sit through a meal, sleep through the night, or complete a chore. They have difficulty accepting direction, discipline, and correction, and are too impulsive to think before they act. They find it hard to wait for things they want or to take turns in a game and are more likely to grab a toy from another child or hit others when upset. ADHD is not just an attention problem, but a problem of impulse control (more on that later). Their urge to act is not being inhibited, so their first reaction becomes their immediate behavior.

As these children grow older, they still have difficulty in starting and completing tasks, making transitions from one thing to another, and interacting with others. They have difficulty following through on directions and organizing multistep tasks and have little goal orientation. New and different stimuli attract their attention and distract them easily.

Still later, other symptoms may appear such as clumsiness, fatigue, listlessness, muscle weakness, aggression, nonstop talking, increased volume of speech, body aches, poor appetite, anxiety, defiance and disobedience, nervousness and depression, wild mood swings, bed wetting, poor hand-eye coordination, swollen neck glands and fluid behind the ear drum, ringing in the ears, excessive sweating, and self-abusive behaviors such as hair pulling.

It's important to realize that children with ADHD usually have a normal or high IQ, but because they cannot control themselves, they often fail at school. It's not that they are unintelligent, it's just that they don't have the self-discipline to learn. They have poor learning skills and underdeveloped social skills that may affect them the rest of their lives.

Adults who have ADHD often have difficulty concentrating for long periods, are impulsive and impatient, and may have short tempers and frequent mood swings. They can have difficulty planning ahead, be overly disorganized, and feel restless and fidgety.

It's believed that many adults with ADHD were never properly diagnosed as children. It was once widely believed that the symptoms would disappear as one got older. However, it's now recognized that these symptoms carry through into adolescent and adult life, giving rise to job performance and interpersonal relationship problems.

According to one 1997 estimate, somewhere between 6.5 and 9 million adults in the U.S. have ADHD – making it as large a problem as drug abuse or clinical depression. In 1997, close to 730,000 adults in the U.S. were taking Ritalin by prescription for ADHD. (5) Ritalin, as we shall explore in depth below, is a psychoactive drug used to treat ADHD.

Food for Thought

I do not intend to exaggerate the problems of ADHD and scare you into thinking that all the possible behaviors mentioned above means your child has a disorder. Kids will be kids, and they have an amazing amount of energy and their attention span is naturally short. But some kids are showing too many of these impulsive and aggressive behaviors, and that is a problem. If something isn't done for them as soon as possible, these behaviors will become more and more ingrained and harder to change as time goes on. There are many simple and natural ways to help children with ADHD (besides using drugs), which we will explore. But please don't get hysterical if your child exhibits some of these behaviors on occasion. Most of them are part of being a child and growing up. It's my personal opinion that unless a number of these behaviors seem out of control, especially the aggressive and violent ones, there's no reason to be overly concerned. If you follow the recommendations in this book, your child will likely recover from these behaviors or never exhibit them.

Attention Deficit and Hyperactivity Disorders

It's estimated that between 10 percent and 15 percent of all school children in the U.S. are affected by ADHD. That's between 1.8 million and 2.7 million children. (6). Since it is difficult to diagnose, it is believed that many cases go undetected. Up to 70 percent of children with ADHD will continue to exhibit symptoms of it in adulthood. (7) Boys are diagnosed with the disorder two to three times as often as girls. (8)

The evidence shows that the ADHD problem is growing. In a medical conference in November 1999, the organizers of the conference estimated that ADHD among children in the U.S. is doubling every three to four years. The use of Ritalin has *quadrupled* between 1990 and 1997. (9)

The traditional medical community considers the cause of ADHD to be unknown even though it is one of the best-researched disorders in medicine. Research does suggest that it has a neurobiological basis. Stewart Mostofsky, M.D., of the Kennedy Krieger Institute and Johns Hopkins School of Medicine in Baltimore, says, "There is a lot of evidence that the brain's right hemisphere is dominant in attentional processes. Abnormalities in the brain's right frontal structure and function may be contributing to the behavioral impairments associated with ADHD." (10) It was also noted that children diagnosed with ADHD often have smaller overall brain volumes than normal children, with significantly less gray matter in their frontal brain region (especially the right frontal part). This study was funded by the National Institutes of Health, and involved 12 boys diagnosed with ADHD and 14 boys without ADHD.

It is also believed that ADHD is caused by a combination of hereditary predisposition and environmental factors. However, there have been some studies of identical twins showing that environmental factors contribute significantly to ADHD (i.e., one twin was normal, the other, exposed to environmental toxins, developed ADHD). (11) So although genetics may contribute to ADHD, it is not the only thing that may trigger it. And you won't be surprised to learn that there is good evidence showing that prenatal exposure to lead, mercury, cadmium, aluminum, fluoride, cigarette byproducts, and alcohol may contribute to its manifestation.

People with ADHD often do poorly in school, may drop out, have low self-esteem, and have difficulty making connections with other people. They are described as messy, disorganized, inattentive, irritable, and aggressive. Because their lives can be unrewarding and frustrating, they may become hostile and violent. In May, 1999, a 15-year-old boy shot six of his schoolmates in Conyers Georgia. At the time, he was taking the prescription drug Ritalin for ADHD.

Peter Montague of the Environmental Research Foundation states, "At a time when Americans are searching for causes of aggression and violence among children, it would make sense to consider malnutrition, food additives, tobacco additives, toxic metals, pesticides, and other endocrine-disrupting industrial toxicants - all of which many U.S. children are exposed to from the moment of conception onward." (12) Let's consider some of these closer.

Food Additives

Food additives such as dyes and colorings have been implicated in ADHD. In 16 out of 23 studies on food additives and ADHD, it was found that these food additives exacerbated the symptoms of ADHD in some children. [13]

Despite these studies (which were double-blind studies) the U.S. Food and Drug Administration has stated in one of its pamphlets "Food Color Facts" that "there is no evidence that food color additives cause hyperactivity or learning disabilities in children." [14]

Food for Thought

It's interesting to note that although the FDA published the pamphlet "Food Color Facts," the publication was actually written by the International Food Information Council. That council is a trade association representing many makers of food additives such as General Mills, Kraft, Pepsi-Cola, Coca-Cola, Procter and Gamble, and others. So it's no wonder the pamphlet says there's no evidence food color additives cause hyperactive or learning disabilities in kids. And then again, some food additives, such as the sulfites we saw in Chapter III, have been known to cause death.

While there has been much research concerning the potential carcinogenicity of artificial colors and flavors, there have been only a few published studies examining their effects on behavioral attributes.

But Ben F. Feingold, M.D., in 1970, claimed that some children showed dramatic improvements in attention deficit and hyperactivity after removing artificial ingredients from their diet. Other researchers subsequently have failed to show this consistently, according to some interpretations of their results. However, these later studies removed only one artificial item from the child's diet, when in actuality, the ADHD child is exposed to many synthetic compounds daily.

To determine if artificial colors specifically can impact a developing organism, Dr. Bennett Shaywitz of Yale University studied young rat pups exposed to a mixture of artificial colors, using amounts that would typically be consumed by American children (1 mg/kg body weight). He reported that the mixture of five dyes (blue, green, red, yellow, and orange) resulted in hyperactivity in the young rat pups. Shaywitz concluded that "...it is apparent that food dyes affect activity levels during the first month of postnatal life." [15]

MSG

MSG (Monosodium Glutamate) is a flavor enhancer used to increase the "perceived" taste of any item it's in. The food industry uses it to save money. Chicken soup made with MSG, for example, requires half the amount of real chicken in it to get the same taste as soup made without MSG. That's a real cost-saver for manufacturers. And it explains why world MSG production in 1976 was 262,000 metric tons.

Food for Thought

I have pointed out how the agricultural practices have changed in the past 60 years from natural growing methods to ones that use chemicals. The nutritional quality of the food has concomitantly decreased (see Chapter XII). Reflective of the quality of the food is how it tastes. It's my opinion that MSG is used in part because our food just doesn't taste like it should and needs flavor-enhancing. Grow more wholesome foods the way nature intended them to be grown, and you wouldn't need any "flavor enhancers."

As discussed in Chapter V, the FDA has stated that MSG is "safe" for most people except for those with serious asthma difficulties. But studies by L. Reif-Lehrer reported that 25 percent of a population sample who have been exposed to Chinese restaurant food (with MSG) exhibit at least some adverse symptoms. (16) MSG was routinely added to baby foods prior to the 1970s, and its use in them was halted following government suggestions.

Dr. Olney, at the department of psychiatry and pediatrics at Washington University School of Medicine, a leading expert concerning MSG, has said:

> According to a NAS [National Academy of Science] subcommittee, in considering the safety of added MSG in baby foods, one must remember that the levels added are small - not higher than 0.6 percent... This means that one small jar of baby food (130 g) would provide about 0.78 g of MSG or 0.13 g/kg of body weight for a human infant weighing 6 kg. Based on our finding that an oral dose of 1 g/kg in the primate or 0.5 g/kg in the mouse is sufficient to destroy hypothalamic neurons, this leaves a 4 to 8 fold margin of safety for a human infant eating 1 jar, a 2 to 4 fold margin if 2 jars are eaten and so forth. This is substantially less than the 100-fold margin generally recommended... in susceptibility of the mechanism of a toxic compound. (17)

The Food Protection Committee of the National Academy of Sciences (NAS) has declared MSG to be a safe food additive requiring no regulation. Despite evidence that MSG causes brain damage in infant rodents, the committee reasoned that the primate infant (humans are primates) was not likely at risk because it has a more mature central nervous system and more highly developed blood-brain barrier at birth.

Subsequent to this ruling, Olney showed that rhesus monkeys (a primate also) exposed to a single dose of MSG developed brain damage (in the hypothalamus). He says, "...it seems unrealistic to deny primate susceptibility to the MSG effect."

Another study using 75 infant mice was done to determine at what level MSG and aspartate could cause brain lesions. All but the very lowest level administered to the mice had harmful observable effects on brain cells. It was found that MSG and aspartate can combine their damage potential when fed to the animals together. [18]

Another Olney study was performed to investigate the possibility of long-term effects from MSG ingestion. Olney examined 38 originally healthy Swiss albino mice from birth to nine months of age. Twenty of these animals received injections of MSG daily. The MSG treated animals appeared stunted in growth and shorter than the controls after 30 days. The average weights of five-month-old animals were significantly less if they did not consume MSG than if they did. And, it's of particular interest to note that the MSG-treated mice actually consumed less food than their thinner control counterparts. This implies damage to the brain area responsible for controlling body weight. [19]

Food for Thought

Could this in part explain the growing obesity pattern in our youth and even our population at large? Have you ever heard someone complain that they continued to gain weight even though they ate practically nothing? I'm sure there are a number of factors responsible for weight gain in children and adults, but could MSG be partly responsible?

Olney also reported that the MSG animals were quite lethargic when they were adults, and they lacked the sleekness of body coat seen in the controls. The reproductive capacity of the MSG females was also modified in that they repeatedly failed to conceive. Olney concludes:

> These observations, linking MSG treatment of the neonatal (the first four weeks after birth) mouse with a syndrome of manifestations, including skeletal stunting, marked adiposity, and sterility of the female, coupled with histopathological findings in several organs associated with endocrine function, suggest a complex endocrine disturbance... The assumption that MSG is an entirely innocuous substance for human consumption has been questioned... the finding that neuronal necrosis can be induced in the immature mouse brain... raises the more specific question whether there is any risk to the developing human nervous system by maternal use of MSG during pregnancy... [20]

One child who was experiencing "innumerable seizures" (100 or more a day) showed dramatic improvements after MSG was removed from his diet. This was reported by Dr. L. Reif-Lehrer of Harvard Medical School in the journal *Federal Proceedings*. The child did not respond to dilantin (a common drug for epilepsy), but had symptoms "Completely alleviated by a diet that excluded exogenously added glutamate." When the child is fed an "MSG meal," the seizures return. Dr. Reif-Lehrer says, "In some individuals, glutamate may be getting through the blood-brain barrier, or to certain areas of the hypothalamus, and may result in undesirable effects..." [21]

It's clearly evident that MSG can have subtle as well as devastating effects on children and adults alike. It's best to avoid it. If you consume nutritious foods, you won't need any flavor enhancers.

Pesticides and Chemicals

Most recently, research has implicated pesticides and exposure to low levels of industrial chemicals to cognitive problems such as ADHD. Undoubtedly, combinations of environmental pollutants may contribute to the problem.

A report entitled "In Harm's Way," by a team of physicians in Cambridge, Massachusetts, says that millions of children in the U.S. exhibit learning disabilities, reduced IQ and destructive, aggressive behavior because of exposures to toxic chemicals. Drs. Ted Schettler and Jill Stein et al. link toxic exposures during early childhood and even before birth, to lifelong disabilities including attention disorders and poorly controlled aggression. As of June 2000, estimates indicate that ADHD, dyslexia, and uncontrollable aggression affects about 12 million children under 18 in the U.S. (almost one in five). The number of children classified with learning disabilities and placed in special education programs increased 191 percent between 1977 and 1994. Experts estimate that autism rates have risen from around four per 10,000 in the early 1980s to between 12 and 210 per 10,000 in the 1990s. [22]

Many pesticides kill insects by killing cells in the nervous system. These pesticides can also disrupt the development and functioning of the human – and child's – nervous system too. Studies show that children in communities that use pesticides a lot score lower on memory, physical stamina and coordination tests, and display more aggressive behavior than children in relatively pesticide-free areas.

Government "safe" exposure levels are based on individual chemicals. But children can be exposed to many chemicals at the same time, which can be far more damaging. One study found that certain combinations of pesticides produce changes in thyroid levels that are not observed when the chemicals are tested individually. Proper thyroid levels are essential for brain development. Other studies show that exposure to a combination of mercury and PCBs, two pollutants that accumulate in fish, can produce even greater effects on neurological development than either pollutant alone. [23]

Of 890 pesticide "active ingredients," the EPA says 140 are neurotoxins and some 20 million U.S. children under age five eat an average of eight different pesticides on their food every day. In addition, there are between 2,400 and 4,000 industrial chemicals now on the market that are neurotoxic. The EPA estimates that nearly a billion pounds of known neurotoxins were released directly into the air and water in 1997.

The authors of "In Harm's Way" write:

We should not need to identify with certainty exactly how much

132

and through what mechanism a neurotoxic pesticide impairs brain development before coming to the conclusion that public health is not protected when the urine of virtually every child in this country contains residues of these chemicals... We do not need to exhaustively understand the mechanism by which methylmercury interferes with normal fetal brain development before concluding that it is not acceptable for freshwater and many ocean fish to be sufficiently contaminated with mercury to threaten developing brains. We know how to reduce the environmental releases of mercury so that fish are once again safe to eat regularly. We can modify manufacturing practices so that lead use in products goes steadily down instead of up. We can eliminate or modify outmoded technologies that produce the dioxin that contaminates fetuses and breast milk. We know how to do these things... In sum, our current regulatory system is like a trial in which the criminal defendant gets to serve on the jury. If we want to have children who can play, think and learn normally, we will have to change corporations and our government so that protecting brain development comes ahead of protecting profits. (24)

Aluminum

High levels of aluminum affect the central nervous system, and are believed to play a role in Alziehimer's disease in the elderly and hyperactivity in children. Aluminum can be ingested from food and water contaminated when cooked in aluminum pans or stored in aluminum foil. Most soft drinks come in aluminum cans and aluminum can be in these beverages. It's also found in coffee, bleached flour (all white flour products and pastas, but not the whole grain kinds), and drinking water. Municipal drinking water plants typically use a chemical called Alum, which contains aluminum, which ends up in the tap water. If someone has a deficiency of magnesium and calcium, the toxic effects of aluminum are increased, so it's necessary to have a diet with sufficient amounts of these two nutrients. (25)

Cadmium

Cadmium is the most toxic heavy metal on the planet (with mercury being the second) and is a highly toxic neurotoxin. It concentrates in the kidneys, liver, and blood and is harmful from the time of conception onward. The half-life of cadmium in the body is from *17 to 30 years*, so it's very difficult to remove it from tissues. Once in, it interferes with the absorption of zinc, which is a vital nutrient necessary for many biochemical reactions in the body. Conversely, adequate levels of zinc in the diet may protect against the adverse effects of cadmium.

Zinc is involved in more than 60 enzymes in the body including those regulating digestion, protein synthesis, vision, the immune system, and prostate health. It's been shown to prevent some birth defects and acts to calm the nervous system (zinc is sometimes called a "sedative" mineral that stabilizes emotions). Our soils are depleted of zinc so getting enough zinc in the diet is sometimes difficult, especially if one is a vegetarian. Zinc is found mainly in animal products, so putting a child on a vegetarian diet may lead to a zinc deficiency. Also, zinc will compete with copper, so if zinc is inadequate, copper toxicity may occur. (26)

Zinc and copper smelters and refiners release more than two million pounds of cadmium into our air every year. Cigarette smoke is the major source of cadmium, coffee is the second largest source, and refined white flour products also contain high amounts. A study of over 150 children showed that those with a high intake of refined carbohydrates (i.e., white flour) had the highest levels of cadmium in their tissues. Since most of the "junk foods" like pretzels, tortilla chips, pizza, etc. contain mostly white flour, it's no surprise that children can accumulate higher than normal levels of cadmium which may contribute to behavioral and learning problems. And if the pregnant mother consumes large quantities of these type foods, some of the cadmium may be passed on to the fetus. (27) Whatever the source of cadmium, studies show that many children with learning disabilities have significantly higher levels of cadmium and lower zinc levels than normal children.

Copper

Like cadmium, excessive copper in the body displaces zinc and contributes to emotional sensitivity, mood swings, and erratic behavior. Other signs of copper toxicity include fatigue, depression, headaches, premenstrual tension, and skin problems. Again, since toxic metals can pass through the placenta, copper toxicity can be passed from mother to child. Junk foods, soda pop, and other non-nutritious foods can lead to copper toxicity. (28) Vegetarian diets are typically high in copper (whereas meats contain more zinc and less copper), so vegetarian diets can also lead to copper toxicity. As the prevalence of vegetarian diets has increased, so has the incidences of copper imbalances. (29)

It's important to realize that toxic metals compete with the beneficial minerals in many biological reactions. Lead will replace calcium, and cadmium can replace zinc. Avoidance of toxic metals and sufficient intake of the good minerals helps to keep these biological reactions functioning normally.

Diet

Poor diet undoubtedly contributes to ADHD, and it's been reported that malnutrition can trigger ADHD. (30) Simply put, if a child does not eat well or has certain food allergies, chances of behavioral and learning problems are increased not to mention compromised overall health.

Certain deficiencies should be watched for, especially zinc deficiencies and essential fatty acid deficiencies. Both have been shown to occur frequently in children with ADHD. Donald Rudin, Ph.D., co-author of *The Omega-3 Phenomenon*, believes that deficiencies of Omega-3 oils (an essential fatty acid) are partly responsible for the increase in emotional and behavioral disorders and wide-spread illnesses. (31)

As you will read in more detail in Chapter XII, the quality and nutritional value of our foods has gone down. They may still look good, but modern chemical fertilizers supply only three basic nutrients (N, P, K – that is, nitrogen, phosphorus, potassium), and the soils our crops are grown on are no longer rich in all the minerals needed to produce healthy, nutritious plants. Instead what we get are exhausted crops not healthy enough to survive natural growing conditions making the heavy use of pesticides and herbicides necessary to grow them. In addition, the chemicals used on crops oftentimes kill the important soil microorganisms that help the plant roots absorb the minerals.

It's not just the plants that have been affected by depleted soils and modern agricultural methods. The animals we eat are now raised in lots and pens and not allowed to roam freely. Their feed is contaminated with metals, hormones and antibiotics, dyes, and additives. Plus, their feed comes from the same fields we grow food for people and has the same depletion of minerals. So it's important you and your child eat as much organically raised food as possible and as much meat from free-roaming, naturally raised animals.

Even though you hear a lot of talk about how bad fat is in the diet, the fact is that we need a fairly good amount of "good" fats to be healthy. These good fats include the essential fatty acids (EFAs), which are building blocks in the membranes of every cell.

If you're worried about gaining weight by eating fat, you don't need to be if you're eating the right kind of fat. Mary Van Elswyk, Ph.D., a leading authority on fat, explains:

> Obesity results when the body is unable to process nutrients. You've got all this stored fat unable to convert to energy, and you're not able to make proper use of it. The cells are literally starving. Then it becomes a vicious cycle: Your body is looking for more energy; you eat more to provide it, but cells don't have access to it and your body holds onto it. If you improve the nutritional status throughout the body with the correct vitamins, minerals and essential fatty acids, cells will function better and be able to access the fat.
> (32)

So eating the right kind of fat and avoiding the bad kind (the kind most of Americans typically eat) can actually help you lose weight because your body will function better.

Although the body needs about twenty different fatty acids to be healthy, it can make all of them except two – Omega-3 (linolenic acid) and Omega-6 (linoleic acid). Since the body can't make them, they must be obtained from the diet or from supplements.

Unfortunately, modern food processing destroys the essential fatty acid content of many foods. Even the fish, chicken, and meat produced has lower levels of EFAs because the feed for these animals is not as nutritious as the food the animal would eat in the wild or as a free-range animal. And, even further, many of the items in our diet such as drugs, sugar, caffeine, and refined carbohydrates tend to block EFA absorption and metabolism. A zinc deficiency that may result from metal toxicity, also adversely affects the functioning of EFAs. (33)

Some research has shown that children with ADHD oftentimes cannot absorb or metabolize EFAs normally, resulting in an EFA deficiency. The requirements for EFAs are thus higher in these children. Hyperactive male children outnumber female children by about three to one. These boys need two to three times more EFAs than the girls, reportedly because they have more difficulty converting EFAs to prostaglandins. (Prostaglandins are tissuelike hormones that control body functioning at the cellular level). Asthma, eczema, and other skin problems are also more prevalent in hyperactive children because of prostaglandin insufficiency. Children with EFA deficiencies usually have abnormally high thirst. Since wheat and pasteurized, commercial milk can block the biochemical conversion of EFAs in the body, these products should be avoided by all children, and especially those with signs of ADHD. (Note: Raw milk is acceptable to feed to children. We will discuss this more in depth later.)

Other things that interfere with EFAs and their metabolism are diets high in hydrogenated oils and food colorings (especially yellow dye), low zinc in the diet, low vitamin E, C, niacin, and vitamin B-6. (34)

Children especially need a diet high in fat. Their nervous system is developing and fat supplies a fair amount of energy production and slows the metabolic rate. Calcium and some vitamins need fat in order to be absorbed, and growth requires the energy of concentrated calories, like those found in fat. The sheathing around nerve fibers is called the "myelin sheath" and is nearly 100 percent fat. It's the insulator and protective cover of the nerve. If we don't have enough of the proper raw fats in our diets, these myelin sheaths will be inadequate and we'll always feel on edge. Children with ADHD often times have faster than normal metabolic and oxidation rates. A diet high in carbohydrates – pasta, chips, pretzels, bread, cereal, and so on – will actually raise the metabolic rate, and fat will lower it, so replacing some of these items with a good natural fat will help the child slow down. (35)

Of course, children (and adults) need the right kind of fat (natural, unheated and uncooked as much as possible), not the fat found in fast food and chips. They also need a consistent supply of EFAs. EFAs can be found in fresh foods such as cold-water fish (salmon, sardines, cod, trout, and mackerel), leafy green vegetables, nuts and seeds, flax seed oil, borage oil, evening primrose oil, avocados, and rice. (36)

Fats to avoid are those that are hydrogenated as found in margarines and shortenings – used extensively in fast foods. Hydrogenation uses chemicals and high heat, which remove most of the vitamins and minerals from the fat and changes the fat into a form that does not spoil as easily. During hydrogenation, polyunsaturated oils (i.e., cis-fatty acids, which are healthy) are changed into oils called trans-fatty acids, which are very detrimental. They alter the permeability of the cell membrane, interfere with certain enzymes and disrupt the vital functions of the EFAs in the body. Avoid products that are hydrogenated (margarine) and also partially hydrogenated oils, which have a high amount of trans-fatty acids. The hydrogenation process changes the oil and strips it of most or all of its beneficial EFAs. The body can't metabolize the trans-fatty acids because they're unnatural and they have been shown to decrease the good cholesterol (HDL) and impede liver function.

Two other fatty acids that are necessary for proper nervous system and overall health are EPA (eicosapentaenoic acid) and DHA (docosahexaenoic acid). They are polyunsaturated fatty acids necessary for proper brain and eye development during pregnancy and proper functioning of the immune, respiratory, circulatory, and reproductive systems. (37) DHA is especially critical in brain development, so it's important for pregnant women and infants to get enough. DHA has been shown to help women carry babies to term. (38)

Although they are produced in the body from Omega-3 fatty acids, it takes a long time, and children with EFA deficiencies may also develop deficiencies in DHA and EPA. A good source of EPA and DHA are fish oils – in fish tissues or cod liver oil. There is not a good vegetarian source of these two fatty acids. The best fish for these are cold-water fish such as salmon, sardines, cod, trout, and mackerel. These fish should be from the ocean or lake, not from fish farms, since farm-raised fish have less Omega-3 fatty acid content.

EPA and DHA are not essential (essential meaning the body must obtain them from outside sources and cannot manufacture it by itself), but are oftentimes difficult for the body to manufacture. Interestingly, people whose ancestors consumed large amounts of meat as a staple in their diets frequently cannot make DHA, EPA, or arachidonic acid (AA), and gamma-linolenic acid (GLA). So these need to be obtained from the diet. Trans-fatty acids, found in commercial vegetable oils and abundant in fast-food products, can interfere with the body's ability to manufacture these fatty acids as well, so obtaining them in the diet is advisable. Consuming egg yolks, liver and other organ meats, fish oils, and organically raised chickens will supply EPA and DHA. GLA can be found in borage oil and evening primrose oils and AA is found in butter and organ meats. (39)

Maybe grandmother's advice of taking your cod liver oil has some merit – though not for infants. Fish oils also contain EPA, which is fine for adults, but in infants it counteracts other EFAs needed for growth. The consumption of DHA alone is best for infants.

Although some researchers might say there is not a good plant source of DHA, there is one product I have found on the market that has been shown to elevate blood levels of DHA in both infants and mothers during pregnancy and lactation. It's called Neuromins Pro, manufactured by MMS Pro (see Resource Guide). This product is highly purified and is believed be less contaminated (especially in mercury) than fish oil DHA. Neuromins does not contain significant amounts of EPA, however.

To understand the importance of fat in the diet, consider what happens when you don't have enough: When your diet no longer supplies the necessary raw materials - many of them derived from fats – lots of things go wrong and the body, and brain, start to shut down. Too many trans-fatty acids and too few essential fatty acids, and you have a recipe for depression.

Trans- or hydrogenated, manmade fats were synthesized originally to extend shelf life of commercial products. The production of trans-fatty acids for human consumption is one of the most devastating nutritional mistakes ever made. In the effort to make foods last longer in the supermarket, all traces of essential fatty acids (such as Omega-3s) are obliterated from processed foods, and trans-fats or partially hydrogenated oils take their place. The absence of omega-3 essential fatty acids in Western diets has contributed to an alarming increase in a number of diseases that appeared only infrequently 100 years ago. A lack of the essential fatty acids and cofactors, such as minerals and vitamins to handle fat, combined with the consumption of trans-fats, is more often the causal factor in obesity and cardiovascular disease than is eating cholesterol-rich foods. After all, the body needs some cholesterol – it's needed to produce crucial hormones that strongly influence mood such as pregnenolone, testosterone, progesterone, estradiol, estrone, and cortisole. [40] Too little cholesterol and you're subject to depression.

Sugar interferes with enzymes that synthesize fatty acids, and aspirin inhibits the enzyme necessary to assimilate Omega-3 fatty acids and may aggravate asthma or allergic disorders. Repeated and prolonged use of aspirin and other non-steroid anti-inflammatory drugs is not recommended. [41,42]

Food Allergies

Allergies to certain foods are another problem, not just for the overall health of children but in the development of ADHD. If a child is being bothered with allergy symptoms, he or she may appear inattentive or have other behavioral problems. It's important to identify and eliminate the offending substance to settle the child down into normal behavior.

Richard E., Layton, M.D., of the Allergy Connection says, "Children who suffer from chronic illnesses or who exhibit certain behavioral difficulties may actually be experiencing allergies. A surprising number of childhood medical conditions can be traced to food allergies. When an allergy is identified as the culprit behind a child's medical or behavioral problems, it can be controlled and even eliminated through several safe and effective treatments resulting in a happier, healthier life." [43]

Symptoms of allergies are not just a runny nose or sneezing. They can include anxiety, depression, hyperactivity, insomnia, irritability, mental confusion, personality changes, joint pain, muscle aches, acne, eczema, fatigue, digestive disturbances, ear infections, hyperglycemia, migraines, and even seizures.

A chemical produced by the body, and also found in many foods, that causes allergic reactions is histamine. It causes rashes, itchiness, and increased mucus production. Most cold, flu, and asthma medications try to block the release of histamines by the white blood cells, thereby stopping the symptoms. This does nothing to eliminate the cause of the problem, however, which, along with a general toxicity of the body, may include eating foods high in naturally occurring histamine. These include tuna, wine, preserves, sausage, sauerkraut, spinach, and tomatoes. Other foods that cause our white blood cells to release excessive histamine include milk, eggs, shellfish, strawberries, bananas, chocolate, papayas, pineapples, some nuts, and alcohol. (44)

Cheese contains high amounts of tyrosine (an amino acid), and children with ADHD have been found to have high levels of this in their blood. Other products that contain tyrosine in high amounts, and to be avoided by children with ADHD, are: chocolate; cream; coffee; citrus fruits; cheese; and yeast extracts. (45)

Other foods that frequently cause allergic reactions are sugar, chocolate, peanuts, apples, carrots, tomatoes, eggs, soy, grapes, corn, oranges, red and yellow dye, and preservatives.

One topic not generally discussed when it comes to allergies is that our brain can be allergic to many things, just like our bodies. In fact, doctors have found that 90 percent of patients admitted to mental hospitals had allergies that affected the brain. When the brain is allergic, swelling and inflammation result, so it's no wonder people suffering from them may have a wide variety of mental disorders. Just about any food, but especially wheat and dairy products, can trigger a brain allergy reaction. Food additives can also be a problem.

The most common symptoms of a brain allergy in children are irritability, mood swings, sleeplessness, depression, anxiety, hyperactivity, learning disorders, lack of concentration, tantrums, fatigue, and muscle weakness. If a child is affected with a brain allergy for an extended period, his or her handwriting may deteriorate and behavior change. Certain smells can also trigger a brain allergy response. Some toxins that can do this are formaldehyde, acetone, methyl ketone, and ethyl ketone. (Check your perfume and nail polish, ladies.) A parent or teacher may jump to the conclusion there's a problem and put the child on Ritalin or other drug, when really it's some kind of allergic reaction. With the high amount of synthetic chemicals, additive, ingredients, and so on in our environment, an allergic reaction of some sort is almost unavoidable.

Two foods that cause many allergic reactions are *pasteurized* milk and wheat products. In fact, by taking a child suffering from allergies off pasteurized milk and wheat products, most allergic reactions usually cease.

Not only can wheat cause allergic reactions by itself, but you and your child may suffer allergic reactions because of the toxic residues in the wheat remaining from its processing. Wheat, when not grown organically, is subjected to: the treatment of the wheat seed with mercury; hormone treatment to increase the size of the seedhead; insecticides; fungicides; and hormone treatment to reduce the length of the stem. All these chemicals can cause allergic or toxic reactions in your child and presumably in a fetus. Oftentimes, just by using organically grown wheat products, you can ameliorate those reactions entirely. (46)

Pasteurized cow's milk is probably the food that causes the most allergic reactions in children. Although mother's milk is by far the perfect food for infants and raw cow's milk is a good second-best, *pasteurized* cow's milk is far from being so for children and adults. (We will discuss why raw milk is not a health hazard in just a bit.) Dr. Julian Whitaker, M.D., writes in his newsletter:

Here are three reasons kids and [pasteurized] milk don't mix. First, [pasteurized] milk is the leading cause of iron-deficiency anemia in infants, and in fact, the American Academy of Pediatrics now discourages giving children [pasteurized] milk before their first birthday. Second, it has been shown that [pasteurized] milk consumption in childhood contributors to the development of Type-I diabetes. Certain proteins in [pasteurized] milk resemble molecules on the beta cells of the pancreas that secrete insulin. In some cases, the immune system makes antibodies to the [pasteurized] milk protein that mistakenly attacks and destroys the beta cells... Third, [pasteurized] milk allergies are very common in children and cause sinus problems, diarrhea, constipation, and fatigue. They are a leading cause of the chronic ear infections that plague up to 40 percent of all children under the age of six. [Pasteurized] Milk allergies are also linked to behavior problems in children and to the disturbing rise of childhood asthma (milk allergies are equally common in adults and produce similar symptoms). Even so august an authority on children as the late Dr. Benjamin Spock changed his recommendations in his later years and discouraged giving children [pasteurized] milk... To start with, knock off drinking [pasteurized] milk altogether. Fluid [pasteurized] milk is likely to be the most highly concentrated, easily absorbed source of growth hormones... be sure to avoid products from hormone-treated cows. A growing number of dairies offer organic or hormone-free diary products. (47) ([pasteurized] added)

Another problem with pasteurized milk is what's called lactose intolerance. Lactose is the sugar found in milk. At about the age of two to three years, children lose most of the enzyme called lactase, which is necessary for digesting the lactose. Most adults have about 5 percent to 10 percent of the lactase they had as in infant. If lactase is missing, the sugar does not get digested, and ends up accumulating in the intestine. This is perfect culture media for bacteria to grow on. This may cause bloating, intestinal pain, gas, and diarrhea. (Raw milk, on the other hand, contains it's own lactase which digests the lactose when you drink the milk. So this is not an issue when you drink raw milk.)

Food for Thought

If pasteurized milk is so bad for you and your child, why do they promote it as being so healthy? The dairy industry has grown, thanks to good advertising and lobbying, to be a major player in the development of dietary recommendations from nutritionists and the government alike. Again, dear reader, the bottom line is money. It's a multibillion-dollar industry.

It all started back in 1935 when a government official of a small dairy in Minnesota named George Pushing discovered he could use pasteurization to prolong the shelf life of milk. (We'll talk about pasteurization and

---

germs in Chapter XII.) He said, "We can buy the milk that dairy farmers cannot sell by themselves, and by applying heat at 155 degrees Fahrenheit, even reject milk will keep for two weeks." (Ch-ching! He could hear that cash register working!) He later admitted that pasteurization was only an economic ploy to increase profits and get control of the dairy industry since pasteurization requires expensive equipment that many small dairies cannot afford. Mr. Pushing later contracted rheumatoid arthritis, a disease that raw milk can prevent, by drinking his pasteurized milk. (48)

Consider what pasteurization (cooking milk at a minimum of 155 degrees Fahrenheit for at least 15 seconds), does to milk:

Pasteurization alters and destroys the beneficial properties of proteins, vitamins, minerals, enzymes, essential fatty acids, and natural antigens. When these substances are altered through heat in this way, they become toxins the body must isolate and eliminate. The body does this by coating these toxins in mucus to transport and eliminate them. Now you know why your child has a runny nose all the time. Minerals often become glass-like and sharp, frequently lacerating liver tissue, blood, and nerve cells. If someone cannot produce enough mucus to eliminate them, they often become the cause of a myriad of allergies. Pasteurized fats become lipid oxides that are known carcinogens, and pasteurized proteins create large amounts of uric acid that can lead to muscular and glandular problems. The heat involved in pasteurization not only creates these toxic substances, but destroys almost all the nutritional value too. It is so lacking in nutrition that if calves are fed pasteurized milk, they die within sixty days! And we'll see in Chapter XII the devastating effects of cooked milk on several generations of cats.

Pasteurization creates degenerative matter in milk on which pathogenic organisms thrive. Many of the reports of the hazards of raw milk have really occurred because of faulty pasteurization, leading to the formation of these harmful micobes and causing sickness and even death. Nutritionist Aajonus Vonderplanitz says, "The microbes that science and medicine term 'pathogenic' are simply the symptom that degenerative matter exists. As soon as the degenerative matter is consumed, the microbes go dormant..." (49)

Here's more proof that pasteurization doesn't even kill all the disease causing microorganisms it's supposed to every time. The January 1974 *Consumer Report* found that one out of six milk samples bought from retail stores had a count of 130,000 bacteria per *milliliter.* In fact, the acceptable standard for pasteurized milk is about 100,000 bacteria per *teaspoon!* (50)

On the other hand, raw milk simply sours, and this microbiological activity is not pathological, as proven by tests in Europe. Conversely, there has never been any scientific studies proving that bacteria in raw milk are dangerous to health. In fact, the souring produces lactic acid and makes milk more easily digestible, especially for people with less than optimum digestion such as infants, the elderly, and infirmed. There have been countless reports of people recovering from many different ailments by consuming raw milk. (51)

Dr. Bieler, a practicing physician for more than 50 years, routinely prescribed raw milk to his patients. He never saw a case of "undulant fever" – which is supposedly caused by unpasteurized milk. (52)

When milk was right from the farm, pure and fresh as it had been for millions of years before 1935 when some greedy dairyman wanted to make more money, it was a good wholesome and nutritious food. And it didn't contain the hormones, pesticides, antibiotics, cancer-promoting substances, and even radioactive particles it does today. All these things are done to and added to milk for one purpose – to make more money! Not to improve it!

With all this toxic material in a glass of "natures perfect food," is it any wonder children have runny noses, ear aches, sinus infections, headaches, sour stomachs, fevers, and so on? These are the reactions of their little bodies trying to get rid of all these poisons. Gabriel Cousens, M.D., says, "I am always amazed how many have their chronic colds, sore throats, and earaches cleared up when I discover they are allergic to dairy and they stop eating diary. Even without an allergy to dairy, the tendency to colds and flu is greatly decreased when diary is eliminated." (53)

Yes, milk does contain a lot of calcium. But if the milk is pasteurized, it's mostly unavailable to the human body because it's trapped within the casein molecule, and pasteurized milk's reaction in the body is acidic. That means in order for the body to maintain the normal blood pH of 7.4, calcium, which neutralizes acid, must be mobilized from its reserves (bones and muscles) to neutralize the acidic effects of pasteurized milk. And to make matters worse, modern dairy cows are now fed feed with a higher protein content than old-time grass-fed cows. This increased protein makes the milk have more protein, which makes it more acidic. This in turn makes your body more acidic when you drink it, which encourages more bone loss due to the necessity of the body to rob calcium from its bones to neutralize the acid.

Although pasteurization doesn't kill all the microorganisms, it does kill some (and the healthy ones at that). Enough to make it last longer on the shelf. And longer shelf life means more money. Is it any wonder the "authorities" make you fear drinking raw milk and have made it a crime to sell it? The more control someone has over a substance, the more money will be made. But raw milk was sold in California for years, and although the health officials kept an eagle eye for problems, there weren't any. They did make raw milk illegal in California in 1990, but now it's my understanding it's back on the market again there. Whereas there had been a dozen illness reports from pasteurized milk in the 1980s and 1990s (*Salmonella, Listeria*), there were none involving raw milk.

On the other hand, raw milk from healthy cows is great for growing children. It is abundant in calcium, has the right kinds of fats their brain and nervous system need to develop normally, is a complete protein with minerals, vitamins C, A, E, and D, B vitamins, and enzymes. All these vital nutrients are easily absorbed and assimilated by the body which allows children to not only avoid the problems with pasteurized milk but to grow into strong, healthy, and well balanced adults.

The bottom line? Stop feeding pasteurized milk to your child. It could be causing a lot of the allergies and other problems he or she is experiencing. But raw milk and raw milk products, loaded with nutrition, can bring them back to health. You'll learn how to find raw milk in the Resource Guide.

An Overlooked Cause of Many Allergies

There are small proteins in our bodies and in the raw food we eat called enzymes. These make biochemical reactions possible and others to proceed at a much faster rate – i.e., they are catalysts. They were first identified in the 1930's, and today over 5,000 have been discovered. If you don't have the proper enzymes or enough of them, things in your body can get sluggish. Nutrients cannot be processed (poor digestion) or transported efficiently (poor assimilation), and waste material cannot be eliminated easily (mucous buildup). This paves the way for congestion, allergies, and even more serious degenerative diseases.

In fact, Maile Pouls, Ph.D., a recognized expert in enzyme therapy, says that between 70 percent and 90 percent of allergies may be caused by the lack of enzymes. (54) The solution is very simple: eat more raw food. Each raw food has the proper enzymes included for it to be properly digested. But when food is heated as in cooking, these precious enzymes are destroyed and digestion becomes problematic.

It's interesting that all enzymes in food are deactivated at a wet-heat temperature of 118 degrees Fahrenheit. That's exactly the temperature you'll feel pain at if you stick your finger in hot water. Anything below this temperature, nature is telling you is fine to eat. Above this temperature, is harmful. (Enzymes are destroyed at a *dry-heat* temperature of about 150 degrees Fahrenheit.) (55)

Another way to address the lack of enzymes is to add some to your diet. They help in digestion and assimilation and thus, overall health. Dr. Pouls has seen many children with allergies, learning and behavioral disabilities, and other problems improve when they received the right enzymes. Adding enzymes to your child's diet, especially if their diet is less than optimal, can be an easy and relatively inexpensive way to help them. The contact information for Dr. Pouls and where to purchase good quality enzymes can be found in the Resource Guide.

Testing for Allergies

There are several ways to test your child for allergies: the skin prick test; blood tests; and a simple one you can do at home called the Elimination Diet. This is where you eliminate from the diet foods that are likely to cause allergic reactions for four to seven days. These foods are milk, soybeans, eggs, wheat, peanuts, nuts, shellfish, corn, and any other your doctor may think a possible cause. More than 80 percent of people who have food allergies get relief when these foods are omitted from the diet. If the symptoms do not go away, more foods are eliminated.

Then, slowly, one food at a time is added back to the diet and you observe whether allergic reactions return. But beware: Common food allergens are "hidden ingredients" in hundreds of packaged or processed foods, and even as filler in some vitamins.

Another way to test if you have an allergy to a certain food is to avoid eating it for at least four days. Then eat a small amount of it on an empty stomach but before you do, test your pulse rate. Check your pulse again immediately after eating the food. If you pulse rises more than a few beats per minute, or if you have any other adverse reaction, you're probably allergic to this food. You can monitor those same reactions in your child – taking care, of course, to seek immediate medical help in the case of severe adverse reaction such as intense wheezing or extreme hives.

Food for Thought

There are certain foods that have a compound in them called "salicylates." These are aspirinlike substances that have been shown to contribute to hyperactivity and asthma in children. These foods are tomatoes, almonds, apricots, peaches, and nectarines. Many children are also allergic to citrus fruits.

How significant can making dietary changes be? Lendon Smith, M.D., a world-renowned pediatrician (now retired), says that 80 percent of children get better from behavioral disorders just by changing their diet and taking vitamins. He believes that food sensitivity is a major factor for many children who have ADHD. William Crook, M.D., studied 182 hyperactive children. He found that most of the children's hyperactivity was definitely related to specific foods. Ninety-four percent of all hyperactive children he has seen are allergic or sensitive to some foods and food colorings. The worst food was sugar, followed by food additives. Other foods such as milk, corn, wheat, and eggs also created problems in many kids. (56)

Dr. Alan Cott, a psychiatrist, reported in his 1977 book, *The Orthomolecular Approach to the Treatment of Children with Behavior Disorders and Learning Disabilities*, that nutritional deficiencies can have a profound effect on learning and behavior. Nutrient deficiencies can stress the body. For example, a vitamin B-12 deficiency may cause severe psychiatric symptoms including mood disorders and paranoid behavior.

In a study performed at the California State University, children placed on vitamin and mineral supplements have been shown to exhibit significantly less violent and antisocial behavior, higher intelligence test scores, and higher academic achievements than children on placebos. (57)

However, nutritional imbalances can cause problems too. If there are excessive amounts of some B vitamins, other vitamins may not work properly. For example, megadoses of vitamin B-6 can induce folic acid deficiency. So a "shotgun" approach of megadoses of vitamins or minerals without proper supervision can cause problems just as deficiencies can. Children who received at least 100 percent of the Recommended Daily Allowance (RDA) of nutrients did better on IQ tests than those receiving 200 percent or 50 percent of the RDA. So excesses, as well as deficiencies, of vitamins or minerals can cause problems. (58) If you do consider supplementing your child's diet with vitamins or minerals, it's important to proceed slowly with proper professional guidance. It's best to start with a low-dose multivitamin/mineral supplement (remember to check for fillers), but an individually tailored supplement program designed by a qualified health care professional is the ideal way to go.

Again, a diet of organically raised foods with no additives, colorings, or sugar will go far in helping your child remain calm and attentive. Since these foods naturally contain more vitamins and minerals than conventionally grown foods, the need for supplementation (especially if these foods are eaten raw) may be reduced or eliminated altogether.

Be aware that vitamin and mineral deficiencies are more likely during growth spurts when nutrient needs are highest. And if children are on drugs for ADHD, their appetite is usually suppressed due to the action of the drugs and they may not want to eat enough. Getting them off the drugs will help their normal appetite to return.

Hypoglycemia

Hypoglycemia is a deficiency of glucose, or blood sugar, in the blood. Medical research indicates that hypo, or low, blood sugar can play a significant roll in mental and emotional disorders including ADHD, antisocial behavior, criminal tendencies, drug addiction and allergies. In one study, 76 percent of 265 children with ADHD were found to have abnormal glucose tolerance tests. (59)

The symptoms associated with impaired glucose metabolism includes the inability to concentrate, mood swings, anxiety, depression, and the tendency to be more emotional than normal. Fatigue, asthma, headaches, hyperactivity, nervousness, insomnia, irritability, restlessness, poor memory, and indecisiveness are also common with hypoglycemia.

Glucose is a kind of sugar the body uses as energy. It is *not* the same as sucrose, which is common cane sugar. There must be a steady supply of glucose in the bloodstream for the body to function normally. The brain is especially dependent on blood glucose and glucose is its sole energy source – so constant and steady supplies of it is essential to normal brain function.

The two most significant factors that contribute to hypoglycemia are diet and emotional stress. Certain foods affect the blood sugar in different ways. For example, simple carbohydrates (eg., white flour) and sugar get absorbed very quickly from the intestines into the bloodstream. This causes insulin to be produced so that the cells of the body can absorb the glucose. If too much sugar is consumed, too much insulin is produced, and a large amount of blood sugar is absorbed in a very short period of time. This quick uptake of blood glucose then leads to a sharp drop in blood sugar – resulting in too low a blood sugar, or hypoglycemia. When this happens, many of the symptoms of hypoglycemia can occur.

As the child senses the drop in blood sugar from this quick absorption due to increased insulin production, they would quite naturally reach for something sweet to replenish the sugar in the blood. These sharp increases and decreases in blood sugar affect the brain and nervous system and the endocrine system as well. Since the pancreas is being over stimulated to produce too much insulin, it is being overworked. Repeated events like this can eventually exhaust the pancreas causing insulin production to be permanently impaired – leading to diabetes. In the short term, the child is on a roller coaster of blood sugar peaks and valleys and experiences emotional and mental instability.

It's important to realize once again that the child thought to have ADHD may simply be suffering from a physiological problem brought on by environmental stressors – in this case, hypoglycemia. Any child experiencing emotional or learning problems should have their blood sugar checked. Simple adjustments in diet could eliminate the cause and preclude the need for any other type of intervention such as drugs.

The modern western diet is probably the best one in the history of the world to promote and cause hypoglycemia. Foods like white bread, sugar, soda pop, sugared cereals, and all other refined carbohydrates are absorbed too quickly into the bloodstream since they require little to no digestion. Even natural products like honey, dried fruit, fruit, and fruit juice can exacerbate the problem. What's the solution?

First off, eliminate or severely restrict all sugar from the child's diet (and yours too). No more soda, no more sugar-filled snacks, no more sugared fruit drinks or Kool-Aid. Although sugar in fruit is a good food, even too much of it can cause problems – so keep fruit consumption low to moderate and be sure to eat the whole fruit by itself along with no other foods (this improves digestion). You should also eliminate or restrict all kinds of refined carbohydrates such as white bread, pasta, pizza, crackers, and so forth. Replace these with their whole-grain counterpart. You can find these products at your local health food store.

Whole grains and vegetables provide slow-release energy. No more peaks and valleys and no more exhaustion of the pancreas. A steady blood glucose level will go far in helping your child maintain concentration, calmness, and emotional stability. You should note that whole grains should be soaked before cooking to make them more digestible. More on that later.

A diet with adequate amounts of protein is also necessary. Cold water fish, chicken, turkey, lamb, and beef – organically raised if possible – are good sources of protein. Other good sources are eggs, leafy green vegetables, sunflower seeds (good for snacking), pumpkin seeds, and almonds. Most dietitians now recommend a diet high in complex carbohydrates like pasta and rice, and little protein and fat. Is this healthy? Historical evidence does not support it. Healthy, primitive cultures ate large quantities of meat, fish, and fat along with vegetables, nuts, and seeds.

And a person with a fast metabolism, will require more protein and fat in the diet. This needs to be kept in mind for children since their metabolism is naturally faster than adults. They undoubtedly need more protein and fat in their diets.

Small frequent meals are also advised for those with blood sugar problems. Five or six small meals are better than three large ones. Between meal-snacks when your child is hungry are also advised, even when overweight is an issue. Just choose carefully. Children will let you know when they're hungry. As long as you provide good, fresh, wholesome, and organically raised foods with no sugar or other additives, letting children eat all they want when they want is fine. Since they are getting nutritious foods, and not addictive foods, their body will operate correctly and natural hunger will arise when food is really needed.

Food for Thought

When I was a kid, I was a hot dog freak. Anytime our family went out to dinner, it's all I would eat and any time I could choose a food, it was hot dogs. Although there are problems with modern-day, regular supermarket hot dogs, I think my body was trying to tell me something. I needed the protein and the fat that was in the meat. Of course, I didn't need the nitrates, additives, and preservatives. But kids need high protein and fat in their diets. Fats will calm them down, and protein is necessary for growth. Of course it should be high-quality protein and fat from organic sources if possible.

Another thing that causes or exacerbates low blood sugar is stress. When stress is encountered, the adrenal glands are activated to mobilize the body's energy reserves of glycogen in the liver and muscles. This in turn causes an increase in blood sugar, which eventually peters out, creating a low blood sugar situation. High stress levels strip the adrenals of vitamin C and the B-vitamins, which will cause them to eventually become exhausted. Caffeine also overstimulates the adrenals leading to blood sugar problems.

Good foods to help deal with sugar cravings are bananas, walnuts, and fresh pineapple. A mineral supplement high in magnesium and trace minerals can also help with sugar cravings. After about a week off refined sugar, the cravings will go away. Getting your child off refined sugar and all the products it's in is one of the best things you can do, not just for your child's health, but your sanity as well.

Food for Thought

As you are discovering, it is my belief that abnormal behavior, be it attention deficits, hyperactivity or aggression is caused by something tangible - that is to say physical/chemical/biological. Although sociologic/psychological conditions may contribute to problems, these sociologic/psychological conditions had to have first arisen themselves out of some sort of biological aberration. Out of this aberration springs forth behaviors inconsistent with a healthy organism. These traits, tendencies, and weaknesses are passed down through the generations and get worse if the original conditions causing the aberration are not reversed. This is not to say that sociologic/psychological programs or strategies are not helpful or necessary – I believe they are. But they are more of a form of damage control and are not getting to the true cause of the problem – that being the degeneration of the human organism physically, chemically, and biologically. Our environment – what we are exposed to, what we eat, and how we exercise are the major determinants to health be it physically, mentally, or emotionally. If we nurture ourselves with the natural things that bring health, we will become more understanding, more loving, and more mentally and emotionally equipped to handle the stresses of life.

Single-Parent Households

One article suggests that the rise in ADHD, and other mental problems in children, are in part due to more single-parent households (up from 15 percent in 1979 to 22 percent in 1996). (60) Divorce is one cause of single-parent households, but also the fact that many women are having children out of wedlock and are forced to raise them largely by themselves. Even when the parents stay together, our fast-paced world, the need for both parents to work to make ends meet, and the resulting lack of attention paid to our children undoubtedly take their toll.

A study of more than 21,000 children between four and 15 years old showed that in 1979, doctors reported psychological problems in 6.8 percent of the children and in 1996, 18.7 percent. (61) Children are almost three times as likely to have an emotional or behavioral disorder today as they were 20 years ago. Emotional problems (other than behavioral problems like ADHD), which include depression and psychosomatic illnesses, went up from 0.2 percent in 1979 to 3.6

percent in 1996. The researchers concluded that living in poverty or in a family with only one parent reflect the increase in the children's psychological problems. Children growing up with only one parent were almost twice as likely to be diagnosed with a psychological disorder. However, Alan Hilfer, a child psychologist, feels that it's a complex problem and that there's other factors that contribute to children's problems such as the tremendous availability of drugs and weapons. "I see children at younger ages being pulled to the dark side," he said. (62)

Another study released by the National Institute of Mental Health says that up to 2.5 percent of children and 8.3 percent of adolescents in the U.S. suffer from depression. (63) Depression onset is occurring earlier in life today than in past decades, and depression in youth may predict more severe mental or physical illness in adult life. Depression in young people often occurs along with other mental disorders such as anxiety, disruptive behavior, substance abuse disorders, and even physical illnesses such as diabetes.

Depression is associated with an increased risk of suicidal behaviors. In 1997, suicide was the third leading cause of death in 10-to 24-year-olds. In adolescents who have major depressive disorders, as many as 7 percent may commit suicide when they are young adults. This risk is higher in adolescent boys than girls. (64)

In childhood, both boys and girls are at equal risk to develop depression disorders. During adolescence, however, girls are twice as likely as boys to develop depression. (65)

Another disorder that warrants mention is called Bipolar Disorder. It's rare in young children, but can appear in older children and adolescents. It involves unusual shifts in mood, energy, and functioning and may begin with either manic and/or depressive symptoms. Symptoms include severe changes in mood – either extremely irritable or overly silly and elated, inflated self-esteem, increased energy and sexual thoughts and feelings, disregard of risk, decreased need for sleep, increased talking, being easily distracted with attention moving constantly from one thing to another. Children who are severely depressed and exhibited ADHD-like symptoms with excessive temper outbursts and mood changes may have Bipolar Disorder. Traditional treatment is usually with drugs – mood-stabilizing medications. One thing to be aware of is if your child is taking drugs for ADHD and has Bipolar Disorder, the drugs may trigger or worsen manic symptoms – perhaps the very symptoms you were hoping to control. (66)

Food for Thought

A sound body, a sound mind. It's no coincidence that people with emotional problems also have some physical problem as well. You know that you're more likely to "snap" when you've had a tough day or not enough sleep or have a headache or whatever. The easiest and surest way to improve one's mental disposition and decrease the likelihood of depression or behavioral problems is to be physically healthy and fit. Our young people are becoming emotional casualties. They are also out of shape and overweight. It's vitally important that we get them outside, away

---

from the TV and computer games, and get them physically active. When one exercises, the body produces natural painkillers – substances called "endorphins." They are very close chemically to drugs such as morphine and opiates. That's why you feel better after a good workout. The bloodstream is flooded with these endorphins, and you can actually get kind of "high." You may have heard the term "runner's high." That's what that is. People can get addicted to this natural high and literally *have* to get out and run or work out. It's the body's natural mechanism to ensure you want to exercise. You simply feel better. Now, our lazy and pampered youngsters get high by using drugs, when really that feeling was meant to ensure that one go out and exercise. Exercise increases oxygenation to the brain, allowing it to function better and be more relaxed. It results in clearer thinking, less stress, less anxiety, better sleep, better digestion, and a better disposition!

Touching and Moving

Recent studies show that the absence of touching, cuddling, and movement for a baby can lead to learning and behavior disorders. In a study of 49 cultures, there was shown to be a direct correlation between the lack of physical affection, especially touching and movement during infancy and childhood, and the amount of adult crimes. The National Institute of Child Health says that early deprivation of touching, contact, and movement results in abnormal social and emotional behaviors later in life. These abnormalities include hyperactivity and depression. (67)

The role of movements such as rocking in a cradle, touching things, crawling, walking upright, running, swinging arms, skipping, and other activities help the brain to develop coordination and balance. Since learning is a sensory process that must be reinforced by proper motor functioning of the brain, its important for babies and children to learn how to move. Movement stimulates the brain cells and helps regulate other brain functions that control physical, mental, psychological, and social development. Not enough movement can cause poor sensory integration, which may cause difficulties in learning to read, write, and do arithmetic. Touching and movement in infancy and childhood is important to help the brain develop normally.

If a child did not get enough touching and movement, it is not too late to help him or her develop the areas of the brain that were adversely affected. One therapy is called sensory integration therapy, which involves increased stimulation in six sensory and motor areas: visual, auditory, touching, mobility, language, and manual skills. Another therapy is writing. One researcher has developed a program to help children integrate their brains by writing in certain ways to music (more on this below).

Food for Thought

As our society becomes more technological, many old-fashioned traditions fall by the wayside. It used to be that babies were kept in cradles and were rocked back and forth throughout the day. Now, children are kept in bassinets, which are stationary and immobile cribs. The fetus gets rocked and moved continually while in the womb and needs to be moved and touched as an infant. But now mothers don't hold their babies as much and carry them around in plastic carriers with no direct physical contact. Touching is as much a nutrient as food. Those who do not get enough develop behavioral and physical deficiencies.

I remember in my college psychology textbook there was a discussion on the importance of touch in early life. There were pictures showing three cages with a baby monkey in each. The first cage was totally empty. The baby monkey died within a day or so. The second cage had a figure of a mother monkey made out of wire. The baby monkey in this cage tried to cuddle, even on this cold wire. It died within a few days. The last cage had the same kind of wire figure covered with soft cloth. The baby monkey in this cage cuddled on this surrogate mother and lived the longest and survived the experiment. It's important to touch and cuddle your baby and child. Do it as much as possible and your chances of a your child developing normally mentally, physically, emotionally, and socially are greatly increased.

Diagnosis of ADHD

The diagnosis of ADHD is not a simple task. As you can see from the list of possible symptoms listed earlier, the determination of ADHD is purely a subjective task. What one person sees as a problem significant enough to classify it as ADHD, another person may not. (68)

There is no positive medical or scientific test such as a blood test or a brain scan that can be used to help determine if someone has the problem. The diagnosis today, as a decade ago, relies totally on behavioral criteria, which are evaluated subjectively. According to the *Diagnostic and Statistical Manual (DSM-IV)*, which establishes the official criteria for testing ADHD, there are 14 activities (such as fidgeting, blurting out answers, interrupting, etc.) that must be evaluated before a diagnosis can be made. Each one depends on the evaluators' perspective, which may not be the same as someone else's. That makes diagnosis particularly difficult and open to debate in each case. And how many evaluators inquire about food sensitivity or heavy metal exposure?

Lawrence H. Diller, M.D., author of *Running on Ritalin: A Physician Reflects on Children, Society and Performance in a Pill* is a highly recognized expert on ADHD. He says that "what often strikes those encountering DSM criteria for the first time is how common these symptoms are among children generally." He adds that diagnosis of ADHD is "very much in the eye of the beholder." (69) In *Driven to*

Distraction by Hallowell and Ratey, the authors said, "There is no clear line of demarcation between ADD and normal behavior." (70)

Mary Eberstadt, in her article "Why Ritalin Rules," recounts performing a nonscientific test on adults using a questionnaire commonly used to help diagnose ADHD. The questionnaire was given to 20 people, all of whom were successful, mostly professional adults. She found that "Apart from the exceedingly anomalous two scores... all the rest of the subjects reported answering 'yes' to at least a quarter of the questions – surely enough to trigger the possibility of an ADD diagnosis..." (71)

Diane McGuinness goes a step further. "The past 25 years has led to a phenomenon almost unique in history. Methodologically rigorous research... indicates that ADD and Hyperactivity as 'syndromes' simply do not exist. We have invented a disease, given it medical sanction, and now must disown it. The major question is how we go about destroying the monster we have created. It is not easy to do this and still save face..." (72)

Richard E. Vatz says, "Attention-deficit disorder is no more a disease than is 'excitability.' It is a psychiatric, pseudomedical term." (73)

In 1998, the National Institutes of Health convened a conference on ADHD with the panel consisting of 13 doctors and educators. Part of the reason for the conference was to help nail down the criteria and evaluations for diagnosing ADHD. As one of the panelists put it, "The diagnosis is a mess." (74)

Considering what's at stake here, that being the health and future of our children, it's simply amazing that the medical community and the public at large are so quick to label a child as having an attention deficit disorder. Especially considering that the diagnosis is "in the eye of the beholder."

The question has arisen whether ADHD is a result of some biological, physical abnormality. Some research has suggested that this is not the case. G.S. Golden, an expert on brain function, says, "Attempts to define a biological basis for ADHD have been consistently unsuccessful. The neuroanatomy of the brain as demonstrated by neuroimaging studies, is normal. No neuropathologic substrate has been demonstrated." (75)

Keep in mind, however, that although there is evidence that strictly biological or anatomical conditions may not cause ADHD, biochemical imbalances may. And, the overall health of the child (or adult) needs to be considered. A medical exam by a physician should be conducted when there is a question whether a child is affected. This should include hearing and vision tests to rule out other medical problems that may be causing symptoms similar to ADHD.

There has also been research that shows that a small number of people with ADHD may have a thyroid dysfunction. (76) Stephen E. Langer, M.D., points out that hypothyroidism can manifest itself in poor short-term memory and difficulty in concentrating. A study at Georgetown University showed that these two symptoms occurred in more than half of 109 cases of hypothyroidism. (77) Nathan Masor reports that in hypothyroidism thinking is slow and memory impaired which often compounds emotional conditions such as listlessness, restlessness, irritability, and miscellaneous body pains. He says that often times these symptoms go away with daily thyroid therapy indicating that in most cases, they were due to hypothyroidism. (78) Besides supplementation with thyroid hormone (which can only be done under a Medical Doctor's prescription and supervision), the diet needs to include all essential nutrients, especially the B vitamins. The lack of thiamin (B-1) and cyanocobalamin (B-12) can slow thinking, cause irritability, and cause memory lapses.

An interesting double-blind study by Dr. Ruth Flinn Herrell was performed where she added just 2 mg of vitamin B-1 to the daily diet of one group of children and a placebo to a second group. The first group's mental and physical abilities rose from 7 percent to 87 percent, while the second group's remained almost the same. (79)

J. MacDonald Holmes, Ph.D., reported in the *British Medical Journal* that a vitamin B-12 deficiency brought on mental and emotional symptoms such as mood disorders, agitated depression, difficulty in thinking and remembering, confusion, visual and auditory hallucinations, epilepsy, and delusions. (80)

In addition to good nutrition, aerobic exercise is important in encouraging brain and memory function, according to Professor Robert Rivera, a memory expert at Valley College in Van Nuys, California. He has found that better blood and oxygen circulation to the brain can cause an increase in a person's IQ as much as thirty points.

This is understandable considering that the gray matter of the brain, where thinking is done, uses 25 percent of our oxygen intake. The blood going to the brain must have an oxygen saturation of 90 percent for us to think efficiently. If it's reduced to 85 percent, the ability of fine concentration and fine muscular coordination decreases. Rivera thinks that oxygen deprivation may also lead to emotional instability. Hypothyroidism can cause oxygen deprivation in the brain because it is usually associated with decreased blood circulation and a general decrease in the rate of metabolism. (81)

Food for Thought

As you already know, our children are less active than ever and their diets are less than optimal. Could it be that many of these learning disabilities and emotional problems are, in large part, brought on simply because our children (and ourselves) are not exercising enough and eating well? More exercise and better nutrition could probably solve many of our young people's problems. A simple solution. But mankind doesn't seem to like simplicity. We must flex our muscles and overcome all those "demons" out there. When really, the demons are all within us.

Treating ADHD

In a 1995 article in the *Journal of College Student Psychotherapy*, Peter R. Breggin, M.D. and Ginger Ross Breggin discuss how to handle children with ADHD:

> The symptoms or manifestations of ADHD often disappear when the children have something interesting to do or when they are given a minimal amount of adult attention... When a small child, perhaps five or six years old, is persistently disrespectful or angry, there is always a stressor in that child's life – something over which the child has little or no control. Sometimes, the child is not being respected because children learn more by example than by anything else. When treated with respect, they tend to respond respectfully. When loved, they tend to be loving... Children do not, on their own, create severe emotional conflict within themselves and with the adults around them. (82)

Breggin says that most so-called ADHD children are not receiving enough attention from their fathers in particular, who may be separated from the family or too preoccupied with work and other things. The treatment that has shown to be most successful is more rational and loving attention from the young person's father. And since many young people are so hungry for the attention of a father-figure, the attention can come from any male adult. He notes that seemingly impulsive, hostile groups of children calm down when a caring, relaxed, yet firm adult male is around.

Studies show that children who receive good and adequate treatment for ADHD in the form of increased attention and caring from adults respond in a very positive manner. Many professionals note that ADHD tends to go away during summer vacation, when the child is in a less structured environment and free to pursue things that interest him.

Smaller schools with smaller class sizes have a dramatic effect on children and their emotions. The teachers can get to know their students better and understand their basic needs. A smaller, more child-oriented school setting can make behavioral problems virtually disappear. (83)

In July 1993, the *New York Times* reported, "students in schools limited to about 400 students have fewer behavior problems, better attendance and graduation rates, and sometimes higher grades and scores. At a time when more children have less support from their families, students in small schools can form close relationships with teachers." Teachers in these schools, said the article, have the opportunity for "building bonds that are particularly vital during the troubled years of adolescence." (84)

When an already troubled student is put into a smaller school, she tends to respond positively. "They are shining stars you thought were dull," said New York City teacher Gregg Staples. Breggin and Breggin say that, "Children respond so quickly to improvements in the way that adults relate to them that most children can be helped without being seen by a professional person." Oftentimes, psychotherapists can help a child without ever seeing the child himself, but rather, working with their parents to help them become more loving or more disciplined, which can indirectly transform the child.

Berggin and Berggin go on to say, "Children can benefit from guidance in learning to be responsible for their own conduct; but they do not gain from being blamed for the trauma and stress that they are exposed to in the environment around them. They need empowerment, not humiliating diagnoses and mind-disabling drugs. Most of all, they thrive when adults show concern and attention to their basic needs as children." (85)

Ritalin

Some drugs that act as stimulants or "speed" in most adults can have a calming effect in children and even in some adults. When a child is diagnosed with ADHD, he or she may be given a drug to keep them under control. The most widely used drug is methylphenidate hydrochloride, or Ritalin – a powerful stimulant, especially to the central nervous system that usually takes effect in 30 minutes and peters out in three to four hours. The use of stimulant drugs such as Ritalin and amphetamines to treat ADHD began in the 1960s. (86)   Ritalin is classified as a Schedule II controlled substance in the same category as cocaine, methadone, and methamphetamine. (87)

Close to four million children in the U.S. are currently prescribed Ritalin. (88) The number of children taking Ritalin for ADHD has approximately doubled every four to seven years since 1971. It's estimated that its use quadrupled between 1990 and 1997, and the *New York Times* reported on January 18, 1999, that the production of Ritalin has increased 700 percent since 1990. Just how much Ritalin is going into our kids? In 1997 U.S children ingested more than 10 tons of Ritalin to control ADHD. (89,90) And the use of the drug is spreading to younger and younger children; in 1995 almost half a million prescriptions were written for children between ages three and six. (91)

The *percentage* of children with behavioral problems being prescribed the drug has increased also. In 1989, 55 percent of children diagnosed as ADHD left the doctor's office with a prescription for Ritalin, and in 1996, that percentage had climbed to 75 percent. Meanwhile, the number receiving psychotherapy fell from 40 percent in 1989 to 25 percent in 1996. Jeff Goodwin, a former pediatrician commented:

> It is easier for physicians to prescribe a drug and categorize a disorder as hyperactivity than it is to deal with the problem. Health services are being cut back, so you have doctors saying, "Take this and live happily ever after. "...The reason Ritalin use has gone up is that we are in an era when psychiatric services are devalued and therapy is not paid for by insurance companies. (92)

It's not just children who are on it. In 1997, between 6.5 million and 9 million adults in the U.S. had been diagnosed with ADHD, and about 730,000 of them were taking Ritalin by prescription. Most of these adults were children diagnosed with ADHD who have continued treatment.

In November 1998, *Time* magazine ran a feature story on Ritalin, which reported:

> For years Ritalin has been a godsend for children who were so hot-wired they were simply unreachable, and unteachable. In severe cases, the benefits of Ritalin (and the family of related drugs) on these children's ability to function and learn and cope are so direct that advocates say withholding the pills is a form of neglect... Some doctors find themselves battling anxious parents who, worried that their child will daydream his future away, demand the drug, and if refused, go off to find a more cooperative physician. Some parents feel pressured to medicate their child just so that his behavior will conform a bit more to other children's, even if they are quite content with their child's conduct – quirks, tantrums and all. (93)

"It's a fixed, stable, low-dose drug," according to Philip Berent, M.D., a consulting psychiatrist. He says that critics who claim diet, exercise or other treatments work just as well as Ritalin are kidding themselves. "The quickest way to end that criticism is to spend a week with a hyperactive child. We aren't talking about kids who ODed on Halloween candy." (94)

However, Lawrence Diller, M.D., author of *Running on Ritalin*, makes an interesting point. "What if Tom Sawyer or Huckleberry Finn were to walk into my office tomorrow? Tom's indifference to schooling and Huck's 'oppositional' behavior would surely have been cause for concern. Would I prescribe Ritalin for them too?" And the disorder is "surprisingly" ill-defined – no one is sure whether it's truly a neurochemical imbalance that can indeed be corrected with medicine, much the way insulin shots help diabetics.

"Let's not deny Ritalin works," said J. Zink, Ph.D., a Manhattan Beach, Calif., family therapist who has written several books on raising children and who lectures extensively around the country. "But why does it work, and what are the consequences of over prescribing? The reality is we don't know."

Scientists don't know why Ritalin seems to help kids with ADHD, but they have some clues: they know which parts of the brain are involved in impulse control and which chemicals in the brain respond to Ritalin. How these two pieces of the puzzle fit together, however, is still unclear. (95)

We do know that amphetamine drugs like Ritalin help the body to produce adrenaline, or they mimic its effects. Low adrenaline levels in children causes the same hyperactive symptoms of ADHD – restlessness, poor attention, and difficulty understanding and solving problems. Consequently, the child cannot filter out all the incoming stimuli to his or her nervous system, which results in excessive activity in the parts of the brain that regulate attention and sleep. If adrenaline is increased, the child will calm down. Ritalin relaxes these low-adrenaline children by helping them produce more adrenaline. (96)

The amount of adrenaline the body produces must be in specific amounts, neither too high nor too low. If too low, the child will have difficulty concentrating and be restless. If too high, the child may become hyperactive. Timothy Jones, M.D., of Yale University found that when children were given the sugar equivalent of two 12-ounce colas, their adrenaline levels were twice as high as adults given the same amount. He suggests that in increase in adrenaline could be why some children become hyperactive after eating sweets and recommends they not eat sweets on an empty stomach. (97)

Ritalin is what is referred to as a psychotropic (mood-altering) or psychostimulant drug. It is pharmacologically classified with amphetamines ("speed") and is very similar chemically to cocaine. In 1995 the Drug Enforcement Administration (DEA) published a report on the drug that said, "Methylphenidate (Ritalin) is a central nervous system (CNS) stimulant and shares many of the pharmacological effects of amphetamine, methamphetamine, and cocaine.... It produces behavioral, psychological, subjective, and reinforcing effects similar to those of d-amphetamine including increases in rating of euphoria..." (98)

Author Richard DeGrandpre in *Ritalin Nation,* quotes a 1995 report in the *Archives of General Psychiatry:* "Cocaine, which is one of the most reinforcing and addicting of the abused drugs, has pharmacological actions that are very similar to those of methylphenidate (Ritalin), which is now the most commonly prescribed psychotropic medicine for children in the U.S." (99) The American Psychiatric Association says that cocaine, amphetamines, and methylphenidate (Ritalin) are "neuropharmacologically alike," that abuse patterns are the same for the three drugs, and that people can't tell their clinical effects apart in laboratory tests. (100) Further, they can substitute for each other and cause similar behavior in addicted animals. The FDA classifies methylphenidate (Ritalin) in the high addiction category (Schedule II) which also includes amphetamines, morphine, opium, and barbiturates. (101) How many parents are told this before the prescription is written for their child?

In the 1980s, methylphenidate (Ritalin) was one of the most commonly used street drugs; youngsters sell their prescribed methylphenidate to classmates who take it for a "high." John Merrow, executive producer of a PBS documentary on ADHD, reported that Ritalin is so plentiful that a black market has developed on the school playground. Ritalin can be crushed and snorted for a cheap and modest buzz, and it has become a "gateway drug" in junior high school, frequently being the first drug a child experiments with. (102,103) The Drug Enforcement Administration reports that as early as 1994 Ritalin was the fastest-growing amphetamine being used "nonmedically" by high school seniors in Texas. DeGrandpre says that in 1991 there were about 25 emergency room visits of children ages 10 to 14 connected with Ritalin abuse. By 1995, the number had climbed to more than 400 visits – about the same number of visits as for cocaine. (104)

Richard DeGrandpre goes on to report that "lab animals given the choice to self-administer comparative doses of cocaine and Ritalin do not favor one over another... a similar study showed monkeys would work in the same fashion for Ritalin as they would for cocaine."

Newsweek, in 1995, reported that "The prescription drug Ritalin is now a popular high on campus..." In *Running on Ritalin,* Diller quotes several undercover narcotics agents who say that "Ritalin is cheaper and easier to purchase at playgrounds than on the street." The 1995 *Time* feature article says that, "more teenagers try Ritalin by grinding it up and snorting it for $5 a pill than get it by prescription." And many teenagers do not consider Ritalin to be anywhere near as dangerous as heroine or cocaine because they think that since their younger brother takes it by prescription, it must be safe. (105) They don't realize it is addictive.

Hallowell and Ratey, in *Driven to Distraction* say that, "people with ADD feel focused when they take cocaine, just as they do when they take Ritalin." (106)

Ritalin works on children the same way cocaine or related stimulants work on adults: It sharpens short-term attention span. This "peak" is followed by a "valley," when the child "rebounds", from its effects. (similar to, as they say on the streets, "coming down" off a drug). One mother comments about her daughter's "Ritalin rebound:" "She'd hold herself together all day, but the minute she got home she'd have this breakdown. You'd be asking the impossible to have my child come home, have a snack and do her homework right away..." (107)

Withdrawal symptoms can include inattention, hyperactivity, and aggression – the very things the drug is supposed to prevent – along with appetite suppression and insomnia (the drug adversely effects children the same way adults are affected by such drugs). (108)

That's why handbooks on ADHD given to parents advise them to see their doctor if they feel their child is losing too much weight, and why some children who take Ritalin are also prescribed sedatives to help them sleep. A catch-22.

Methylphenidate can cause permanent disfiguring tics and suppress growth (height and weight). Much of the brain's development takes place during the years in which children are given this drug, and thus the brain's size could be reduced. Although there have been no consistent brain abnormalities found in children with ADHD, one study found brain shrinkage in adults labeled ADHD who have been taking methylphenidate for years. The authors of this study suggest "cortical atrophy may be a long-term adverse effect of this [methylphenidate] treatment." (101) Michael F. Jacobson and David Schardt in *Diet, ADHD & Behavior; A Quarter-Century Review,* found that Ritalin causes liver cancer in mice (although not in rats). (109) The DEA also says:

> Most of the ADHD literature prepared for public consumption and available to parents does not address the abuse liability or actual abuse of methylphenidate. Instead, methylphenidate is routinely portrayed as a benign, mild stimulant that is not associated with abuse or serious effects. In reality, however, there is an abundance of scientific literature which indicates that methylphenidate shares the same abuse potential as other Schedule II stimulants... Abuse data indicate a growing problem among school-age children... ADHD adults have a high incidence of substance disorders, and that with three to five percent of today's youth being administered methylphenidate on a chronic basis, these issues are of great concern. (110)

Doctors do not always warn of these dangers. And they do not tell parents that there are almost guaranteed non-drug methods to improve the conduct of nearly all so-called ADHD children through more interesting and engaging schools and a more loving, attentive family, let alone changes to diet and physical health. Nor do they discuss what diagnosis and treatment might do to a child's self-esteem. Once labeled with ADHD, a child is viewed differently, and even normal behavior could be interpreted as problem behavior requiring drugging. This diagnosis can follow the child through his school years and even throughout life. Side effects (both short-term and long-term) of taking prescription drugs can wreak havoc on the child's mental as well as physical health.

Our children are not only getting attention disorders and learning disabilities, they're getting depressed too. It's estimated that 3.4 million Americans under 18 are said to be "seriously" depressed. In 1997, approximately 800,000 antidepressant prescriptions were written for drugs such as Prozac, Zoloft, and Paxil, for children, some as young as 5 years old. Many of these kids were also taking Ritalin – not surprisingly since depression can be a by-product of the drug and ADHD. Antidepressants can lead to agitation and nervousness in anyone, but in children they can trigger full-blown manic episodes. Doctors are not sure how these drugs affect a young, still elastic brain. (111)

It's interesting to note that healthy adults respond in the same way children do to these drugs (methylphenidate and other stimulants such as cocaine and amphetamines), regardless of whether they are diagnosed with ADHD or hyperactivity. Diller says that methylphenidate "potentially improves the performance of anyone – child or not, ADD-diagnosed or not." And, psychologist Ken Livingston says, "studies conducted during the mid-seventies to early eighties by Judith Rapaport of the National Institute of Mental Health... clearly showed that stimulant drugs improve the performance of most people, regardless of whether they have a diagnosis of ADHD, on tasks requiring good attention. Indeed, this probably explains the high levels of "self-medicating around the world" with "stimulants like caffeine and nicotine." (112)

Food for Thought

So what has taken place is this: A "disease" – ADHD – is "created" with such a nebulous, subjective, broad scope of symptoms that almost anyone can be diagnosed as having it – especially kids who are naturally full of energy and have short attention spans. Then, a drug is called upon that will "improve the performance of most people" (can't-miss prognosis!) to get the child into "compliance," settle down and not be a threat or bother to anyone. It's very clever, don't you think? So clever that more than 10 tons of Ritalin are ingested by kids all across the country every year. Just think of the profits! I think we're on to something!

How could such a potentially harmful substance be foisted upon our children with the consent and even encouragement of the parents? Here's something to consider:

In 1991, the U.S. Department of Education formally recognized ADHD as a handicap (under the Individuals with Disabilities Education Act and Section 504 of the 1973 Rehabilitation Act). The department then directed all state education officers to make sure that local school districts establish procedures to screen and identify ADHD children. Those children would then be given special educational and psychological services. New funding to the schools was then possible.

The U.S Department of Education told school superintendents that there are "three ways in which children labeled ADHD could qualify for special education services in public school under existing laws." In 1990, the Individuals with Disabilities Education Act mandated that... "Eligible children receive access to special education and/or related services, and that this education be designed to meet each child's unique educational needs" through an individualized program.

So, ADHD children are now entitled by law to a long list of services including separate special-education classrooms, learning specialists, special equipment, tailored homework assignments, social services, mental health care, speech therapy, counseling, and psychological services. So, it's in the interest of the school to have children with ADHD because it will get better funding for services they think are necessary in areas directly related to ADHD and also other areas not necessarily related to ADHD. And what school doesn't want more "free money"? (113)

Children are regularly tested by teachers for emotional, social, mental, and physical disorders (especially ADHD) inside public schools. As stated earlier, the diagnosis of ADHD can be made by a nonphysician. Once a child is diagnosed and labeled with ADHD, school health officials have the authority to treat them by prescribing and administering Ritalin (a Schedule II drug, remember). Other drugs that may be used are Valium, Lorazepam, and Prozac.

CHAAD (Children and Adults with Attention-Deficit/Hyperactivity Disorder), a nationwide ADHD support group, mounted a campaign in 1995 to have Ritalin changed from a Schedule II drug to a Schedule III drug, which would have made it far easier to obtain. CHADD considers itself the leading information center for ADHD. (In 1993, 35,000 families were members, with 600 chapters across the country.)

CHADD's petition to the DEA to reclassify Ritalin as a Schedule III drug was cosigned by the American Academy of Neurology and was supported by other distinguished medical bodies including the American Academy of Pediatrics, the American Psychological Association, and the American Academy of Child and Adolescent Psychiatry. However, it was uncovered that Novartis (then called Ciba-Geigy – the pharmaceutical giant that manufactures Ritalin) had contributed nearly $900,000 to CHADD over five years and that CHADD had failed to disclose this.

The DEA stated it had concerns over "the depth of the financial relationship between CHADD and Ciba-Geigy." They said that Ciba-Geigy "stands to benefit from a change in scheduling of methylphenidate." They expressed concerns over the use of methylphenidate and that nongovernmental organizations and that parental association in the U.S. were actively lobbying for the medical use of methylphenidate, not to mention that "Methylphenidate shares the same abuse potential as other Schedule II stimulants." When it learned of the DEA's concerns, CHADD withdrew its petition to decontrol Ritalin. (114)

Food for Thought

When an individual or organization with credentials says something, people tend to listen and believe. If a group like the American Academy of Pediatrics wanted Ritalin decontrolled, it's easy for someone not informed to take it for granted that they must know what they're talking about and that the substance is not that dangerous or harmful. But, as evidenced, there were perhaps other reasons these associations wanted it decontrolled – and an open checkbook could easily sway them to agree with their pharmaceutical friends.

Approximately 90 percent of Ritalin production is consumed in the United States. But not every nation sees it as a godsend. Sweden, for example, had methylphenidate withdrawn from the market back in 1968 after a number of abuse cases. And for good reason that country has not sought to reintroduce it in order to keep kids in line.

Alternative Ways of Treating ADHD

First, please realize that ADHD is a very loosely diagnosed problem. What one person may see as ADHD, another may not. Oftentimes the diagnoses is made simply so that an unruly but "normal" child can be silenced and easier to handle. Remember, children are bundles of energy, and their attention span is naturally short. But in our fast-paced, "both-parents-working-let's-put-the-child-in-day-care" world, it's easy to understand why parents don't have the patience with their little Tom Sawyer and why a more easily controlled child is an attractive alternative – even if drugged. But is a little peace and quiet now worth the possible nightmare later?

Food for Thought

It's a good thing that Ritalin wasn't around when I was a kid. I surely would have been put on it. I drove my mother crazy. Although I could sit quietly in a chair if I was given a reward, I ran around and never stopped until I worked myself into a state of near exhaustion. When I was about two or three, I would somehow unlock the front door early in the morning before

---

my parents were up and bolt out into the neighborhood with no clothes on whatsoever. I'd scoot around the neighborhood in my little push-pedal Chevy car going 100 kiddie miles and hour. My parents were awakened many times by the neighbor down the street knocking on the door with naked little Bobby in his arms. This was in Queens, New York, in the early 1960s. Try that today and see what happens. (I also remember going "Trick or Treating" with a friend when I was seven, all alone, past dark. In Queens! My, have things changed!)

The first thing a parent should do if a child is difficult to handle is to pay him more attention and give him as loving an atmosphere as possible. A prominent male figure is important. Ask the child questions, pay attention to him, take an interest. If at all possible, move the child into a school with smaller class sizes.

Improve the child's diet. Eliminate or minimize processed foods, foods with additives, coloring and foods containing sugar or "sugarlike" ingredients (i.e., high fructose corn syrup). Sugar was discussed in detail in the section on diabetes in this book and how it relates to mental health. Buy organic foods as much as possible since they are free of pesticides and their nutritional value is greater. Also, encourage your child to eat as much raw, uncooked food as possible.

Since our water supply is greatly compromised, either buy a good bottled water or get a water purification system. The fewer pollutants going into your little loved ones, the better their brains will be able to function.

Limit your child's exposure to television. Leonard Shalin, M.D., says that since TV is "image based" only, it puts the brain into an alpha brainwave pattern, fostering right-brain dominance, whereas reading a book requires the left brain's beta brainwave functioning. Shalin says that the detrimental influence of TV is from its passive influence as it precludes interactive neural stimulation. When a child is at play, this neural stimulation is present, and thus the brain develops as it should. (115)

Russell Barkley, author of *ADHD and the Nature of Self Control* says that ADHD is now considered a "developmental issue of self-control." Lack of impulse control is the inability to regulate the emotional energy flow which is required to focus. It causes an "act now, think later" behavior that results in increased emotional agitation and a feeling of being like a "cat on a hot tin roof" – agitated and restless. (116)

While Ritalin may control the symptoms of ADHD, it does nothing to change the underlying condition. That condition, no matter the cause, is one of lack of impulse control and the inability to focus – which leads to agitation and frustration.

Jeanette Farmer has an interesting perspective on ADHD and impulse control. She is a certified handwriting movement specialist, and contends that the lack of impulse control is in large part due to a lack of proper brain and neural development. She says that this can be corrected or avoided by teaching children correct penmanship – which helps develop the neural pathways that lead to learning and impulse control. Impulse control, reading, and learning are inextricably, linked, and they depend on the proper balanced development of the two hemispheres of the brain. (117)

The brain is divided into two hemispheres – left and right. Each has its own unique and specific function. The left hemisphere does what is called "hard thinking" and is mostly concerned with conscious awareness. It uses logic and reason, thinks in words, plans, is ordered, controlled, and structured and its focus is external and narrow. The right hemisphere does what is called "soft thinking" and is mostly concerned with unconscious awareness. It uses emotions, intuition and creativity, thinks in pictures, is spontaneous, is unstructured, has an internal focus, is holistic, diffuse, and unfocused (covering a wide area). Impulse control is tied to the emotionally influenced right brain, while the ability to focus and stay on task is tied to the left brain. Farmer says:

> The child is born in a natural right-brain state, a state primarily motivated by the intertwined factors of instant gratification and lack of impulse control. Normally, the child gradually matures out of that state by gaining some degree of impulse control, influencing a gradual shift in dominance to the left brain for the vast majority of the population. That is, when all goes well – but any number of environmental, nutritional, medical, educational, parental influences or conditions may preclude that normal and natural transition. Due to the increased stimulation in multi-sensory handwriting training, it can play a powerful role in aiding that transition. (118)

Handwriting with the right hand activates the left hemisphere (since the nerves from the body cross over to the opposite side of the brain) and stimulates the left hemisphere's language capacities. By activating and using the left hemisphere, it becomes increasingly less submissive and more dominant in the overall functioning of the brain. That is to say that as the left brain is used, the impulsiveness of the right brain is subdued. It is brought under control and the child or person can function more out of a "thinking" than "reacting" way. Leonard Shalin, M.D., in his book *The Alphabet versus the Goddess*, says that any form of writing influences left-brain dominance.

Farmer continues:

> Impulses are the essence of the emotional life force that drive behaviors. Learning to control impulses has profound implications for future success in life. No psychological skill is more valuable than the ability to resist impulses, the root of self-control. Lack of impulse control and instant gratification are linked. Research in 1960 nearly 40 years ago with four-year-olds and marshmallows deliver a telling message about impulse control as a predictor of future success.
>
> A group of four-year-olds were gathered around a table with some marshmallows on it. The researcher told them that he had to go do an errand and if they could wait until he got back they could have two marshmallows. If not, they could have one right then. This proved to be a dramatic telling test. These students were tracked

down when they graduated from high school. Those who could delay gratification and endure frustration were more socially competent, personally effective, self assertive and better able to cope with frustration of life. They could better direct their energies to achieve functional productivity. Moreover, it predicted a 210-point advantage in SAT scores some 17 years later. Clearly impulse control should be a major educational concern...

I have found that when the right brain dominant child is thrown into a left brain system and expected to perform using processing skill not yet in place, it immediately sets up stress and anxiety in trying to meet expectations. Stress has such a negative impact on the brain that it can easily shut down the learning process and the ability to lock information into the working memory... A neurophysiologist and well experience teacher, Hannaford believes that movement is essential for learning and thought... My personal experience leads me to believe that learning disabilities are made, not born. I believe it is learning styles and a dominance issue which should be rightly called "learning differently." While research clearly supports handwriting's role in helping establish dominance, failure to sufficiently stress the process is an underlying factor that has subtly influenced achieving the educational crisis... Obviously, if I can use handwriting, as a fine motor process, to "retrain the brain," (a shift in dominance pattern) then it must have the inherent capacity to "train the brain" (develop impulse control and cause a shift in dominance) in the first place... Fine motor control (as needed in writing) and emotional control are deeply intertwined - it capitalizes on the left brain-right hand connection... Intentional movement taps the unconscious (i.e., emotional) mind. As impulse control is an "act first and think later" factor, training the brain impacts behavior. It can't be gained by just wanting it, simply "trying harder" or by straining, willing it or coercing the mind to function. A specific game plan is necessary to develop that innate potential – it comes from repetitive actions that imprint the brain. (119)

Carla Hannaford, Ph.D., says that hemispheric dominance is an educational issue that is vastly ignored. In Hannaford's book *Smart Moves - Why Learning is Not All in Your Head* she contends that learning disabilities are a brain dominance issue. Hannaford says that "up to 80 percent of all American school children could be diagnosed as learning-disabled." She found that 78 percent of left-brain dominant children were considered "gifted and talented" while 78 percent of right-brain dominant children were in special education (dyslexia, learning disabled, etc.). This underscores the importance of activating the left hemisphere. Not only does the left hemisphere deal with concepts that are largely factual and logical (which would show up on test scores), but its activity and activation subdues the right hemisphere's tendency to be impulsive, disorderly and out of control. (120)

Food for Thought

Often creative people are seen as a little "loose in the head." The "absent- minded professor" types. These creative people are often not very well organized or neat and have a difficult time completing tasks. Hey – I can relate to that! (Although I've been called messy much more often than genius!) I contacted certified handwriting movement specialist Jeannette Farmer to see if her handwriting exercises could help adults, and if these symptoms had to do with a brain dominance imbalance. She told me that yes, by consistently activating the left hemisphere, the right hemisphere's impulsiveness can be subdued even in adults. She said that: "Adults with unremediated ADD create a number of life changing problems such as difficulties in maintaining long term relationships or even holding a job. Self-defeating behaviors require 'retraining the brain.' Current research finds that humans operate out of a 'comfort zone' by sheer habit and automatic responses over 90 percent of the time. Without changing automatic responses, it's as the old saying goes, 'if you continue to do what you've always done, you will get what you have always got.' To make positive behavioral changes, one must get out of that well established 'comfort zone.' Handwriting movement exercises provide a fast track to creating change by 'retraining the brain' due to increased neural stimulation, offering potential for new habits and responses."

Interesting, I thought. So I started to do the handwriting exercise she recommends in her manual *Training the Brain to Pay Attention the Write Way*. In this manual she also recommends doing the writing movements to music (which she supplies) with a beat of 60 beats per minute which also has the capacity to "entrain" the brain and make learning more efficient. Upon doing the exercise, I felt an immediate difference. I seemed to calm down, although I hadn't noticed I was anxious, and I felt more at peace. The rest of my day, when I do these exercises, is easier, flows more smoothly and I'm not as prone to getting upset.

Although I do not have ADHD, I did benefit from these exercises – but I must confess that I have had problems with neatness, organization and memory, all left-brain functions which are enhanced with these exercises. It's nice to know that adults with ADHD need not become victims of the drug trap. If they were to devote a few minutes a day to these exercises, I feel sure they would see improvements. The exercises are painless, cost nothing (other than the initial price of the manual and tape) and certainly do no harm. I figure it's worth a try. I personally have not seen the results of these exercise with children, but Farmer assures me that children who do them consistently not only make tremendous leaps in their learning abilities, but are calmer, more centered and have greater self-esteem. You can order the manual and tape by calling (303) 740-6161 or on line at www.retrainthe-brain.com.

The bottom line of all this is that perhaps one of the reasons so many children are fidgety and have learning and self control problems is that they are not practicing their writing! I know it sounds simple, but by activating the brain in the way that writing does, it most definitely changes not only its function, but also its physiology – that being it creates new neural pathways and actually can grow new neurons. When Albert Einstein died, researchers removed his brain and examined it to see if they could determine if there were any distinct differences in his brain compared to a person of normal intellect. What they found was that his brain was no larger than normal (it was even a little smaller), and it did not weigh more. But, it had an amazing number of "neural pathways" in it. There were lots more "connections" in Einstein's brain than a normal person's. Research has shown that these neural pathways develop as the brain is used. That is, the more you flex your noggin', the stronger it gets – and the smarter you are.

Experiments in rats bear this out too. A rat that is in a rich and diverse environment will develop more neurons than a rat in a sterile, boring environment. The less our children are encouraged to learn, the easier we make it for them, the lower the standards become – the dumber they will be. And the more impulsive they will be. As our school systems have become more lackadaisical, so has the insistence on good handwriting skills, and so has the intellect of our children declined and their impulsiveness increased.

Literacy in America

It's appropriate here to take a look at the literacy in America. Unfortunately, it's not an encouraging picture. In 20 years, from 1972 to 1992, the literacy rate in America fell from 13th worldwide to 49th. In 1992, according to government statistics: 2.5 million young adults graduated from high school with one million of them being functionally illiterate; 22 percent, or 42 million adults are functionally illiterate; only 5 percent of 17-year-olds can read at an advanced level; 57 percent of California's 4th graders, 58 percent of Hawaii's and 75 percent of Washington, D.C.'s read below basic grade level - and several other states were not far behind. Only 13 percent of today's 16- to 25-year-olds read at Level 4 or 5, the highest proficiency levels. During the 1990s, there's been a 30 percent increase in the need for special education services. (121)

Diane McGinnis, Ph.D., in her book, *Why Our Children Can't Read and What We Can Do About It*, points out that illiteracy correlates with school dropout rates. A large percentage of adolescent criminal offenders are functionally illiterate. She sums up her research by saying, "The truth provided by these statistics is that children's reading problems, and ultimately adults' reading problems, are caused by the school system, and not because there is something wrong with poor readers. It is impossible that 30 percent to 60 percent of all schoolchildren have an inherent or 'brain-based' deficit leading to reading failure." (122)

McGinnis's research identified four essential principles of successful reading. Neither the "whole language" approach or the "phonics" approach was based on any of these principles. Rather, she says "that when the sequence of reading and spelling instruction is compatible with the logic of the alphabet code and the child's linguistic and logical development, learning to read and spell proceeds rapidly and smoothly for all children and is equally effective for poor readers of all ages."

In short, the good old-fashioned way of learning to spell and read is the way that works best in the long run. It is the sequential, step-by-step processing style of this form of learning that activates the left hemisphere of the brain, forcing it to develop. As the left hemisphere develops, so does impulse control, since the right hemisphere's spontaneity is subdued.

Neuropsychologist R. Joseph suggests that repetition is the essence of learning. Children thrive on repetition since it promotes self-mastery, which is closely tied to developing the powers of self-control. He says that physiologically, repetitive movement hones the neural pathways, where nerve cells in a particular experience become more complex, more sensitive, and more easily activated. In short, repetition is necessary in learning. In fact, it's been determined that for a child to learn something new, it needs to be repeated an average of eight times. And, to unlearn an old behavior, and replace it with a new one, the action needs to be repeated an average of 28 times – 20 times to eliminate the old behavior and eight to learn the new one. Repetition ensures that an action becomes "habitual," and in so doing it requires less energy and can be performed with less effort. (123)

Repetitive exercises by-pass the "thinking" brain (the cortex) and influence the deeper levels of our emotional brain. The "conditioning process" stimulates neural pathways which in turn create new dendrites and synapses (i.e., nerve cells or neurons). Remember Einstein's brain - extremely rich in neurons and neural pathways. And repetitive movement allows a better balance between the "thinking" brain and "feeling" or emotional brain, which promotes the integration of the right and left hemisphere. This process is called sensory-motor integration. Repetitive movements, like those in Jeanette Farmer's writing manual, stabilize and regulate the emotional energy flow, and the dynamics of emotional release, while honing the neural pathways.

Handwriting has the power to tap the emotions. James Pennebaker, M.D., did research at SMU which found that just 20 minutes a day for one week spent writing to ventilate emotional issues produced a measurable influence on the immune system. And rhythmic movement gives us a sense of well being. (124)

Multi-sensory experiences greatly enrich the learning process. By combining music with movement, more of the brain is stimulated and the brain functions in a more balanced and powerful way.

Sound in itself can have a dramatic effect on us. Alfred Tomatis, a French physician, has done pioneering research on sound and the human body. He found that hearing and touch are closely related and that every neural process passes through or relates to the nucleus of the inner-ear cochlea's system as the principle congregating point for all our senses. He contends that every cell in our body registers sound (it "feels" the sound) and passes the information on to higher centers for processing. (No wonder people like to dance!)

Don Campbell of the Mozart Effect Resource Center says that music impacts the mind, body, and spirit simultaneously. Heart patients derive the same benefits from listening to 30 minutes of classical music as they did from taking Valium. The right music can lower heart rate and blood pressure because the heart tends to speed up and slow down to match the pace of the music. (125) No wonder "rock & roll" can incite riots!

Food for Thought

Since sound and touch are closely linked – that is, sound has an actual physical impact – extremes of loud rock music could be sought after just as much if not more for this physical-impact stimulation than for the music itself. In our "touch-starved" society, could this be why loud, raucous music is so popular among children and teenagers? It's a substitute for the touch they didn't get at day care or because mom and dad were too busy working or they were put in a plastic carrier as babies because it was more convenient.

The rhythm of the music can alter brainwaves and breathing patterns. And, music can affect intelligence and productivity. Students who listened to 10 minutes of Mozart prior to taking SATs generally scored higher than those students who were not exposed to the music.

Rhythm and movement stimulate the frontal lobes of the brain and enrich language and motor development. Young children especially need this stimulation that movement and rhythm provide to establish a pattern of recognition for learning in the future. Exercise along with calm music can do wonders for children who have emotional problems and learning disabilities. As these movements are repeated, the brain creates new neural pathways and the child's mind improves. As this occurs, the left and right hemisphere's activities become more balanced and the child learns, at the root level, self-control. And, since the movements and music will calm the child, their stress level goes down.

High stress levels tend to impair reason and logical thinking. As reason and logic are reduced, so are the choices a person can make confronting a given situation. One who cannot think clearly cannot see the solution, or the choice of taking a specific action, which could logically lead to a solution. Thus, as choices decrease, the level of functioning the brain uses goes down to the lower levels – more along the lines of the "fight or flight" reaction. As a person thinks on this lower level of awareness, the chances of a reactive, aggressive reaction increases.

Simply put, as stress increases (i.e., environmental or physiological), judgment, reason, and choice are reduced, leading to reactive, possibly aggressive behavior.

Cheryl Beckett, Ph.D., in her book *Growing Up Inside Out*, reveals that children's stress levels (in elementary and junior high school) were found to be as high as those for top executives. Stress overload is a major problem for those with ADHD. They struggle to cope with educational demands that require specific information processing which is not yet in place - possibly because they were not forced to learn to write and read correctly. That is because their brains were not nurtured and exercised to develop the neural pathways necessary for the kind of learning that is now expected of them at a higher level. (126)

The child then gets anxious, feels like he is "dumb and stupid," with a resultant increase in stress and anxiety. As this stress level increases, the child is more likely to rebel and be aggressive because they are now operating not out of reason, logic, and impulse control, but from an imbalance, right-brain dominated, "fight or flight" mode. Try as he might, the learning just won't sink in simply because the brain is not trained to process the information yet.

So he is labeled ADHD or learning disabled. And if he finds out he has such a label, he get even more stressed out because now he is "different." More stress leads to more reaction without thinking. Another vicious cycle.

Further suggestions to help a child (or adult) to handle and even diminish their ADHD, learning disability or aggressive nature are to encourage learning to write and read the old-fashioned way – and perhaps with the help of Jeanette Farmer's writing programs. At first this may be difficult because the child's attention span is so short. But as that child practices, neural pathways are developing and the right hemisphere's impulsiveness is being subdued, thus making it easier the next time. If the movements or exercise are done to slow music, classical perhaps, this further encourages neural development and self-control.

ADHD and other similar disabilities are fairly recent phenomena in our society and ones that indicate a system that has gone awry. A growing number of children are being affected, and this trend will only continue unless things change. Drugging them with Ritalin and other phamaceuticals is not the answer and in the long run only compounds the problems. A return to the basics is needed to allow the mind and body to function as nature intended. Clean, nutritious foods, and a clean, nurturing environment will allow future generations to eliminate these disabilities and allow children and adults alike to learn and act normally.

CHAPTER VII
Birth Defects

A birth defect can be defined as "an abnormality of structure, function or body metabolism (inborn error of body chemistry) present at birth that results in physical or mental disability, or is fatal." (1) Simply put, a birth defect is a "congenital malformation."

There are more than 4,000 known birth defects, and they are the leading cause of infant mortality in the U.S., accounting for more than 20 percent of all infant deaths. Of the 120,000 babies born each year with a birth defect, 8,000 die during their first year of life. In addition, birth defects contribute substantially to childhood morbidity and long-term disability. (2)

Although birth defects can be caused by genetic and environmental factors, it's estimated that the causes of approximately 60 percent to 70 percent of birth defects remain unknown.

The National Research Council of the National Academies reports:

> Approximately half of all pregnancies in the United States result in prenatal or postnatal death or an otherwise less than healthy baby. And major developmental defects, such as neural tube and heart deformities, occur in approximately 120,000 of the 4 million infants born here each year. Exposure to toxic chemicals, both manufactured and natural, cause about 3 percent of all developmental defects, and at least 25 percent might be the result of a combination of genetic and environmental factors. (3)

Birth defects arising from genetic causes are dependent on random variability – that is, plain old luck. (Except in instances where a mother or father has a birth defect passed on to the child. In these cases the likelihood of an offspring having a birth defect is higher.) So the percentage of birth defects caused by genetic problems should, everything else remaining equal, be about the same over generations. Given that fact, the percentages of birth defects in our population should be remaining stable. Is this happening?

Let's take a look at the National Vital Statistics reports. In 1900, there were 12.0 deaths per 100,000 live births due to congenital deformities. By 1948, the number was 13.2. But in 1997, there were 159.2 deaths per 100,000 live births. (4,5) This is over a hundred fold increase. Is this reasonable, or is something else besides genetics causing an increase in birth defects?

These statistics can be helpful, but having read this far, you should realize that there are many reasons to suspect them. For one, the reporting of birth defects over the years is less than consistent. Surveillance methods have improved since the 1960s, spurred by the serious and widespread birth defects because of the drug thalidomide given to pregnant mothers (which caused babies to be born with flippers instead of arms and legs). So the numbers have tended to go up simply because they are being reported better. Also, prenatal care has improved over the years resulting in more live births and therefore more potentially "imperfect" (rather than merely dead) babies. I could understand a slight to moderate increase in reported birth defect deaths because of these factors, but a hundredfold increase? My contention is that something other than genetics is causing this increase.

And more recent data shows a similar trend. The Centers for Disease Control started the Birth Defects Monitoring Program (BDMP) in 1973 to monitor birth defects as an early warning system of an emerging birth defects problem and to correlate the occurrences of birth defects with possible human teratogens. A teratogen (from the Greek words meaning, "monster producing") is anything that causes birth defects. From 1979 to 1987, the BDMP showed of the 38 types of birth defects monitored, 29 increased, two decreased and seven remained stable (less than 2 percent change per year). Some of the increases were dramatic – one doubled during this period, and another was estimated to be doubling every 14 years. The BDMP was discontinued during the mid-1990s and was eventually replaced by a new program comprising eight Centers for Birth Defects Research and Prevention (CBDRP). [6]

Food for Thought

I remember in my college genetics class, we did an exercise to determine if the actions the Nazis took on the Jews during the Holocaust would have a significant impact on the gene pool (the genetics of a whole population), and if those mass murders would ultimately get rid of or significantly decrease the genes of Jews in the overall population of the world (as the Nazis were intending). What we discovered was that even with this mass killing-off of the Jewish population, it was not significant in changing the gene pool, and even if the numbers were increased to the point of absurdity, the genetic pool would basically remain the same.

My point is this: under normal conditions, a change in the gene pool of a population takes thousands, if not millions of years. The alarming rate of birth defects in the last 50 years or so is not because of genetic probability or variability – it's because of a drastic and dramatic degeneration of the human organism which make it more susceptible to abnormal defects. This degeneration, since genetics don't change that quickly, must then be due to mostly environmental factors.

Although changes in human genetics cannot account for the dramatic increase in birth defects in recent years, inheritance of birth defects can certainly occur. The likelihood of a parent with a birth defect having a child with a birth defect is greater than for parents with no birth defects. A study published in *The New England Journal of Medicine* found "...a definite tendency for women with birth defects to also have children with birth defects." The study also found that women with birth defects were less likely to survive to adulthood, and if they did reach adulthood, they were less likely than other women to bear children. (7) Another study reported in the *Journal of the American Medical Association* showed that offspring of men with birth defects are twice as likely to have defects too. Allen J. Wilcox, M.D., Ph.D., co-author of the study, said, "What surprised us is that the children of the affected fathers had a higher risk of all kinds of defects, not just the same defect as their father." In the study, boys with birth defects had a lower-than-normal survival rate to age 20. Even if they survived to adulthood, they were 30 percent less likely to be able to father a child than other men. (8)

Food for Thought

The two studies just cited clearly show that birth defects can increase through the generations and that offspring of parents with birth defects are less likely to survive and reproduce themselves. This is most significant. In these cases what is happening is that there is a degeneration of the organisms from one generation to the next – so much so that they may not be able to reproduce. I suspect that if this study were to be continued into the third generation, we would see a further decline in reproductive capability to the point of near extinction. This, taken with the fact that birth defects are increasing in the population in general, paints a less than cheery picture. If the occurrence of birth defects continues to increase and the inability for people with birth defects to have babies (in this or subsequent generations) is true, in a short time, having to use birth control could be a thing of the past!

Birth defects will continue to increase, mainly because of the increased prevalence of teratogens. There are more than 500 new chemicals introduced into commercial use each year, added to the more than 75,000 chemicals already in commercial use. We tend to believe these chemicals are "innocent until proven guilty," so a chemical will be used until significant damage is shown to have occurred. That, along with the fact that there's not enough time or money to test all these chemicals for toxicity and teratogenicity, makes our world a very hazardous place.

Besides chemicals, the environmental agents that could potentially cause birth defects are many: heavy metals such as mercury; lead; cadmium; X-rays; pesticides such as DDT; alcohol; tobacco; recreational drugs; poor nutrition; and pharmaceutical drugs such as thalidomide. (9)

Many of these agents have already been discussed. But a special mention of thalidomide is in order here since it is a known teratogen and, according to a recent survey, two thirds of people of childbearing age are not familiar with it – a shocking fact given the tragic and widely publicized results of its use in generations past. Considering that the FDA gave approval in 1998 for thalidomide to be marketed in the U.S. again, it's very important women know about it and understand its risks.

Thalidomide was first used in the late 1950s as a sleeping pill and to treat morning sickness during pregnancy. Of course, no one knew it caused birth defects. But in 1961 scientists discovered that the medication stunted the growth of fetal arms and legs. Taking only one dose of thalidomide early in pregnancy can severely affect the growth of fetal limbs (arms, legs, hands, feet) causing them to look like flippers instead of arms or legs (Figure 5). It wasn't until more than 10,000 children around the world were born with these major malformations that it was withdrawn from the market in the early 1960s. (10)

Figure 5

The dangers of thalidomide – what a baby may look like if his mother takes this medication during pregnancy.

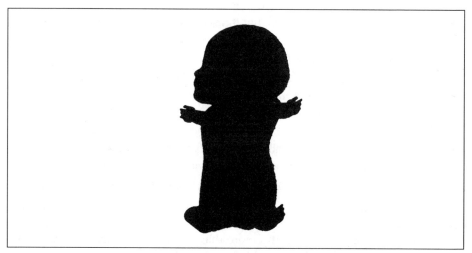

The recent FDA approval of the drug is for the treatment of a complication of leprosy, a disfiguring skin disorder involving loss of feeling that can lead to paralysis. This disease affects only a few thousand people in the U.S. – but even so, thalidomide has been approved, giving physicians the ability to prescribe it for many more people with other conditions. That includes women of childbearing age. It's extremely important young women realize the dangers of this drug.

The FDA, recognizing the potential dangers of thalidomide, has taken special safeguards never before imposed with any drug. This underscores how bad it can be. Only physicians who are registered may prescribe thalidomide to patients, and those patients – both male and female – must comply with mandatory contraceptive measures, patient registration and patient surveys. That's all well and good, but the chances of someone misusing it or going off their contraceptives is there. My advice is to leave it alone all together. You can heal yourself in other ways.

You may be wondering if you can take measures to prevent birth defects. Naturally, following a wholesome lifestyle will go a long way in this regard. But there is one specific nutrient that should be mentioned here because of its importance in preventing a common form of birth defect called neural tube defect (NTD).

The neural tube is the embryonic structure that develops into the brain and spinal cord. It starts out as a tiny ribbon of tissue that normally folds inward to form a tube by the 28th day after conception. When this doesn't happen correctly and the neural tube does not close completely, defects in the brain and spinal cord can result. In the U.S., about 2,500 babies are born with NTDs each year, and many other affected pregnancies end in miscarriage or stillbirth. (11)

The most common NTDs are spina bifida and anencephaly. Spina bifida (open spine), affects the backbone and sometimes the spinal cord. Children with severe spina bifida have some degree of leg paralysis and bladder and bowel control problems. Anencephaly is a fatal condition in which a baby is born with a severely underdeveloped brain and skull. Women with diabetes or epilepsy are at increased risk of having a baby with an NTD and should consult their physician prior to pregnancy.

A certain B vitamin called folic acid, or folate, has been shown to greatly reduce the risk of a woman having a baby with an NTD. (Other studies also suggest folic acid may help prevent cleft lip and palate malformations.) The U.S. Public Health Service, March of Dimes, CDC, and the Institute of Medicine all recommend that all women of childbearing age get at least 400 micrograms (or 0.4 mg) of folic acid every day – and no more than 1,000 micrograms per day. An adequate folate intake could prevent up to 70 percent of these types of birth defects. Women must realize that they need folic acid even before they get pregnant because by the time they realize they are pregnant, much of the neural tube formation has already occurred. (12)

Women can take a vitamin with folic acid in it to be sure they get enough. This is recommended just to be safe, considering that the body more readily absorbs folic acid from vitamin supplements than from food. But there are many foods that have healthy amounts of folate: orange juice and other citrus fruits and juices; leafy green vegetables; beans; broccoli; asparagus; peas; lentils; and whole grain products. Synthetic folic acid is added to certain grain products including flour, rice, pasta, cornmeal, bread, and cereals.

Considering about half of all pregnancies are not planned, it's wise for women to make sure they're getting enough folic acid every day. It could prevent a lifetime of misery. Taking this a step further, women of childbearing age should strive to lead as healthy a lifestyle as possible. Avoid smoking, drinking, street drugs, medications and over-the-counter medicines for starters. Eat as clean a diet as possible. This ideally goes for the father too. Healthy parents give rise to healthy children. Like begets like – a simple law of nature. Although the chance of having a child with a birth defect is always there just because of plain old luck, that chance can be reduced to virtually nonexistent if the parents are healthy and have healthy and vital eggs and sperm.

The Truth About Children's Health

CHAPTER VIII
Infertility

Although fertility may not seem to directly impact children, the ramifications of the growing fertility problem in the United States do affect the yet-to-be-born child. With fertility problems on the rise, we have reason for concern – protecting our children assumes that there are children to protect. If things continue to degenerate, there soon may not be.

"Infertility is defined as the inability to conceive a child despite trying for one year. The condition affects about 5.3 million Americans, or 9 percent of the reproductive age population [anyone of reproductive age]," according to the American Society for Reproductive Medicine. (1)

A report from the National Center for Health Statistics says the percentage of infertile *couples* in 1995 was 18.5 percent, compared with 14.4 percent in 1965. (2) Dr. Marc Goldstein, director of the Center for Male Reproductive Medicine at New York Hospitals, said, "Infertility is definitely going up. I see it in my practice. There is a decline in fertility in men and an increase in infertility in older couples. Studies show an increase in infertility from 11 percent to 16 percent in all married couples." He believes the cause to stem in part from lifestyles that include alcohol, marijuana, and cocaine. (3)

Interestingly, there also have been numerous reports of reproductive problems in wildlife, which doesn't use drugs or alcohol. Some believe the problems are due to the presence of chlorinated chemicals that are now ubiquitous in our environment and tend to mimic estrogen. Others believe they are happening because many industrial pollutants mimic hormones, thus upsetting the delicate reproductive system. Dioxin is a chlorinated chemical that does not mimic hormones, yet Earl Gray, a senior research biologist with the EPA, testified before Congress in 1993 that, "Our studies (in rats) show that a single dose of dioxin administered during pregnancy permanently reduces sperm counts in the male [offspring in adulthood] by about 60 percent." (4) Another effect of estrogen-mimicking chemicals is that they appear to cause girls to enter puberty sooner, developing breasts and pubic hair before the age of eight – for some at as young as three years of age. (5) The authors of this study said that PCBs and DDE (a breakdown product of the pesticide DDT) may indeed be associated with early sexual development in girls.

Infertility can be due to a problem with the man, women or both. It's estimated that 40 percent of couple infertility is due to the male. Not only does a lower sperm count increase the chances of having difficulty conceiving, it also increases the risk of miscarriages and birth defects.

In 1938, one half of 1 percent (that's one man in 200) of men were functionally sterile. Today, it's between 8 percent to 12 percent (between eight and 12 men in one hundred). (6) ("Functionally sterile" is defined as a sperm count below 20 million per milliliter of semen.) The expected sperm count of a man born in Paris in 1945 was 102 million, whereas in 1962 it was exactly half that. Pierre Jouannet, a French researcher, projects a further decline in the future. He said in 1996, "It will take 70 or 80 years before it (sperm count) goes to zero." (7) (Again, difficulty in conceiving occurs at sperm counts of 20 million or less, and sterility at five million. So effective species infertility would occur sooner than the 70 or 80 years projected for '0' sperm counts.) Not only are sperm counts going down, but cancer of the testicles has increased over threefold from 1940 to 1980. (8)

The important observation here is that infertility is increasing and increasing significantly. As I already mentioned, one estimate is that by the year 2020, people living in industrialized countries will not be able to reproduce - we will be infertile. Considering the above estimate, it may take until 2070. Still, a chilling thought.

The odds of having a miscarriage or child with birth defects rise dramatically when fathers have lower sperm counts. In a study at the University of Arkansas, it was determined that when the fathers' sperm counts were above 80 million/ml, they had only a 1 percent birth defect rate, compared with 6 percent for the general population. Miscarriages were also lower for the fathers with higher sperm counts (6 percent compared with 12 percent for the general population). (9)

Another study, in Sweden, reported in the *International Journal of Fertility*, found that married women experiencing miscarriages typically had husbands with lower sperm counts. In those men, on the average, 48 percent of their sperm appeared "abnormal" (i.e., two heads, two tails, etc.). Men who fathered normal pregnancies had a 25 percent higher sperm count and only 5 percent visually abnormal sperm. (10)

In a study on sperm counts and testicle abnormalities at the University of Copenhagen, Denmark, the researchers concluded that: "Recent data clearly indicate that the semen quality has markedly decreased during the period 1938 - 1990, and concomitantly the incidence of some genitourinary abnormalities including hypospadias [an abnormality of the male urinary opening], [testicle] maldescent, and cancer has increased. Such a remarkable increment in the occurrence of gonadal abnormalities over a relatively short period of time is more likely to be due to environmental rather than genetic factors. Generally, it is believed that pollution, smoking, alcohol... play a role." (11)

The British Medical Journal analyzed 61 previous sperm studies conducted in 20 countries. The report concluded that the average sperm counts had declined from 113 million sperm per milliliter of semen to 66 million during the past 50 years (from 1940 to 1990) – a 42 percent decline. (12) Remember, a man's fertility becomes questionable when sperm counts get down to 20 million sperm per milliliter. When the count drops to 5 million, he is considered sterile. One reference made note that the number of normally shaped sperm produced by the average man has dropped below the level of that of a hamster, which has testicles a fraction the size of a man's. (13) As early as 1981 sperm banks in the U.S. were having difficulty acquiring good-quality sperm. If the decline continued at the same rate sperm banks would soon start having great difficulty finding sperm donors whose sperm met the recommended standards. Similar observations about declining sperm quality have been noted in Denmark. (14)

It requires between 65 and 74 days for the male to make the sperm that will get his partner pregnant. Any exposure to toxins during this time can impact the health of the sperm and thus the eventual fetus and baby. Men exposed to toxic chemicals on the job or at home for two months prior to their partner's conceiving have a greater likelihood of their child's being born with health disorders including learning and behavior problems. (15)

A common misunderstanding of the process involved in producing sperm (spermatogenesis) is that the male manufactures millions of sperm daily, and that those are the sperm ejaculated that same day during sex. However, since it takes over two months to "build" a sperm from start to finish in the testicle, that is not the case. It follows that the environment it is created in determines whether it's normal or abnormal. Therefore, "all chemical exposures experienced by the man (from alcohol to pesticides) have the ability to weaken or damage this process, thereby resulting in offspring of lowered genetic potential." (16)

Food for Thought

A lower sperm count means increased chances of infertility and miscarriages and less healthy babies. Less healthy babies lead to less healthy children. The less healthy a child is, the less content he or she is. The less content, the more prone to violence, behavior problems, and substance abuse later in life. The less healthy a child, the more likely he or she will be learning-impaired, hyperactive,and unmanageable. My point is that some of the problems we are experiencing with today's children can be traced back to conditions present even before they were conceived. It's not just the environment the fetus experiences that in large part determines the state of health of the baby, but it's the state of health of the sperm and the egg that play a large part too. If you are of reproductive age, that is vitally important to realize because the health of your future baby in large part depends upon the health of your sperm or egg which depends on the health of *YOU*.

To return to the subject of alcohol for a moment, a study at the University of Michigan showed that fathers who drank an average of two drinks a day had babies that weighed more than one third of a pound less than babies whose fathers were only "occasional" drinkers – independent of the mother's alcohol, tobacco, or marijuana use during pregnancy. (17)

At the Institute of Sterility in Vienna, Austria, physicians compared 103 consecutive couples who had sought artificial insemination with donor sperm to 103 consecutive couples who had sought help due to female fertility problems. It was found that the men in these couples who worked in the agriculture industry were more than 10 times more likely to be infertile. They noted in this study that:

What was particularly noteworthy was that the concentrations of

Infertility   179 some environmental toxins were generally clearly higher in those semen specimens which did not lead to fertilization as opposed to those specimens from which a pregnancy resulted. [This study] has unequivocally confirmed this observation, the number of farmers being remarkably higher in the group seeking AID (Artificial Insemination with Donor Sperm) than in the control group within the same time period. This conspicuously high prevalence can probably be explained by the increased exposure to chemical sprays... These toxic chemicals probably have a detrimental effect on male fertility and therefore we suggest more caution in the way they are handled. [18]

Studies in rats in Japan tested the effects that the pesticide DBCP (dibromochloropropane) and some chemically similar industrial chemicals had on fertility and sperm morphology (structure). The results showed drastic reductions in sperm counts in exposed rats compared with unexposed rats. Many sperm in the pesticide-exposed rats were missing a tail (865 per 1000), which helps explain the infertility from these chemicals. [19] No tail, no travel.

It's not too surprising that pesticides or chemicals could directly cause male infertility, but its also been shown that the way the food itself is grown could be a factor. At the Royal Free Hospital School of Medicine in London, groups of rats were fed either a diet of totally organically raised food, food grown with chemical fertilizers or food grown with some chemical fertilizers and some manure. Of the rats fed the chemically grown food, only 11 percent had normal testicular structures. Forty-eight percent had normal structure when fed the food raised with chemicals/manure or with nothing but manure. The researchers noted that "reproductive performance was a sensitive indicator of differences between diets which had hardly shown significant differences in comparative growth tests." [20]

Essentially what they are saying is that the reproductive system is more vulnerable and more sensitive to harmful effects from chemicals than other systems in the body. Most previous studies on pesticides determine only whether lab animals die after exposure. Clearly, more research is needed to examine what effects might be realized at more subtle levels – reproductive, neurological, and immunological.

Another point to consider is that food grown organically has been shown to have higher levels of trace minerals than foods grown commercially. Organic farmers often use fertilizers such as rock powders, compost, and marine byproduct fertilizers that have higher mineral content than commercial chemical fertilizers. Chemical fertilizers typically have only nitrogen, phosphorous, and potassium (as in 10-10-10 fertilizer) and maybe five to 10 core minerals. But medical experts are now realizing the importance of "trace minerals" (such as selenium, boron, chromium, etc.) in maintaining health. Therefore it is highly recommended that couples wishing to have children consume mostly if not all organically raised foods.

Food for Thought

Consuming nothing but organically raised food is actually a good thing to do for anybody. If you were truly concerned with your own health and the health of your children, that's what you'd do. Sorry if this makes you feel guilty, but there's really no denying the research and your common sense. Which do YOU think is better – food raised naturally in harmony with nature, or food treated with harmful chemicals and pesticides born out of chemical warfare? If you think this is a radical suggestion, here's another: I believe that the chemical fertilizer plants and the pesticide plants should be totally dismantled and outlawed. I know it would take some time and effort and money to adjust. But remember back in the 1930s, the government had all these WPA projects it funded to help get the nation working again and out of the depression? Why couldn't our government institute a project to help farmers switch from chemicals to natural fertilizers – from chemical pesticides to natural pest deterrents? I don't know – call me optimistic. It could be done. And you know what? If it were, America would raise future generations of super-kids and super-people. Not to mention the improved health and well being of people living now. It all starts with a strong foundation. Good food = sound minds and sound bodies = good societies.

Other environmental factors also affect sperm counts. Marilyn F. Vine, Ph.D., at the University of North Carolina reported that men who smoke had sperm counts on the average of 13 percent to 17 percent lower than nonsmokers. Three of the men in this study who smoked and then quit were found to have an increase in sperm counts from 50 percent to 800 percent. The article suggested that the toxic chemicals in the smoke are responsible for the decreased sperm counts and that by quitting the reduction in sperm count is reversible. (21) It's also not surprising that smokers have more abnormal sperm. "Male smokers have an increase in sperm abnormalities, thereby suggesting a mutagenic effect." (22) A chemical found in marijuana (THC) has been found to be directly toxic to the developing egg. (23)

The research has shown that sperm counts have decreased and infertility has increased markedly since 1940. There are a couple of reasons cited in the literature that, among others, stand out as being most significant. One is that cigarette consumption in the U.S. has increased three-to-four fold from 1940 to the early 1980s. Another is that the agricultural industry switched from natural growing methods to chemical fertilizers and pesticides in the early 1960s.

As for other chemical exposures, consider that painters are more likely to father children with defects of the central nervous system. Men who work in the aircraft industry or handle paints or chemical solvents have a higher risk of producing children with brain tumors. Paternal exposure to paints has been linked to childhood leukemias. Firemen appear to have an unusually high number of abnormal sperm and are less fertile, probably because of the toxic smoke they are exposed to (from burning carpets, paint, etc.) Dental workers (i.e., dentists and dental assistants) are more prone to spontaneous abortions, stillbirths, and congenital defects. Animal studies suggest that paternal (father) exposure to recreational drugs and industrial chemicals can contribute to problems such as miscarriage, stillbirths, and diminished aptitude for learning in the offspring. (24)

When it comes to conceiving and giving birth to a healthy child, the environment can be a determining factor in success or failure, health or disease. In fact, Wolfram Notten, Ph.D., of the University of Wisconsin, says that "20 percent of all cases where the male is the only contributing factor to infertility can be corrected by lifestyle." (25)

Although we have focused on men to this point, women are also vulnerable to environmental stresses and toxins when it comes to infertility and reproductive problems. The most common female factor to contribute to infertility is ovulation disorders. Without ovulation, the eggs are not available for fertilization. Problems with ovulation are often signaled by irregular menstrual periods or lack of periods altogether (called amenorrhea). Stress, diet, and athletic training can affect a woman's hormonal balance, which in turn affects her ovulation. And blockages of the fallopian tubes also can cause infertility.

Oftentimes, fertility drugs are prescribed to women to increase ovulation. Eighty to 90 percent of infertility cases are treated with drugs or surgery. But using those drugs does not come without risks. Multiple births occur in 10 percent to 20 percent of births resulting from fertility drug use. (26) And it's believed that fertility treatments may have a direct effect on the development of ovarian cancer due to the raised concentrations of estrogens and persistent stimulation of the ovary by the drugs. (27)

In one study, John A. Collins, M.D., found that fertility treatments result in only a 6 percent improvement in achieving pregnancy over "infertile" couples who just "kept trying." In a second study, Collins tracked the pregnancy rates of 2,000 couples; rates between the treated couples and the nontreated couples were the same. Why are treatments so staunchly advocated? Infertility treatments are a $1 billion-a-year industry. (28)

The dietary habits of the mother can play a big part in whether she gets pregnant and has a healthy child. And here's where caffeine comes in again. In a 1988 study by Allen Wilcox of the National Institute of Environmental Health Sciences in North Carolina, it was found that women who drank just one cup of regular coffee a day were half as likely to become pregnant. (29) Most other studies had this at three or more cups a day. At Johns Hopkins University a study showed that women who consumed more than 300 milligrams of caffeine a day reduced their chances of pregnancy by 17 percent in any given month. A more recent study at Yale University school of Medicine stated that the risk of not conceiving for 12 months (the usual definition of infertility), was 55 percent higher for women drinking one cup of coffee a day, 100 percent higher when they drank one and a half to three cups, and 176 percent higher for women drinking more than three cups of coffee per day. (30) Mark Klebanoff of the National Institute of Child Health and Human Development says "it's probably prudent for women who are trying to become pregnant, and especially for those having trouble, to cut back on caffeine." (31)

Coffee drinking before and during pregnancy has been associated with more than twice the risk of miscarriage when the mother drank two to three cups per day. Smoking is another impediment to conception. It's been shown that women who smoke have less chance of getting pregnant by about 10 percent. Smokers are three to four times more likely than nonsmokers to have taken greater than a year to conceive. (32)

MSG was found to cause infertility problems in test animals. (33) Other food additives such as dyes and flavorings have also been implicated in fertility problems as well as some cosmetic chemicals.

The effects of alcohol will be discussed at some length in the chapter on pregnancy, but as far as its effect on fertility, a study at the Washington University School of Medicine showed that there was a 50 percent reduction in conception in test animals after "intoxicating" doses of alcohol were given 24 hours prior to mating. The *Harvard Health Letter* reported in October 1992 that in the ancient cities of Carthage and Sparta, there were laws prohibiting the use of alcohol by newlyweds, due to the belief that a child conceived by intoxicated parents would be unhealthy. (34)

The effects of chemicals on fertility and miscarriages can be profound. Women who are consistently exposed to chemical solvents (including xylene, acetone, trichlorethylene, petroleum distillates, and others) have a more than four-fold increase in spontaneous abortions. (35) It was reported in *Time* magazine that pregnant mothers exposed to two solvent chemicals had a 33 percent miscarriage rate. (The normal miscarriage rate is 15 percent.) (36)

Birth defects occurred almost three times more often in nurse-anesthetists (nurses who help with anesthesia preparation). As far back as 1860, it was observed that wives of men who worked with lead were less likely to become pregnant, and if they did, they were more prone to miscarrying. Boguslaw Baranski, M.D., of the Institute of Occupational Medicine in Denmark has observed that "Risk of infertility increased in females who reported exposures to textile dyes, dry cleaning chemicals... lead, mercury and cadmium. There was a significant risk of increased time to conception among women exposed to anti-rust agents, welding, plastic manufacturing, lead, mercury, cadmium or anesthetic agents." As far as men are concerned, Baranski says, "There was also an increased risk of delay to conception following male exposure to textile dyes, plastic manufacturing, and welding. Those who unpacked or handled antibiotics had a significant association with delayed pregnancy of at least 12 months." (37)

Miscarriage risks after exposure to the following chemicals was: 4.7 times greater for perchlorethylene (from dry cleaning); 3.1 times greater for trichloroethylene (from dry cleaning); 2.1 times greater for paint thinners and strippers; 2.9 times greater for glycol ethers (found in paints). Women working in rubber, plastics or synthetics industries have a 80 percent greater chance of having a stillbirth, according to a study funded by the March of Dimes. This study also showed that women whose husbands worked in the textile industry (chemical dyes, plastics, formaldehyde etc.) had a 90 percent greater risk of stillbirth. (38)

There are many chemicals in our environment (as well as some foods such as soy - see Chapter XIII) that mimic the female hormone estrogen and/or otherwise may disrupt the human hormonal system. Several currently used pesticides commonly found in food mimic the female hormone estrogen, and others clearly interfere with normal hormone function. Recent studies show that the effect of estrogenic pesticides are additive, and that exposure to estrogenic mixtures at low levels can cause the same effect produced by a single chemical when administered at a higher dose. (39) Childhood exposure to these chemicals can have harmful effects later on in life. The British medical journal *The Lancet* said: "The various facets of declining male reproductive health seem to have a common origin in childhood, and defects that may be induced in the current birth cohort by xeno-estrogens [estrogens from sources other than the human body] or other compounds may not become apparent for a further 20 to 40 years." (40)

For all the potential risks associated with them, little is known about most chemicals - even chemicals that are produced and used in great amounts. Of the several thousand chemicals that are produced in amounts of more than 1,000 tons per year (and many at 10,000 tons per year), toxicological data of any kind exists for only a few hundred, and reproductive toxicology data exists for probably a hundred or so.

David La Roche, the secretary of the International Joint Commission, was quoted in *Esquire* magazine concerning chemicals that can harm reproduction (which number in the hundreds if not thousands), "The responsibility should not be on the people exposed to chemicals to prove they have been hurt. The responsibility should be on industry to prove that chemicals cause no harm." (41)

Food for Thought

Clearly, more research is desperately needed in this area. It may be hard to find funding for it though, since there is always resistance from manufacturers to showing the products they produce are harmful. The improvements in our lifestyle due to chemicals, plastics, and so on are undeniable. But we need to be aware of their hazards and how to avoid having them come back to harm us. If we don't, we may literally be facing extinction.

CHAPTER IX
A Delicate Time –
How Conditions During
Pregnancy Can Influence
Your Future Child

A fetus is a particularly unique and vulnerable life form. It is growing at a fast rate and is totally dependent on what its environment is and what is passed to it via the umbilical cord. If the substances the mother passes on to it are detrimental in any way, the growth and development of the fetus may be delayed, interrupted, slowed or otherwise altered. Consequently, the child may be adversely affected either temporarily or permanently.

Numerous environmental agents have been shown to affect the developing fetus in a variety of ways. In this chapter, I have attempted to address many of the most important and prevalent things that may affect a fetus and discuss each topic briefly. Some of them have already been touched on, and some have not been addressed yet and may come as something of a surprise.

Aspirin

Children born to mothers who took aspirin during pregnancy were found to have lower intelligence scores and increases in attention deficit problems, according to a study of 421 predominantly middle-income families conducted by the Department of Psychiatry and Behavioral Science at the University of Washington. Pregnant woman who used aspirin "several times per week" had children whose IQ scores were 10.1 points lower for girls and 1.3 points lower for boys. The testing was done at age four using the Weschler Preschool & Primary Scale of Intelligence (WPPSI) and a standard "vigilance" testing procedure for attention deficit problems. One of the researchers noted:

> IQ scores by age four years have a good predictive validity for later intellectual function. A 10-point IQ decrement is about two-thirds of a standard deviation, a sizable magnitude considering the number of related variables that have been adjusted for in this analysis. The finding that IQ was more differentially affected for girls compared to boys was a surprise and not a usual finding in behavioral teratology studies, in our experience. Attention decrements of the type measured in this study have been associated with learning disabilities in school-age children and with attentional deficits in the classroom, but only further follow-up of this sample would reveal the degree to which these children will sustain long-term behavioral and performance deficits associated with maternal aspirin use during pregnancy. (1)

Forty percent of women take aspirin during pregnancy. Forty-one percent of women take acetaminophen *(Tylenol)* during pregnancy, but IQ problems or attention problems were not found with the acetaminophen use. The authors of this study cited three other studies that found that exposure to aspirin during pregnancy inhibited learning, increased activity, and caused developmental delays in test animals. The authors concluded "The effects could be due to exposure at a very specific time in early pregnancy when the central nervous system was at a critical developmental state." (2)

The effects of alcohol on the developing fetus are well documented. But taking aspirin while drinking is even worse. Indeed, the combination appears to greatly increase the amount of damage to the developing brain – this according to a report from the Alcohol and Brain Research Laboratory at the University of Iowa. Their testing involved 15 groups of pregnant rats and results showed that the mean total brain weight was 29.5 percent less for the rats given alcohol and aspirin compared with the control group. Alcohol alone caused mean brain reduction of 19.8 percent. The researchers said "...the worsening of the alcohol-induced microencephaly [small brain size] by aspirin appears to have been due to an interaction between aspirin and alcohol rather than merely an additive effect..." (3)

Alcohol

Many physicians believe that low levels of alcohol will not harm the fetus. A glass of wine with dinner, they say, should not cause any physical abnormalities; some even recommend it as a treatment to alleviate Braxton-Hicks contractions. However, other neurological defects can occur from occasional and low alcohol consumption. These "defects" may include behavior problems, learning disabilities, attention deficit disorders, hyperactivity, aggression, violent tendencies, impassivity, "reduced" personality, and increased shyness.

Nancy L. Day, Ph.D., of the University of Pittsburgh reports that in 1964 what could be defined as "heavy" alcohol drinking in pregnant women occurred in 4 percent of the population; by 1988 the number had risen to 5 percent. The percentage of pregnant women who are "binge drinkers" (more than five drinks in a day) has risen 50 percent in just 20 years, going from 4 percent of all pregnant women in 1964 to 6 percent in 1984. Fetal alcohol exposure may have even farther-reaching effects, perhaps interfering with cognitive function long after that fetus becomes an adult. Even one episode of binge drinking can damage a child's developing brain. (4)

In 1973 the term Fetal Alcohol Syndrome (FAS) was coined to describe the pattern of birth defects occurring in children whose mothers consumed large amounts of alcohol during pregnancy: one in 1,500 babies are born with in FAS. FAS is characterized by congenital birth defects including prenatal and postnatal growth deficiency; small head circumference; flattened midface; sunken nasal bridge; flattened and elongated philtrum (the groove between the nose and upper lip); central nervous system dysfunction; and varying degrees of major organ system malformations. (5)

Alcohol can also cause the loss of nerve-cell connections in the hippocampus – an area of the brain important for learning and memory. Behavioral and bio-chemical abnormalities occur in test animals exposed to alcohol during pregnancy, findings borne out in studies of humans. For example, Jones et al. found that among the offspring of 23 pregnant women classified as heavy drinkers, 44 percent of the surviving children had borderline or moderate mental deficiency at age seven years. (6) In a study at the University or Washington School of Medicine, four children born to drinking mothers were studied for abnormalities after their deaths. One child was stillborn, the other children died at three days, six weeks, and 10 weeks – all the deaths were due to complications caused by the mothers' alcohol drinking. In three of the four cases, the brain was shown to have grown abnormally; the fourth child had been born two months prematurely. The researchers wrote, "The mechanisms through which alcohol might interfere with brain morphogenesis are not yet understood, but it would appear that intermittent high peak doses of ethanol (alcohol) can cause damage. The severity in effect probably relates not only to dosage but to gestational timing and individual fetal response as well." (7)

Research from the University of North Carolina at Chapel Hill suggests that even one drinking session of five or six drinks early in the pregnancy could be enough to cause mental retardation and many of the facial defects associated with FAS. (8) Another study of 163 middle-class, predominantly white children determined that there is a 10 percent risk of having an abnormal or FAS child if drinking ranged from one to two ounces of absolute alcohol per day (two to four drinks) and a 19 percent risk of having an abnormal or FAS child, if the drinking ranged above two ounces of alcohol daily (more than four drinks). In other words, if a mother has two to four drinks per day, she has a one in 10 chance of having an abnormal or FAS child and if she consumes more than four drinks daily she has nearly a one in five chance of having an abnormal or FAS child. Other research has shown that having more than five to six drinks a day means the risk of having a clinically abnormal child is as high as 40 percent. (9)

An important conclusion of these studies is that drinking in the very early stages of pregnancy has extremely important implications for fetal growth and development. The earliest stages of pregnancy seem to be most critical. The researchers stated that "This observation is of vital importance in counseling, since a woman may not be aware she is pregnant for two weeks or more... At the present time, it seems prudent to advise women to reduce their alcohol intake prior to starting a pregnancy."

A study of 475 young school age children determined that impulsivity, attention, and distraction problems were found to occur more often in children whose mothers drank moderate amounts of alcohol (a few drinks a week) during pregnancy. The number of errors in a simple test given to the children were shown to increase the more the mothers drank during pregnancy. (10)

A study headed by Ann P. Streissguth, Department of Psychiatry and Behavioral Sciences, University of Washington, showed a variety of neurological and school problems among 500 children of primarily white, middle-class, well-educated women – women who are considered at low risk for adverse pregnancy outcomes. But approximately 80 percent of this group were drinking during pregnancy, which changes things considerably. Streissguth concluded:

1. The effects of prenatal alcohol exposure caused behavioral problems at all ages from birth to seven years old.

2. Binge drinking caused more serious consequences than steady drinking, and drinking early in pregnancy has more serious consequences than drinking in mid- pregnancy.

3. The effects of alcohol-related scholastic and neurobehavioral deficits are evident by the second grade. By age 11, problems from prenatal alcohol exposure surfaced as behavioral problems and lower academic performance – especially in arithmetic. At 14 years, prenatal alcohol effects continued, with effects on attention and memory as well as on measures of phonological processing and numerical reasoning. (11)

The impairment to brain function may show up later in life. One study found that a single large dose of alcohol to pregnant rats resulted in memory loss to their offspring, but only after the offspring reached two years of age (equivalent of a middle-aged human). This may explain why some adults could develop learning/memory problems at ages younger than what would normally be expected. (12)

A study by the Emory University School of Medicine and Georgia Mental Health Institute found that in mothers who drank, head circumference was much lower than in nondrinking mothers. Scores for math were significantly lower – 96.5 percent for children whose mothers never drank, compared with 84.8 percent for children who drank consistently during pregnancy. Reading scores were significantly lower for the "continued to drink" group, suggesting the importance of neurological growth in the reading areas of the brain, which develop during the last three months of pregnancy. Short-term memory processing was also shown to be significantly affected. "Taken together," the researchers wrote, "these reports suggest that third-trimester exposure may affect the developing hippocampus or allied structures, leading to deficits in the ability to encode visual or auditory information. Math skills and prereading identification of words and letters are significantly lower in both alcohol groups. These findings suggest that alcohol-exposed children are likely to experience academic difficulties, and it is possible that some of these children will develop specific learning disabilities." (13)

In a study of 15 children at the Yale Learning Disorders Unit whose mothers were known to have a history of heavy drinking during pregnancy, not only it showed that these children generally had smaller head circumferences than normal, but also suffered from learning problems. The researchers said,

> Our findings provide further support for the belief that milder degrees of central nervous system dysfunction are frequently encountered in the offspring of alcoholic women... An increasing body of evidence suggests a relationship between parental alcohol abuse and development of disorders of activity and learning in their offsprings as, for example, in... attention deficit disorder. Alcohol exposure in utero (during pregnancy) may be an important, prevent-

able determinant of attention deficit syndromes in childhood. (14)

So, if a mother drinks during early pregnancy, attention, behavioral problems, and impulsivity may result; while drinking later in the pregnancy may affect reading, math, and other cognitive skills.

At the Department of Psychology at the Carleton University in Ottawa, Canada, Joanne L. Gusella and P.A. Fried found that among 84 children at 13 months of age whose mothers drank an average of 0.24 ounces of absolute alcohol per day (about one-half drink per day), verbal comprehension and spoken language scores were significantly lower. (15)

To summarize these studies and findings, pregnant mothers who drink can cause a number of developmental, behavioral, and learning problems in their offspring. Timing and amount of drinking are important determinants to the type and severity of difficulties the child may experience. Ideally, the mother should not drink during any part of her pregnancy – and that's well within her control, especially if she stops consuming alcohol before attempting to become pregnant. Not only will the child be healthier, smarter and better behaved, but the mother will have an easier time raising him or her.

Cigarette Smoking

By now, virtually all Americans are aware of the Surgeon General's warnings printed on every pack of cigarettes sold in the United States. We know cigarette smoking can harm a developing fetus. Let's examine the nature of that harm.

Overall, smoking increased three- to fourfold from 1940 to the beginning of the 1980s and since then has decreased somewhat. (16) Although the percentage of smoking in the general population is declining, the rate of that decrease is slowest among women of childbearing age. The National Household Survey on Drug Abuse reported that among women of reproductive age, about one-third smoke cigarettes on a regular basis. The percentage of heavy smokers has increased, especially so in women during the past decade, and this is particularly significant since the relationship between the consequences of maternal smoking and the effects on the offspring appears to be dose-related. Even nonsmokers are at risk, however. The U.S. Office of Smoking and Health says that about one third to one half of nonsmoking pregnant women are exposed to significant levels of involuntary or secondhand smoke.

Maternal smoking is causing an increase in hyperactivity in our children. A study at the University of Saskatchewan, Canada, reported in the *Canadian Psychiatric Association Journal* notes:

> [The] apparent increase in prevalence (of hyperactivity) during the past thirty years has coincided with a wide expansion of cigarette smoking, particularly cigarette smoking by women. The child of smoking parents is continually exposed to the products of tobacco combustion and some of these are able to disrupt the normal activity of the central nervous system. Therefore, it seemed appropriate to investigate the prenatal and postnatal exposure of hyperkinetic

children to tobacco smoke, and to compare it with the exposure of non-hyperkinetic control groups. [17]

Before smoking became pervasive, ADHD was uncommon. Back in the 1940s and 1950s textbooks very rarely mentioned the "hyperkinetic syndrome" as it was called back then (i.e., ADHD), in school-age children. Henderson and Gillespie in *A Textbook of Psychiatry for Students and Practitioners; 6th Edition*, state that "hyperkinetic disease" is one of the "very rare" psychoses of childhood. [18] In another earlier textbook, Kanner gave only five sentences to "the restless, fidgety, hyperkinetic child," and did not even discuss hyperactivity as a possible cause for scholastic problems. [19] How times have changed. By the 1990s textbooks routinely estimated that hyperactivity occurs in from 5 percent to 10 percent of North American elementary school children, and one textbook even said that hyperactivity is "The single most common behavioral disorder seen by child psychiatrists." [20]

The Canadian study also noted that mothers of "hyperkinetic" children were found to have smoked an average of 14 cigarettes a day during pregnancy, compared with six cigarettes on average for mothers of "normal" children. The researchers speculate that the accumulation of carbon monoxide in the fetal bloodstream could lead to serious reductions in oxygen to the developing infant. The levels of carbon monoxide-carrying hemoglobin (rather than oxygen-carrying hemoglobin) were twice as high in the fetus than in the mother's blood – showing a concentrating effect.

Food for Thought

As an added point of interest, cigarettes have a significant amount of sugar in them. About 5 percent sugar is added to cigarettes (20 percent in cigars and as much as 40 percent in pipe tobacco). [21] And, due to the flue-curing processes typically employed, the natural sugars found in the tobacco leaf are left intact, resulting in (with the additional sugar added), cigarettes containing as much as 20 percent sugar by weight. The old-style air-curing methods used by the Native American Indians and early on in Westerners' tobacco use allowed the natural tobacco sugars to ferment away. In 1972, *The London Sunday Times* cited studies that showed that British cigarettes (flue-dried with high sugar content) may increase the risk of serious lung disease, even though the tar and nicotine ratings are relatively low. And in countries where air-cured cigarettes with low sugar content were smoked (Russia, China and Formosa), researchers have found no correlation between smoking and lung cancer. Could it be that the worst thing about a cigarette is the sugar? Could it be that this sugar may be a major reason cigarette smoking by a pregnant mother is so bad for the fetus and has contributed to the correlation between women smoking and hyperactivity in children? Something to think about.

The Truth About Children's Health

Secondhand smoke may also contribute to behavioral problems. The mothers of hyperactive children were shown to smoke an average of 23 cigarettes a day compared with eight cigarettes a day for the normal children's mothers. (22)

A hallmark study of over 9,000 children undertaken in Britain as part of the National Child Development Study highlighted the real dangers of smoking during pregnancy. Children of mothers smoking either zero, 10, or more than 10 cigarettes per day during pregnancy were tested at seven and 11 years. Results showed that children of mothers who smoked 10 or more cigarettes a day are on the average 1.0 centimeters shorter and between three and five months behind in reading, math and general ability when compared with the offspring of non-smoking mothers. (23)

One hundred ten six- to 11-year-old children were studied by Dr. Joel S. McCartney of the Department of Psychology, Carleton University, Ottawa, Canada, for their ability to process auditory information (the ability to listen, follow directions and remember what a teacher has said). He found that maternal smoking during pregnancy was linearly associated with the poorer performance on overall testing. He also found that children exposed to passive cigarette smoke or "light" prenatal smoking performed more poorly than children of non-smokers in auditory processing, aspects of memory, and word discrimination. (24)

In another study at the Department of Psychology, Carleton University, 91 children between the ages of six and nine years were tested for developmental, academic, and behavioral skills. The children were divided into three groups: children of nonsmoking mothers, children of mothers who experienced passive smoke during pregnancy, and children of mothers who actively smoked while pregnant. The children of nonsmoking mothers were found to perform better than the two smoking groups on tests of math ability, speech and language skills, intelligence, visual/spatial abilities, and on the mother's rating of behavior. This is in agreement with other studies showing children of active smokers have a higher incidence of misbehavior, poorer adjustment at school, and increased activity levels. The children of nonsmoking mothers were shown to have the best attention and cooperation. (25)

There are actual physiological changes to the cerebral cortex (i.e., the brain) in rats after prenatal nicotine exposure. Animals exposed to nicotine showed significantly reduced thickness of the cerebral cortex, smaller cerebral cortex neurons, and reduced brain weight. There was also an overall decrease in "dendritic branching" (connections to other brain cells). The greater the dose of nicotine, the greater the biological effects were upon the offspring. This supports the many other studies linking increased hyperactivity, attention deficits, lower IQ and learning disabilities in children with parents who smoked during pregnancy. (26) Figure 6 shows the difference in nerve cells of a baby born to a smoker and to a nonsmoker.

Figure 6

Dendrites of one baby born to a smoker and another born to a nonsmoker

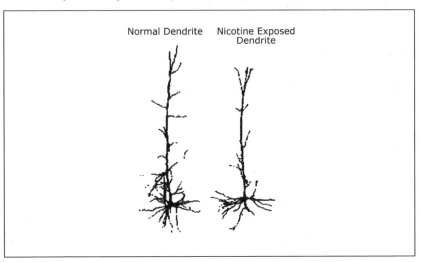

Normal Dendrite   Nicotine Exposed Dendrite

Food for Thought

I previously mentioned that when Einstein's brain was examined, the only noteworthy difference between his brain and brains of other people of normal intelligence was the degree of connections between the nerve cells. These studies show that smoking by the mother during pregnancy or even exposure to secondhand smoke during pregnancy will decrease these "dendritic branches," thus leading to a less intelligent child. I don't know whether Einstein's mother smoked, but I would bet she did not.

Michael Weitzman, Ph.D., conducted a study that showed that the more cigarettes a mother smoked during pregnancy, the greater the likelihood her child would demonstrate severe behavior problems as the child became older. Women who smoked at least a pack a day had children with twice the rate of extreme behavior problems such as anxiety, conflict with others, and disobedience. Weitzman's study, funded by the Labor Department, interviewed parents of 2,256 children ages four to 11. Smoking less than a pack a day during pregnancy was shown to increase behavior problems, although the rates of behavior problems were not as high as for children of heavier smokers. (27)

In a journal article in the *Archives of General Psychiatry*, a study was published which again linked maternal smoking to behavioral problems. One hundred seventy-seven boys, ages seven to 12 years, were assessed for six years. Mothers who smoked more than half a pack of cigarettes a day during pregnancy were more likely to have a child with a conduct disorder than mothers who did not smoke during pregnancy. The researches stated that prenatal exposure to nicotine is associated with adverse reproductive outcomes including altered neural structure and functioning, cognitive deficits, and behavior problems in the offspring. (28)

And, from the Department of Public Health, University of Oulu, Oulu, Finland, it was reported that 14-year-old children of mothers who smoked during pregnancy were found to have more health and academic problems than children of nonsmoking mothers. This study assessed over 11,000 children. The researchers concluded that:

> ...school performance of the smokers' children was poorer than that of their controls when measured in terms of their mean ability on theoretical subjects... this trend being seen among both the boys and the girls and in all social classes. The children of the smokers were more prone to respiratory diseases than the others. They were also shorter in height by nearly 1 centimeter [a little less than half an inch] and their mean ability at school was poorer than among the controls... This differences remained significant after adjusting for mother's height and age, social class as determined by the father's occupation, number of older and younger children in the family and the sex of the child. (29)

Loving parents have high hopes for their children, wishing them a nurturing early life, a stimulating period of development from elementary through high school and beyond. Prenatal and childhood exposure to poisons such as nicotine compromises not only a child's early life, but also – and permanently – his prospects for a happy, healthy future as a productive and fulfilled adult. A tragic – and preventable – consequence.

Coffee and Caffeine

In 1980, the FDA published a warning advising pregnant women to restrict or even eliminate the consumption of coffee due to its teratogenic effect (the ability to cause birth defects). A review of over 200 medical journal articles by Dr. Astrid Nehlig in the 1994 journal *Neurotoxicology and Teratology* reiterated significant hazards of caffeine intake for pregnant women and their developing fetuses. (30)

Coffee and caffeine consumption from other sources has also been associated with a higher incidence of spontaneous abortions (miscarriage). (31)

Food for Thought

A typical cup of coffee contains about 90 mg of caffeine. Instant coffee has about 63 mg of caffeine. Even decaffeinated coffee contains about 3 mg of caffeine. Tea has 32 mg to 42 mg of caffeine. A cola drink typically has about 16 mg. The average daily consumption of caffeine in the general population ranges from 202 to 283 mg of caffeine. It was reported that the number of cups of coffee per consumer per day has increased from 1980 to 1991.

The effects of caffeine on the fetus are more pronounced than for an adult because the fetal hepatic (liver) enzyme systems are not yet mature and cannot metabolize and eliminate the caffeine as effectively. Whereas the half-life (amount of time half of it stays in the system) of caffeine is from 2.5 to six hours in adults, the half-life in newborn infants is from 40 to 130 hours.

The absorption of caffeine has been shown to have a vasoconstrictive effect on placental circulation – restricting blood flow to the developing fetus. Indeed, placental blood flow is significantly diminished after the mother drinks just two cups of coffee. "This decrease in blood flow along with increased concentration of noradrenaline induced by caffeine in the maternal serum could represent a potential risk of the fetus," says Nehlig. (32)

It's been shown that caffeine diffuses through the placenta and accumulates in the brain of the fetus. Exposing female rats to caffeine during pregnancy caused proportionally greater loss in fetal brain weight than in body weight. Maternal intake of caffeine during gestation and lactation can induce modification in various amino acids, nucleic acids, and serotonin, which can cause behavioral abnormalities, mood disorders, and learning problems. The behavioral effects induced by prenatal caffeine exposure could be related to the "hyperactive" child syndrome. That cup of "java" not only juices you up, but your soon-to-be child as well!

Also, the risk of congenital abnormalities is greater for infants whose mother's drank caffeine during pregnancy – 3.7 percent versus only 1.7 percent in mothers who did not consume caffeine. In 1983 at Carleton University, Canada, 286 pregnant women who consumed caffeine (from all sources) were studied. It was shown that the most significant effect of heavy caffeine users (more than 300 mg per day) was reduced birth weight (379 grams) and smaller head circumference (1.1 cm). The researchers concluded that "It is during the last trimester of pregnancy that the greatest spurt in fetal growth occurs. The present results suggest that daily caffeine intake of 300 mg or more can interfere with normal fetal growth..." (33)

Clearly, the caffeine a woman may have relied on before her pregnancy is simply not an option when she's eating – and drinking – for two. Anyone worried about "withdrawal" from caffeine addiction should phase out her intake before becoming pregnant. There are many good herbal teas and natural coffee substitutes you may try, available at health food stores. Don't switch to regular tea, since it too is loaded with caffeine.

Although not directly related to fertility, a study at Vanderbilt University showed that coffee drinking caused a 20 percent to 25 percent reduction in blood flow to the brains of healthy college volunteers 30 minutes after drinking 250 milligrams – about one cup. (34) Lower blood flow means lower intelligence.

Pesticides

Although the literature abounds with studies on the effects of pesticides on adults, and some on children, studies focusing on the effects of pesticides on the pregnant mother and her fetus (human or animal) are sorely lacking. This area most definitely needs to be studied more. It would not be surprising to discover that fetal pesticide exposure during gestation leads to an increase in physical birth defects and long-term learning, memory, and behavioral problems in children.

A research team headed by D. Machera, Ph.D., at the Laboratory of Pesticide Toxicology in Athens, Greece, found that a common fungicide, cyproconazole, which is widely used in agriculture, increased test animals' risks of lower birth weight and lower body length as well as strongly increasing the risk of cleft palate and hydrocephalus. (35)

Pesticides are intentionally designed to damage the nervous system. Of course, they are intended to damage the nervous system of the target pest, not people, babies, or fetuses. But they damage humans too, causing health and learning problems.

Currently, manufacturers are required to test pesticides to determine their links to such conditions as cancer, skin irritation, fatality risk, and major birth defects. But they are not required to tested for more subtle neurological effects such as changes in memory, learning, and behavior. It will take years if not decades of research to learn the effects these chemicals may have on children and a developing fetus. But there's a simple way around all the time and expense of testing these deadly chemicals – stop using them and switch to organic farming! (I recently saw a bumper sticker advising: "Die Healthy – Eat Organic!")

MSG

Monosodium Glutamate (MSG), used as a flavor enhancer, is another compound that may affect the developing fetus. John Olney, M.D., and his colleagues at the Department of Psychiatry and Pediatrics at Washington University School of Medicine have done extensive research into the possible health effects of MSG. He reports,

> The assumption that MSG is an entirely innocuous substance for human consumption has been questioned recently in view of its role in the Chinese restaurant syndrome. The finding that neuronal necrosis can be induced in the immature mouse brain by 0.5 mg/kg of MSG raises the more specific question whether there is any risk to the developing human nervous system by maternal use of MSG during pregnancy. The primate placenta maintains amino acids in consistently higher concentration in the fetal circulation than those found in the maternal circulation, the ratio of glutamic acid being greater than 2:1... The possibility that brain lesions could occur in the developing primate embryo in response to increased glutamic acid concentrations in the maternal circulation, therefore, warrants investigation. (36)

The Federation of American Societies For Experimental Biology echoes Olney's findings:

> It is prudent to avoid the use of dietary supplements of L-glutam-

ic acid by pregnant women, infants, and children. The existence of evidence of potential endocrine responses, i.e., elevated cortisol and prolactin, and differential responses between males and females, would also suggest a neuroendocrine link and that supplemental L-glutamic acid should be avoided by women of childbearing age and individuals with affective disorder. (37)

Food for Thought

Perhaps they should have warning signs on Chinese restaurant menus and any other restaurant that uses MSG:

"Warning : Ingestion of food with MSG may cause nervous system problems in developing fetuses and resulting children. Pregnant women should avoid eating food with MSG added."

Better yet, why don't restaurants stop using it? (Answer: It saves them money.)

Mercury

In a study at the University of Minnesota Medical School, the researchers concluded, "We found that... offspring from mercury-exposed mice behaved significantly different from controls when tested for subtle deviations during postnatal development." (38)

Thus, another substance that can adversely affect the developing fetus. But again, studies on mercury effects on developing human fetuses is lacking. Knowing what we know about mercury poisoning, however, doesn't it make sense to avoid exposure to it before, during, and after pregnancy?

Ultrasound

Ultrasound is routinely used once or twice during most pregnancies in the United States; some physicians even provide it with every visit. Ultrasound uses sound waves that are above the range of human hearing to "see" objects – similar to the way radar or sonar "sees" objects. Most physicians believe it is safe based on early studies showing no adverse effects on the human fetus. But as technology and testing procedures have improved, now there are questions as to its safety.

Studies show the possibility of lower birth weight and dyslexia in the children who were exposed to ultrasound during pregnancy. One study concluded that the most consistent effect of ultrasound exposure was low birth weight, although other studies do not support that finding. Such discrepancies could indicate that the ultrasound safety tests need to be more sophisticated and that the timing of the ultrasound exposure during pregnancy could be critical for determining whether or not it is harmful.

A study performed by Dr. M. Prakash Hande attempted to determine ultrasound effects on test animals if exposed during two specific fetal periods (6th and 11th day of pregnancy). The offspring were allowed to develop normally and then tested for detrimental effects at three and six months. According to the study, "The results indicate that repeated exposures to ultrasound or its combination with X-rays could be detrimental to the embryonic development and can impair adult brain function when administered at certain stages of organ growth." After birth, the exposed animal (while in the womb) experienced hypoactivity and impairment in learning as a result of the ultrasound exposure. At birth, the head length and brain weight of the exposed group did not show any statistically significant differences from the control group, although the exposed group had an 8.6 percent growth retardation rate compared with 3.3 percent for the nonexposed control group. (39)

The health of our children in part depends upon the environment they encounter in the womb during their development. Remember, children are more sensitive to environmental stresses than adults. It's likely that the fetus is even more sensitive. More information is desperately needed in this area, and it may be up to us to demand testing and regulations that protect our children, born or yet to be.

CHAPTER X
Breastfeeding, Formulas, and Baby Food

To ensure an infant will grow into a healthy, responsible adult, proper nutrition is crucial. Undoubtedly, the best way to do this is by breastfeeding. Breast milk is created by nature to give a baby perfect nutrition – and the act of breastfeeding is important for the baby's emotional development.

"Human milk," the American Academy of Pediatrics says, "is the preferred feeding for all infants, including premature and sick newborns... It is recommended that breastfeeding continue for at lease the first 12 months, and thereafter for as long as mutually desired." (1) The World Health Organization goes even further and recommends breastfeeding for at least two years.

Despite these recommendations, only slightly more than half of all mothers offer their newborns any breast milk at all, and fewer than 22 percent of American babies are still breastfed at five months of age. That figure drops to under 10 percent by 12 months. This means that the vast majority of American babies rely solely on synthetic infant formula for most of their critical first year of life. (2) Although a federal survey found in 1995 that 58 percent of American mothers started off breastfeeding their babies, which is the same percentage as in 1985, 20 percent fewer mothers today are still breastfeeding after three months. (3)

There are many reasons to breastfeed. The academy also says, "Human milk is uniquely superior for infant feeding and is species-specific; all substitute feeding options differ markedly from it." And those differences can deprive your baby of health and vitality. "...Infant formula can never duplicate human milk," write researchers John D. Benson, Ph.D. and Mark L. Masor, Ph.D. "Human milk contains living cells, hormones, active enzymes, immunoglobins and compounds with unique structures that cannot be replicated in infant formula." (4) These two scientists, who are both pediatric nutrition researchers at infant formula manufacturer Abbott Laboratories, believe that creating formula that duplicates human milk is impossible. (And if the manufacturers' own scientists conclude that, you can bet the evidence must be overwhelming!) M. Walker, R.N., International Board-Certified Lactation Consultant, says, "Formula-fed infants depend on products which can be quite different from each other, but which are continually being found deficient in essential nutrients... These nutrients are then added, usually after damage has occurred in infants or overwhelming market pressure forces the issue." (5)

Breast milk provides immune factors to many diseases and aids in the development of the baby's immune system. It's more digestible than formula because it contains an enzyme that aids in that process. Breast milk forms softer curds in the infant's stomach than cow's milk and is more quickly assimilated into the body. Virtually all the protein in breast milk is available to the baby, whereas even though cow's milk has more protein, about half passes right through the baby's body as a waste product. Similarly, iron and zinc are absorbed better by breast-fed babies.

And iron is of particular concern. William J. Klish, M.D., chairman of the American Academy of Pediatrics (AAP) Committee on Nutrition, says, "There should not be a low-iron formula on the market for the average child because a low-iron formula is a nutritionally deficient formula. It doesn't provide enough iron to maintain proper blood cell counts or proper hemoglobin." (Hemoglobin is a blood protein that carries oxygen from the lungs to the tissues, and carbon dioxide from the tissues to the lungs.) Studies have shown that children who had good iron status as infants performed better on standardized developmental tests than children with poor iron status. Yet, the FDA permits low-iron formulas to be sold under the assumption that a physician is monitoring iron status and prescribing iron supplements when appropriate; but when was the last time your pediatrician discussed your baby's iron status with you?

Although human breast milk contains less than 1 milligram of iron per liter, it is virtually 100 percent absorbed by the baby. The baby does not absorb iron nearly so efficiently from formula even though iron-fortified formulas contain about 12 milligrams of iron per liter. Currently, the FDA is evaluating what level of iron in formula is best, which is an important piece of the puzzle, since too much iron could lead to abdominal discomfort, constipation, diarrhea, colic, and irritability. (6)

Breast milk always contains the right proportions of fat, carbohydrates, and protein. Formula companies are constantly adjusting these proportions looking for the best composition. Interestingly, a mother's milk composition changes from feeding to feeding depending on the needs of the child. So standardized formulas can never be totally correct.

Jack Newman, M.D., a Canadian pediatrician who has been a UNICEF infant nutrition consultant in Africa and has published articles on breastfeeding in medical journals, says:

> Modern formulas are only superficially similar to breast milk. Every correction of a deficiency in formulas is advertised as an advance. Fundamentally they are inexact copies based on outdated and incomplete knowledge of what breast milk is. Formulas contain no antibodies, no living cells, no enzymes, no hormones. They contain much more aluminum, manganese, cadmium, and iron than breast milk. They contain significantly more protein than breast milk. The proteins and fats are fundamentally different from those in breast milk. (7)

Martha Neuringer, a professor of clinical nutrition, says, "Human milk is an incredibly complicated substance. It contains proteins we haven't even identified yet, much less know the function of." (8)

Part of the reason for the ineffectiveness of formula is that it is always pasteurized. Pasteurization kills microorganisms, but also changes the structures of proteins, carbohydrates and fats significantly. It also kills enzymes, which are necessary for complete and efficient digestion. In an experiment with baby calves, some were fed raw milk from their mother, and others fed pasteurized milk from their mother. The ones fed pasteurized milk died within six weeks. That shows the importance of the milk being raw, as it is, straight from the breast of the mother. Pasteurization also completely destroys the enzyme phosphatase. In fact, this is one of the tests to see if the product was adequately pasteurized – if phosphatase is not present, the pasteurization process was a success. Problem is, phosphatase is essential for the absorption of calcium in the human body! So, the calcium in pasteurized milk products is, due to this fact – largely unavailable. (9) And, by the way, human breast milk is never contaminated with bacteria. In fact, it has antibacterial properties.

Some mothers may fear that their breast milk is deficient in nutrients. There have been scary stories in the media in which a baby dies because the mother breastfed and the baby did not receive adequate nutrition. One such case involved Tabitha Waldron and her seven-week-old infant. The national headlines read "Breastfeeding can kill?" and "Nursed to Death." However, upon closer scrutiny, it was discovered that the problem with Tabitha and her baby, as with most cases of problems with breastfeeding, was that the milk was not being effectively transferred from breast to baby. It was not that the milk was deficient, but rather the baby was simply not getting enough. (10) That can occur if the mother is uninformed on the correct way to breastfeed. Although malnutrition from breastfeeding may be possible, it's not very likely if done correctly. Of course, the breastfeeding mother needs to be in fairly good health and she needs to take care of herself during pregnancy and while breastfeeding.

That makes good intuitive sense, doesn't it? The so-called primitive cultures of the globe show us it's right. Weston Price, D.D.S., traveled the world examining native cultures to determine their dietary habits. He discovered that in many cultures, young women who were hoping to conceive, pregnant women, and women nursing were fed exceedingly rich diets. Although these peoples did not know all the science behind nutrition, pregnancy, and breastfeeding, they instinctively knew that it puts high demands on the mother's body, and that the nutrients the fetus and baby need drain her of those nutrients. (This explains why pregnant women are drawn to certain foods. These compulsions are her body crying out for certain nutrients found in those foods. If the mother-to-be is wise, she will choose the most healthy, wholesome variety of these foods.) So a nutritionally adequate diet for the mother is essential for nutritious breast milk.

Food for Thought

Concerning the sale of baby formula, it's an amazingly profitable business. The average bottle-feeding family in the U.S. spends $1,500 to $2,000 per year on infant formula – so every time a mother chooses to breastfeed, the industry loses that money. According to the Attorney General of Florida, for each dollar charged for infant formula, the manufacturer spends only 16 cents on production and delivery. Infant formula companies make $3 billion a year, up 54 percent since 1989. (11) The same

---

Breastfeeding, Formulas, and Baby Food

companies that make formula make other medical supplies. Abbot Laboratories, for example which makes Similac and Isomil, two popular baby formulas, also makes Pediasure, an oral rehydrating solution for infants and young children with diarrheal disease, and antibiotics used to treat infant infections.

As you are learning, infants who are bottle-fed are much more likely to have health problems. Not only are these pharmaceutical companies making money on the formula, but they are also selling more of their other products to help "fix" the kids who get sick because of them. There's a lot of money involved here. Is it any wonder that the companies who manufacture baby formula have enlisted the assistance of the trusted health care provider - doctors – to help them sell their products? (12)

Traditional medical doctors rarely encourage mothers to breastfeed, and when asked if breastfeeding is better than formula feeding, they are oftentimes indifferent. Only 37 percent of pediatricians recommend breast-feeding for the first year – even though their own association (AAP) recommends it. In a recent American Academy of Pediatrics survey, 45 percent of pediatricians responded say they see formula-feeding and breast-feeding as equally acceptable methods for feeding an infant. These doctors also are split in opinion as to whether breastfed babies are healthier than bottle-fed babies, even though there is much and decisive evidence showing that they are. (13)

And the government is involved too. The U.S. government's food program for Women, Infants and Children (WIC) serves the nutritional needs of low-income mothers and their kids. It is the single greatest purchaser of commercial infant formula, providing free infant formula to 37 percent of all infants born in the U.S. That costs $500 million annually. (14) Guess where that money comes from? Your tax dollars. You would think our benevolent, caring government would be encouraging breastfeeding because – according to its own agency, the FDA - it provides the best nutrition for the baby. (Not to mention that it's free!) But then consider that the infant formula industry contributes $1 million annually to the AAP, and that the U.S. pharmaceutical industry spends $6,000 to $8,000 per doctor per year in promoting formula, using these "incentives" that sometimes include gifts, office supplies, meals, a year's supply of free formula for themselves or a relative, lavish parties and receptions, and even vacations. (15)

Researcher Katie Allison Granju says, "Obviously, marketing and product giveaways on this scale cost infant-formula companies millions and millions of dollars each year. But it pays off. Their own market research, as well as medical literature and anecdotal observations by lactation professionals, have demonstrated that these tactics make it statistically less likely

The Truth About Children's Health

that a women will breast-feed without supplementation or breastfeed at all. And once a woman stops nursing and begins feeding infant formula, these companies know that they likely have her "hooked" on their product, since even a brief interruption in the nursing relationship can cause a woman's own milk supply to dwindle or the baby to begin refusing breast in favor of bottle... Many Americans are under the mistaken impression that today's commercial infant formulas are nearly identical to human milk. And because of this, parents who routinely approach other important infant health and safety issues in a thoughtful, deliberate way are largely unaware that in epidemiological terms, the decision to formula-feed when breast-feeding is an option places their child at demonstrably higher risk for a wide variety of ailments." (16)

Back to the headlines. Can you imagine reading a headline proclaim-ing: "Mother's Choice to Formula-Feed Leads to Preemie Dying!" And yet, that's what can happen much more often for formula fed vs. breastfed pre-mature babies. Necrotizing enterocolitis is an inflammation of the large and small intestine that is fatal in 20 percent to 40 percent of the premature infants who become ill with it. And formula-fed preemies are 10 times more likely to get it than breastfed. An already concerned new mother may be hesitant to breastfeed a premature baby. But preterm milk is specially designed for premature infants, differing from milk produced after a full-term pregnancy; mother's milk is custom-made! Isn't nature amazing?

Here's an instance that illustrates the influence of big business on the mindset of the American public. During the 1998 - 1999 television sea-son, in an episode of "Chicago Hope," the plot revolved around the death of a breastfed infant due to malnutrition. Is it a coincidence that this episode, as was the entire last season of "Chicago Hope," was sponsored in part by the Pharmaceutical Research and Manufacturers of America? The episode was so blatantly anti-breastfeeding that the Baby-Friendly Hospital Initiative (a pro-breastfeeding organization) and a manufacturer of breast pumps issued formal complaints and said the program was a "gross misrepresentation." But millions of Americans saw the show and went away fearing breastfeeding.

Breastfeeding also satisfies the baby's emotional needs. All babies need to be held and cuddled. Studies have shown that premature babies are more likely to die if they are not held or stroked. Bottle-feeding oftentimes does not provide the same degree of intimacy and warmth. Breastfeeding also promotes bonding between mother and baby. Part of this is because breastfeeding stimulates the release of the hormone oxytocin in the mother's body. "It is now well established that oxytocin, as well as stimulating uterine contractions and milk ejection, promotes the development of maternal behavior and also bonding between mother and offspring." (17)

Other advantages of breastfeeding, according to the 1998 Policy Statement on Breastfeeding and the Use of Human Milk by the AAP include: protection against Crohn's disease for the baby; decrease risk of baby developing Type I diabetes; decreased risk of developing allergies and asthma; decreased risk of sudden infant death syndrome (SIDS); protection against diarrheal infections; bacterial meningitis; respiratory infections; ear infections (19 percent to 80 percent less); botulism; urinary tract infection; childhood lymphomas; juvenile rheumatoid arthritis; Hodgkins disease; and vision defects. (18) The benefits of breastfeeding last into adulthood: Women breastfed as infants, for example, have a 25 percent lower chance of developing breast cancer later in life. Breastfed babies are healthier overall, are less likely to die before their third birthday, require fewer doctor visits, get fewer cavities, and have better speech development. (19)

"More than 1,000 childhood deaths per year in the United States could be prevented through breastfeeding," says author Allan Cunningham, M.D., associate professor of pediatrics and the State University of New York Health Science Center in Syracuse, N.Y. "This includes infants who die from a wide variety of illnesses such as diarrheal diseases like rotavirus, as well as pneumonia and bacterial meningitis... My estimate is that you roughly double the statistical risk of a baby dying of SIDS if you formula-feed. This is something parents just aren't made aware of." (20) Cunningham has shown that for every 1,000 bottle-fed infants, 77 hospital admissions would result, vs. just five for breastfed infants. In another survey, bottle-fed infants were 14 times more likely to be hospitalized than breastfed infants. (21) Formula-fed babies averaged more than $1,400 more per year in additional health care costs than breastfed infants in a 1995 survey. (22)

"When overall health of formula-fed infants in the U.S. is compared to that of breastfed infants – even after controlling for variables such as parents' socioeconomic backgrounds – it becomes clear that formula-fed babies are sicker, sick more often, and are more likely to die in infancy or childhood. " Cunningham says. (23)

Breast milk may not be magic, but it certainly has properties that seem that way. One protein found in breast milk, called alpha-lactalbumin, has been found to literally destroy every cancer cell with which it comes in contact. Swedish and British researchers discovered this while trying to determine why "the relative risk of childhood lymphoma is nine times higher in bottle-fed infants, and the risk for carcinoma is also elevated." They go on to say, "This [alpha-lactalbumin] is a substance that kills lots of tumor cells, every cancer we test it against – lung cancer, throat cancer, kidney cancer, colon cancer, bladder cancer, lymphoma, leukemia, and pheumococcus bacteria too." (24) (I think now you know one of the reasons children are getting cancer younger and younger. Most of them have not been breastfed and are thus more vulnerable not just early in life, but later in life too.)

Another vital substance found in mother's milk but not found in formulas sold in the U.S. is the fatty acid called docosahexaenoic acid (DHA), and it is a crucial component of the brain and nervous system. Deficiencies have been linked to depression, aggression, Alzheimer's disease, schizophrenia, and multiple sclerosis in adults, and learning disabilities in children.

An excellent source of DHA is good old-fashioned Cod liver oil, which also contains high amounts of vitamins A and D. Sally Fallon, a noted researcher and author, comments on DHA:

> Adequate DHA in the mother's diet is necessary for the proper development of the retina in the infant she carries. DHA in mother's milk helps prevent learning disabilities and vision problems. Cod liver oil and foods like liver and egg yolk supply this essential nutrient to the developing fetus, to nursing infants and to growing children. Saturated fats help the body put the DHA in the tissues where it belongs. (25)

William Campbell Douglass, M.D., an eminent physician and former author of a popular newsletter called "Second Opinion" has some important things to say about DHA, formula, and children. The title of his article is: "A Substance Found in Breast Milk Helps Depression, Alzheimer's." I am going to be brave and quote the entire article for several reasons: Although this book is about kids, most of you reading this are adults, and Campbell gives several recommendations aimed at us. In addition, I want you to see that I am not the only one with a healthy skepticism of our government agencies, and I also like his spunky attitude, which would be lost by paraphrasing.)

> Depression and Alzheimer's disease are reaching epidemic proportions in America, and, as a result, Prozac and other pharmaceuticals that supposedly treat these ailments are selling like hotcakes.

> The good news, though, is that recent studies are now indicating low levels of a fatty acid called docosahexaenoic acid (DHA) contribute to the many major physical and psychological disorders in adults. These ailments include depression, aggression, Alzheimer's disease, schizophrenia and multiple sclerosis. (To avoid any confusion, DHA is unrelated to DHEA. DHA is a fatty acid and DHEA is a hormone.)

> Approximately 60 percent of the human brain is composed of fatty material, and 25 percent of that material is made up of DHA. While DHA is the primary structural fatty acid in the brain, humans cannot produce it- they must consume it.

> Studies show that the DHA levels of women in America today are comparable to those women in Third-World countries. This is attributed to the trend against eating DHA-rich foods such as fish (tuna, salmon, trout, and sardines), liver, brain and other animal organs, and eggs.

> Despite a growing body of evidence that DHA is the essential structural ingredient of breast milk and is lacking in infant formulas, the Food and Drug Administration continues to ban its use in the U.S. Even the National Institutes of Health have endorsed the addi-

tion of DHA to infant formula with no visible effect on the FDA.

I know you're not an infant, but it's not too late for you to benefit from the brain- and mood-boosting benefits of this wonderful supplement. It is important that you understand how this fatty acid benefits infants, though, because it directly relates to how it affects you. Hang with me on this for a little bit.

Breastfed babies have an IQ six to 10 points higher than formula-fed babies. Scientists and nutritional experts attribute this to DHA, an omega-3 fatty acid that's an essential structural component of the brain and retina. It's found naturally in mother's milk. In case it will impress you, the World Health Organization and the Food and Agricultural Organization of the United Nations also endorse the addition of DHA to infant formula.

During the last trimester of a pregnancy is when the mother transfers to her baby much of the DHA needed for the development of his or her brain and nervous system. The DHA content in the mother's diet reflects in the amount of DHA passed on to the baby. If the baby is not breastfed at all, it receives no DHA after birth and is short-changed in neurological development, thus impairing mental and visual acuity. DHA levels of premature infants are especially low, since they miss much of that last trimester and when born, haven't developed the sucking mechanism - so they are usually bottle-fed. It's a wonder they live at all, and it's a crime they aren't getting DHA in their bottle from birth.

Many European and Asian countries are producing infant formula with DHA and making recommendations of daily allowances. The American company, Wyeth Nutritional, does make infant formula that contains DHA; however, it's only available in Hong Kong, the middle East, and Australia, since distribution is banned in the U.S.

Dr. David Kyle, chief of research at Martek Biosciences Corporation, has been involved in several studies involving DHA. He has consistently observed that formula-fed babies have far lower levels of visual and intellectual acuity than do their breastfed peers.

As I mentioned at the outset, DHA has uses beyond the newborn. Studies show that low DHA intake in infancy can lead or contribute to Attention Deficit Disorder (ADD) and Attention Deficit Hyperactivity Disorder (ADHD). We're moving up the age ladder - don't give up - we'll get to you in a minute.

The government is under pressure from prominent drug companies (such as Novartis, which manufactures Ritalin) to keep DHA out of the information bank of the average consumer. If Ritalin could be replaced by a simple and safe fatty acid, Novartis would be in trouble, people might have to be laid off, and profits would tumble. Do you think a drug company could be that heartless and put profits ahead of the lives of children? Maybe you don't but I've seen it happen more than a few times.

Bill Taylor is a retired engineer who teaches elementary-aged ADD children as a volunteer and is on the forefront of the infant formula debate. He said: "There is a lot of money at stake. Scientists are dependent on drug companies for research grants." Drug companies aren't interested in a simple cure for anything and certainly not a cash cow like the ADD/Ritalin market.

A study done on Japanese students during the high-stress period of final exams showed that students supplemented with DHA were significantly less aggressive than students who were not supplemented with DHA. Now we get to you, my patient reader. You are no longer a baby, that's for sure, so why am I giving you all this infant-formula information? First, you probably have children – or even grandchildren – and they need to know about DHA for their children. But more relevant to you personally, consider the following:

- Studies show that symptoms of multiple sclerosis, such as muscular weakness, loss of coordination, and speech and visual disturbances, are linked to sub normal levels of omega-3 fatty acids such as DHA.

- DHA helps supply the brain with serotonin, which regulates moods, thus making one less vulnerable to stress and depression.

- Over 1,200 patients participated in an epidemiological study that showed people with high DHA levels were 45 percent less likely to develop dementia than people with low DHA levels. This suggests that proper DHA intake may reduce the risk of developing Alzheimer's disease.

- A 1997 study showed that schizophrenic patients were less likely to have been breastfed in infancy, and the lack of DHA during early brain development contributes to the development of schizophrenia.

While these last two areas need more research, science is already starting to bear witness to the desperate need of people of all ages to consume plenty of DHA. Obviously, diet plays an important part in the consumption of DHA. And while taking a gel cap of DHA is great, you've got to fix your diet, as many people are consuming foods that actually contribute to depression, Alzheimer's, and some of the other problems we've discussed.

I've preached for years about the dangers of eating margarine as a substitute for real butter. Now the devastating results are starting to hit hard. In addition to it being nutrient-free, margarine is saturated hydrogenated fat (a.k.a. trans-fatty acids) that causes our neurochemistry to go into a tailspin. You don't have to be a brain surgeon to understand the brain runs every system in the body. So when the neurochemistry is messed up, the rest of the body is messed up.

In contrast, essential fatty acids are just that, essential. The difference between trans-fatty acids and essential fatty acids is the exact difference between depression and a normal emotional state of mind. It's also a major factor that needs to be considered in greater detail in Alzheimer's and other brain illnesses.

Action to Take:

1) As you age, it's terribly important that you avoid any and all dairy products that aren't real or have been altered by processing. That means you can toss out any margarine, EggBeaters, and low-fat or no-fat dairy products. It also means you need to get milk that's not homogenized or pasteurized. All of these fake fats and processed products accelerate the aging process and cause your brain to malfunction.

2) At the same time, you need to increase your intake of good, fatty animal meats. I know this goes against the grain of current medical dogma, but the evidence of their benefits is growing increasingly indisputable.

3) I can also recommend that you begin taking a capsule or two of DHA each day. It's not as good of a source as the fatty meats, but it's the next best thing (and essential if you're a vegetarian). You can probably find DHA at your local health food store.

If not, you can order Neuromins, a DHA supplement made by Martek Bioscience Corp. (see Resource Guide). Martek is one of the leading manufacturers of DHA supplements, and it claims that its algae-based product provides DHA in its "purest possible form." (26)

Food for Thought

It seems I'm not the only one suspicious of drug companies. They have us coming and going, since their tentacles reach deep into our government. Since the addition of DHA to infant formula is banned in the U.S., thanks to our friendly FDA, we are raising a generation of aggressive morons. After a few years of a diet insufficient in DHA and other nutrients not found in formula, the children are more likely to develop learning disabilities, attention deficits, and behavioral problems. The solution? Drug them with Substance II drugs such as Ritalin. First they sell the deficient formula, then they sell the drugs later. Very tricky.

Speaking of the FDA, although it may sometimes seem to be in alliance with the drug companies, it does offer some valuable information even though most of the time it doesn't know what to do with it. In an article by Isadora B. Stehlin on the FDA internet homepage, she writes, "More than half the calories in breast milk come from fat, and the same is true for

---

today's infant formulas. This may be alarming to many American adults watching their intake of fat and cholesterol, especially when sources of saturated fats, such as coconut oil, are used in formulas... But the low-fat diet recommended for adults doesn't apply to infants." (27)

In a study of 1,000 children over 18 years in New Zealand, those children who were breastfed as infants had both better intelligence and greater academic achievement than children who were formula-fed. (28) It's also been shown that psychomotor and social development of breastfed babies is significantly better than bottle-fed ones. (29) This means the child is less likely to have behavioral problems later in life since he or she are more socially adept.

How important is breastfeeding? Lawrence Gartner, M.D., F.A.A.P., is a respected medical authority on infant feeding. He says that parents today aren't fully aware that deciding to breast- or bottle-feed is so important. "Compared to other equally important child safety issues like car seat use or babies' sleep position, parents should understand that the decision whether to breast- or bottle-feed ranks right up on top when it comes to protecting babies. The AAP certainly puts it in that category." (30) Katherine Detwyler, Ph.D., an associate professor at Texas A&M and world renowned expert on infant nutrition, agrees: "I would rank the decision of how to feed your baby as the No.1 safety issue in this country." Detwyler also commented on the marketing of formula: "Infant formula should be seen for what it is: a pharmaceutical product, not for routine use. The way these companies market it as equivalent to breast milk and just one equal choice among several is wrong." (31)

Breastfeeding is not just good for the baby, but for the mother too. A mother who breastfeeds her child is less likely, compared with those who bottle-feed, to get breast cancer, ovarian cancer, or endometrial cancer. It helps shrink the mother's uterus after childbirth, and the baby's suckling actually helps prevent postpartum hemorrhage. Nursing helps the mom lose weight after the baby is born and decreases the mother's insulin requirements. It even decreases the chances of maternal osteoporosis later in life.

If a mother cannot breastfeed, the World Health Organization says, the second choice is the mother's own milk expressed and given to the infant in some way. The third choice is the milk of another human mother. The fourth and last choice is artificial baby milk.

There is a small network of human milk banks in the U.S. for mothers who are unable to breastfeed their own babies. Though an uncommon practice in today's western society, sharing human milk has been common throughout human history. The first U.S. milk bank opened in Boston in 1911. The current milk banks in the United States follow strict health and safety guidelines (similar to that of a blood bank) and are available for use by prescription only. As the awareness of the importance of human milk is growing, the demand is greater than the supply at these milk banks, even though the price for the human milk is expensive. But some insurance companies will pay, and even Medicaid pays in some states.

Breastfeeding, Formulas, and Baby Food   211

You may think that breastfeeding your baby correctly is simple, and it is. But it can be done wrong, and your baby may not get enough milk. The following are signs that will tell you if your baby is getting enough breast milk: Make sure you monitor yourself and your baby to avoid any nutritional deficiencies.

- Baby should feed at least every two to three hours – at least eight times in 24 hours during the first two to three weeks of life.
- Your breasts should feel emptied and softer after feeds.
- Baby should have a healthy color and firm skin – which should bounce right back after being pinched. If the baby is dehydrated, the skin will stay puckered for a few seconds.
- The number of wet diapers should start increasing by the fifth day to total at least eight wet diapers in a 24-hour period.
- You should be able to hear him swallow while breastfeeding in a quite room.
- At first you will see yellowy-mustard stools or frequent dark stools. They should begin to lighten in color by the fifth day after birth.

Signs your baby isn't getting enough breast milk:

- Baby stops feeding after 10 minutes or less.
- You rarely hear the baby swallow.
- Your breasts don't feel softer after feedings.
- Baby is unsettled or lethargic most of the time.
- Baby makes clicking noises while breastfeeding or has dimples in his cheeks while breastfeeding.
- Baby wets fewer than six diapers in a 24-hour period after the fifth day.
- Baby doesn't have a bowel movement at least once a day or is having small, dark stools five days or more after birth.
- Baby becomes more yellow, instead of less, after the first week.
- Baby's skin remains wrinkled after the first week. (32)

If any of these signs appear, contact your health care provider immediately. You may be feeding the wrong way or your milk could be deficient in nutrients and need supplementation.

Please note that if the mother supplements breastfeeding with formula, she may make less milk. Breast milk is made in response to the baby's sucking. If you feel you don't have enough milk to keep your baby satisfied and growing, then try feeding more often at the breast and be sure your baby is well positioned so he or she feeds effectively.

Formula Problems

Most formula on the market these days is either pasteurized cow's-milk based or soy-based – both of which can pose problems for the developing infant.

Again, the following discussions concerning the problems with milk have to do with commercial, pasteurized milk. Whole, raw milk – the way nature intended it – is a good food and suited for feeding to children. But modern processing methods, as well as the way the cows are fed and treated, have made commercial milk a disease-producing food.

Pasteurization destroys the valuable enzymes in milk. Without these enzymes, milk is difficult to impossible to digest completely. For example, lactase, the enzyme that digests the milk sugar lactose, is destroyed. Since infants cannot produce significant amounts of lactase, lactose intolerance can occur resulting in excessive gas, abdominal distention and pain, and diarrhea.

The enzyme phosphatase is also destroyed. This enzyme is necessary for the assimilation of calcium. That's why consumption of commercial milk may lead to the calcification of joints and arteries. Raw milk has this enzyme intact, so proper assimilation of calcium occurs.

Commercial milk is homogenized which turns it rancid. The butterfat, a nutritious ingredient and a great source of preformed vitamin A and natural vitamin D, is removed, which makes the assimilation of fat-soluble vitamins difficult. Synthetic vitamin D is added to commercial milk to make up for its removal which is in the butterfat. But it has been shown to be toxic to the liver and have little beneficial effect. Skim milk is touted as a health food, but it is really anything but that and best left alone by children and adults alike.

The protein in milk (casein) is also harmed during pasteurization making it very difficult to digest. As we will see, many allergies and other illnesses can be attributed to this potentially harmful substance.

But raw milk (as is the case in all raw foods), the necessary enzymes to digest the sugars, fats and proteins, are already in the milk. So the nutrients in the milk are digested and absorbed with ease, eliminating the problems normally associated with pasteurized milk.

Many infants are allergic to pasteurized cow's milk, and newborns are seven times more likely to experience allergies related to cow's-milk proteins than to any other allergen. There are both immediate and delayed patterns of milk allergies. The immediate kind tend to be obvious and show up on skin tests. The delayed patterns are not so obvious and tend to produce chronic disease that is seldom diagnosed. Milk problems may be due to intolerance to the sugar found in milk (called lactose) or to the proteins found in milk. Symptoms that may indicate an adverse reaction to cow's-milk protein also include vomiting, diarrhea, abdominal pain, and rash. Later in life, symptoms may include asthma, sinus problems, eczema, hives, inflammation of the middle ear, intestinal problems, headaches, attention deficit/hyperactivity disorder, Crohn's disease, anemia, rheumatoid arthritis, and insulin-dependent diabetes mellitus. Lactose intolerance, as this condition is called, will produce acidic stools that contain glucose, whereas if protein is the problem the stools will be nonacidic and have flecks of blood.

Milk allergy, as opposed to lactose intolerance, is a protein problem and is not improved by changing the milk sugar. And although infant milk allergy is thought to be a specific and limited condition that children "outgrow," that can be misleading since many children continue to have chronic symptoms from milk (i.e. ear infections, sinus problems, skin problems). And even though the original problem may disappear, the pattern of illness merely changes and confuses parents and physicians.

Children with immediate anaphylactic reactions (severe reactions to a foreign protein) to cow's milk as infants, may exhibit a prolonged pattern of hypersensitivity with the development of multiple food and inhalant allergies, multiple hospitalizations, and frequent episodes of drug reactions. These children may continue to be hypersensitive and grow into adults with immune-sensitive diseases. There's enough evidence to suggest that pasteurized milk proteins play a major role in human disease at all ages. In fact, an Australian study of children who developed diabetes found that those given cow's milk formula in the first three months of life were 52 percent more likely to develop diabetes than those not fed milk. Overall, children who were breastfed had a 34 percent lower incidence of developing diabetes than formulafed infants. (33) Other studies corroborate these findings. (34,35,36)

There are at least 30 antigenic (producing an immune response) primary proteins in milk, and digestion probably increases this number to over 100. Casein is the most commonly used milk protein in the food industry, while others include lactalbumin, lactoglobulin, bovine albumin, and gamma globulin. These proteins tend to stay intact as milk is converted to dairy products of all types during food processing and are thus still present in the food. During digestion, milk proteins may induce the production of antibodies, which may trigger complex and variable immune responses. So even when milk allergy is suspected, simple skin tests with whole milk proteins may be misleading. (37)

Robert Cade, M.D., and his colleagues have now identified a milk protein, casomorphin, as a probable cause of attention deficit disorder and autism. They found Beta-casomorphin-7 in high concentrations in the blood and urine of patients with autism (and also patients with schizophrenia). In another study it was observed that casomorphin aggravated the symptoms of autism. Since brain allergies have been observed in ADHD, depression and schizophrenia, pasteurized milk, with its highly allergic tendencies, truly seems a likely potential cause of these conditions. (38) Other researchers have made similar conclusions. (39,40) In fact, the Autism Research Unit of the School of Health Sciences says on their website, "The quantities of these compounds [casomorphin byproducts from pasteurized milk], as found in the urine, are much too large to be of central nervous system origin. The quantities are such that they can only have been derived from the incomplete breakdown of certain foods." (i.e., pasteurized milk and pasteurized dairy products.)

Another problem with feeding cow's-milk products to your child is that cows are now treated with recombinant bovine growth hormone (rbGH). Although approved for use by the FDA, which says it has no metabolic effect on humans, the studies conducted to support its safety are suspect, and there are other studies that suggest that milk from cows treated with rbGH is a key factor in prostate cancer, breast cancer, and lung cancer. (41,42,43)

A popular alternative to cow's-milk-based formula is soy formula. The United States government promotes its use among recipients of WIC funds. Pediatricians frequently suggest it as an alternative for colicky babies whose tinny bodies cannot tolerate pasteurized cow's milk. But did you know that some consumer groups are calling for a ban on soy formula? That's right: because of the overwhelming evidence that soy is not good food for babies (or anyone else for that matter), consumer groups in New Zealand and Canada have called for a ban on the sale of soy infant formula.

Soy-based formula accounts for about 20 percent of the formula sold in the U.S., with about 25 percent of bottle-fed babies in the U.S. receive it. (44,45) Proponents of it say that the carbohydrates in most soy formulas are easily digested and absorbed by infants, and since it doesn't contain lactose, it does not cause milk-sugar problems. Over the past several years, soy has become more popular and widespread owing to promotions touting it as a good, healthy food.

However, soy is not a very good source of protein and babies who consume it don't absorb some of the minerals such as calcium very effectively. According to the American Academy of Pediatrics (AAP), "Healthy full-term infants should be given soy formula only when medically necessary." (46) Early exposure to soy through commercial infant formulas may be a leading cause of allergies among older children and adults. (47)

Another problem with soy-based formula and soy foods in general is that they contain high levels of isoflavones (sometimes called phytoestrogens), which act like estrogens (female sex hormones) in the body, thus upsetting hormonal balance. A 1998 study showed that hormonal effects on an infant exposed to isoflavones in soy formula are six to 11 times greater (based on body weight) than that same dose given to an adult consuming soy. Put another way, babies fed only on soy formula receive the estrogen equivalent of at least five birth control pills per day. What possible problems can this lead to?

First, let's consider how a normal baby develops. In males, there is a testosterone surge during the first few months of life (testosterone is the male sex hormone). If a male baby is taking in estrogen, this will upset the balance and possibly cause problems later in life. This is when the template for the expression of male sex characteristics and male behavior is set. A lack of testosterone impairs spatial perception, learning ability and tasks such as reading. Sexual orientation may also be affected during this time by improper hormonal balance.

In females, too much estrogen early in life may be contributing to the alarming increase in sexual abnormalities. In the journal *Pediatrics*, a survey found that 1 percent of all girls now show signs of puberty (such as breast development and pubic hair) by the age of three. By age eight, 14.7 percent of Caucasian girls and nearly 50 percent of African-American girls showed signs of puberty. Interestingly, soy formula is more commonly given to African-American babies because of a fear of milk allergy in these children. Early onset of puberty in girls has been associated with failure to menstruate, infertility, and breast cancer. (48)

There is other evidence that soy formula is harmful. Parents of babies fed soy have noticed symptoms such as extreme emotional behavior, asthma, immune system problems, pituitary insufficiency, thyroid disorders, and irritable bowel syndrome. Even after stopping consumption of soy, impaired thyroid function can last for up to three months. Soy formulas started becoming popular in the 1970s. Since then, learning disabilities and behavioral problems have reached epidemic proportions. (49)

Goiter and hypothyroidism were reported in infants fed soybean diets as early as 1960. Recent reports indicate that the plethora of adult thyroid disorders may be attributed to feeding soy-based infant formulas. A study of 37 adults showed that diffuse goiter and hypothyroidism appeared in half of the subjects after consuming 30 grams per day of pickled roasted soybeans for three months. Some researchers believe that soy isoflavones interfere with thyroid hormone synthesis. (50)

Soy contains a substance called goitrogens, which depress thyroid functioning. This in turn can cause growth retardation and sexual malfunctioning. Could this be why pediatricians are noticing greater numbers of boys whose physical maturation is delayed, or does not occur at all, including lack of development of the sexual organs?

Food for Thought

Remember, thyroid problems have been linked to the development of ADHD. And adults can be affected too in other more personal ways: celibate monks in Japan will intentionally eat large quantities of soy to dampen

---

their libido. It's no wonder it would do this because of all the estrogen it contains. I wonder if any of them ever developed enlarged breasts? My editor (the lovely and talented Amy), upon reading these comments, noted, "A friend of mine was receiving an herbal treatment to fight his prostate cancer. He later learned that the 'cocktail' contained large amounts of 'natural' estrogen. You guessed it – no sex drive. And breasts! Poor guy won't wear a T-shirt anymore..." Men, if you want a better sex life, don't eat the tofu! (With all the soy-foods foisted upon us, it's no wonder so many men have erectile dysfunction!) And men are not alone: as already noted, there's been a corresponding dramatic rise in early menarche (menstruation) in girls – a departure from the timetable nature set-up – and something that can be considered unhealthy.

Soy formulas, as all soy foods, are high in protein, but it's not well absorbed. This is because there are also potent enzyme inhibitors in soybeans as well. The most notable enzyme inhibitor blocks the action of trypsin, a protein necessary for protein digestion. In test animals, diets high in trypsin inhibitors depress overall growth and cause enlargement and pathological conditions of the pancreas, including cancer. Even in low amounts trypsin inhibitors prevent normal growth in rats. (51)

Although the soy industry knows this is a problem and has spent millions of dollars to determine the best way to remove trypsin inhibitors, they have not been completely successful. One way to get them out is to subject the soy to considerable periods of heat treatment. But this in turn over-denatures other proteins in soy, especially lysine, and excessive heat also makes these proteins difficult to digest and possibly toxic.

Soybeans also contain high levels of phytic acid, also called phytates, an organic acid that blocks the uptake of essential minerals such as calcium, magnesium, iron, and especially zinc. In 1967, researchers were aware that phytates found in soy formula caused a negative zinc balance in every infant to whom soy formula was given. Research has also shown a strong correlation between phytate content in formula and poor growth, even when the diets were additionally supplemented with zinc. (52)

Food for Thought

One popular "health-food" way of eating is called the "macrobiotic" diet, which stresses the consumption of a lot of grains and soy foods. (Grains also contain phytic acid, as do seeds.) Children on this kind of diet have consistently shown retarded growth. And in infants this is especially problematic because it causes a delay in the accumulation of lipids (fats) in the myelin (the nerve's protective sheath) and hence jeopardizes the development of the brain and nervous system. One way to decrease the phytates in grains, nuts, and seeds is to soak them overnight in water. This deactivates the phytates and thus allows more efficient mineral absorption. So if you're making a rice dinner, for example, soak the rice overnight in water. It will be better for you and your children.

"Soy protein isolate" (SPI) is the main ingredient in soy formula. It's a powder extracted from soybeans through a process that involves not only high temperatures but also caustic chemicals. The alkaline soaking solution produces a carcinogen lysinealine, and reduces the cystine content (already low in the soybean) necessary for proper growth. Other carcinogens called nitrosamines are formed during high-temperature spray drying and are often found in soy protein foods. If that's not enough, a number of other substances of questionable safety are added to soy formulas, including BHA, BHT and sodium hydroxide (caustic soda).

Scientific studies of soy's deleterious effects find it to be quite dangerous. Test animals fed SPI develop enlarged organs, particularly the pancreas and thyroid gland, and increased deposition of fatty acids in the liver. (53) Aluminum is 10 times greater in soy formula than milk-based formula. It has a toxic effect on the kidneys of infants and has been implicated as causing Alzheimer's in adults. Soy formulas also lack cholesterol, another nutrient that is essential for the development of the brain and nervous system. And soy formulas lack lactose and galactose, sugars that play an important role in the development of the nervous system as well. Soy increases the requirements for vitamins E,K,D, and B-12, a nutrient vital for good health and can create deficiency symptoms of calcium, magnesium, manganese, molybdenum, copper, iron, and zinc. And early studies showed that soy blocks the uptake of fats, vitally necessary for the growing infant and child. (54)

If all this about soy isn't enough, consider this: soy infant formula is loaded with manganese – up to 200 times the amount found in breast milk. Can this be harmful? You bet. Researchers at the University of California at Irvine, noted that scalp hair of hyperactive children and youths detained for felony crimes had elevated levels of manganese. Francis M. Crinella, one of these researchers says, "Manganese ingested during a period of rapid brain growth [that is, infancy] and deposited in the critical [areas of the brain] may affect behavior during puberty when powerful stresses are unleashed... and altered behavioral patterns appear." (55)

Infants' FDA daily requirements for manganese are excessively high and were determined by calculating backwards from adolescent requirements. This does not take into the account of the unique characteristics of the infant's digestive tract, which acts like a sponge with manganese. It does this because human milk is so low in it, and the baby must absorb most of the manganese it ingests in order to get enough. Excess manganese is not only harmful to the developing brain, but can be outright toxic to the baby. Researchers theorize that part of the increase in ADHD and adolescent violence may be due to the high manganese content of the soy formulas they were raised on. (56)

The Truth About Children's Health

Soy's influence begins even before a baby is born. There's now evidence that indicates consuming the phytoestrogens found in soy may impact a developing fetus. Phytoestrogens have estrogenic effects on the human body, and although they may help women who are past their childbearing years deal with unpleasant symptoms of menopause, they are dangerous for pregnant women, having been shown to affect the organization of tissues in utero. (58) So if mom is eating something that acts like a sex hormone (i.e. phytoestrogen), it's logical to conclude that it could change the baby's development.

Phytoestrogens influence the way the brain is organized, the way the reproductive organs and cells develop, and the way the immune function develops. That has been shown in animal studies and in pregnant women as well. In a study in Los Angeles, it was found that about 80 percent of the fetuses of pregnant women were exposed to estrogenic isoflavones at concentrations from 20 to 180 times the levels of naturally occurring female sex hormones in the amniotic fluid. Since this happened during critical stages of the baby's development, various organs might be adversely effected. (59)

Female rats fed genistein (an isoflavone that is known to have significant estrogenic properties) during pregnancy produced pups that were more masculine than usual. This was due to the fact that the genistein actually caused the mother's hormonal system to alter its hormones, thus changing the kind of hormones transferred to the developing fetus. The rat pups also showed early onset of puberty (which is what we're currently seeing in children). (60) In similar studies, genistein has been shown to cause irreversible damage to the enzymes that synthesize thyroid hormones (in rat studies). (61)

Soy formulas started becoming popular in the 1970s. Since then, learning disabilities and behavioral problems have reached epidemic proportions. Given soy's proven adverse effects – in utero, infancy, during childhood, and beyond – it seems more than just a coincidence.

Formula Recalls

Between 1982 and 1994 alone, there were 22 significant infant formula recalls in the United States – of products made by well-known companies including Nestle (Carnation), Abbott, Mead Johnson, Wyeth, and Nutricia. At least seven of these were classified by the Food and Drug Administration as Class I, meaning health problems could be life-threatening to babies who were fed the tainted formula. (62). Why the recall? Products were recalled for such things as contamination by salmonella, klebsiella pneumoniae, and bits of glass. (63)

- In early June 1999, Mead Johnson, makers of the infant formula brands Enfamil and Prosobee, reported that 120,000 cans of formula shipped to stores were being recalled due to a labeling mistake that could lead to "severe medical problems" in some babies. Company officials said cans labeled as infant formula could actually contain the adult nutritional supplement Vanilla Sustacal!

- In April 1999, 75,000 32-ounce cans of Nestle's Carnation Good Start brand infant formula were recalled due to the product's having curdled. No mention of this recall was made on Carnation's promotional web site for parents.

- In June 1993, 102,048 cans of Nutramigen brand infant formula were recalled from the U.S. and Canada because the product was contaminated with glass particles.

- In June 1997, 104 cases of Isomil brand soy protein infant formula with iron were recalled because they did not contain the labeled amount of inositol, a nutrient required by law.

- In September 1996, 2,764 cases of Alsoy soy formula were recalled because the lids stated "Do Not Add Water," when in fact the formula was supposed to be diluted.

- In July 1993, Soylac Powder infant formula was recalled because it was contaminated with salmonella. (64,65)

You may be under the impression that the FDA closely and carefully monitors infant formula, considering its prevalence in our children's diets. But the FDA sets only minimal standards regarding the production and sale of synthetic milks. The mandated nutrient requirements for formula are contained in the outdated Infant Formula Act of 1980, which the U.S. Congress passed in reaction to a formula-manufacturing error that flooded the market with chloride-deficient formula. Today, manufacturers are required simply to include an insignificant number of mandated ingredients and to list them on the package. (66)

As you can see there are many problems associated with infant formula, whether cow's-milk based or soy-based. There's a simple way to get around all these problems: Breastfeed your baby! You'll even save money. But, if you must use formula, I would definitely stay away from the soy-based ones. Pasteurized cow's milk has its problems, but soy to me seems far more damaging. Also, check frequently to see if there have been any recalls, go to the FDA website: (www.fda.gov).

What to Feed Your Baby

So now that we've examined the wrong way to feed your infant, let's take a look at the right way. First, let's go over what your baby needs from the very beginning – even before he is conceived.

As previously mentioned, Weston Price, D.D.S., traveled the world examining the dietary habits of primitive peoples. He found that a common practice among these isolated groups was that special foods were customarily fed to both men and women for a period of time before conception to ensure the healthiest egg and sperm. These foods were very rich in fat-soluble vitamins A and D as well as macro and trace minerals.

The importance of fat-soluble vitamins, especially vitamin A, cannot be overemphasized. Vitamin A is considered to be the catalyst on which all other biological processes depend. It is vital for efficient mineral uptake and the utilization of water-soluble vitamins. Price demonstrated that generous amounts of vitamin A will help ensure healthy reproductive capabilities and healthy offspring. He found that the healthy "primitive" peoples' diets oftentimes contained 10 times more vitamin A than the typical American diet. When these people went on the "white-man's" diet, which included refined grains and sugar and less natural food, Price found that among other problems, vitamin A deficiencies resulted. This contributed to high infant mortality, blindness, stunting, bone deformities, and susceptibility to infection. (67)

Foods rich in vitamin A include organ meats (liver, heart, kidney, etc.), cod liver oil, and butter. The foods that pregnant and nursing mothers received in these primitive cultures included fish heads, fish eggs, shellfish, insects, organ meats, and animal fats – all rich in vitamins A and D. (You may want to leave out the insects!) And primitive man ate much of his animal foods uncooked which preserved much of its nutrition.

Sally Fallon, nutrition researcher and author, advises:

> Couples planning to have children should eat liberally of organic liver and other organ meats, fish eggs and other seafood, eggs and the best quality butter, cream, and fermented milk products they can obtain for at least six months before conception. A daily cod liver oil supplement is also advised. Organic meats, vegetables, grains and legumes should round out the diet, with a special emphasis on the leafy green vegetables rich in folic acid, which is necessary for the prevention of birth defects like spina bifida... A good rule of thumb for pregnant women is liver once a week, at least two eggs per day [preferably raw] and 1 tablespoon cod liver oil daily. A daily ration of superfoods, such as evening primrose oil, bee pollen, mineral powder, wheat germ oil, and acerola will provide optimal amounts of nutrients for your unborn child... (68)

It's important for your growing child to get enough fat in the diet. Newborns must derive 50 percent of the calories they consume from dietary fat. Fat is essential for normal growth from infancy on, since fats provide fatty acids, the building block children need for critical metabolic programming of brain growth and development.

The brain is 60 percent fat. Most brain tissue is formed after a child is born. When very young, children go through a process called myelination. This is when the brain and nerve cells are coated with a fatty myelin sheath that permits electrical transmission and chemical messages between the brain and nerve cells. Processed cow's milk doesn't contain enough linoleic acid, so it's not advisable to feed it to a child younger than 12 months old. (69)

The Truth About Children's Health

Never feed your baby anything that contains trans-fatty acids. This includes margarine, shortening, and baked goods containing these products. Trans-fatty acids inhibit the interconversion of fatty acids needed for normal brain growth. They may impair or delay essential developmental processes in your child. Read the labels. Most "junk foods" including chips, pretzels, and fast foods are made with trans-fatty acids. (70)

Food for Thought

A couple notes on cod liver oil are in order here. First, high doses of cod liver oil are not advisable, since it has been shown to be toxic in high amounts. One to two tablespoon a day for adults and a half-teaspoon a day for babies and children is all that's needed. Buy cod liver oil in dark bottles and store in a cool, dark place. A good brand of cod liver oil is the "Dale Alexander" brand. It comes straight or in orange or cherry flavors. The orange flavor doesn't taste bad at all. Also, Dr. Price found that cod liver oil worked best when butter was included in the diet – he always gave cod liver oil with butter. Get the best raw organic butter you can find – you may want to find a local farmer or dairy who makes his own butter from pasture-fed cows.

It's important to consume nutrient-dense foods during six months before conception and nine months of pregnancy. Ms. Fallon also recommends a "cleansing fast" to be taken six months or more before conception: Avoid all sugar, white flour, hydrogenated and rancid vegetable oils, tobacco, caffeine and alcohol, and oral contraceptives should be avoided during this "fasting" period. (Oral contraceptives deplete the body of zinc, the "intelligence mineral.") Once the baby is born. "It must be emphasized, however, that the quality of mother's milk depends greatly on her diet. Sufficient animal products will ensure proper amounts of vitamin B-12, A, and D as well as all-important minerals like zinc in her milk. Lactating women should continue with a diet that emphasizes liver, eggs, and cod liver oil. Whole raw milk products and stock made from bones will ensure that her baby receives adequate calcium." (71)

Food for Thought

Vegetarians reading this are probably ready to throw this book out the window. It's understandable to feel resistance when one's personal beliefs are challenged. If vegetarianism works for you, fine. But please remember that your child really needs fats and animal products to develop a fully wired nervous system. Once they are adults, they don't need the same amounts of fat and fatty acids quite so much – that is to say, it's not so important for development (but still important for maintenance – remember the study that showed adults supplementing with DHA had improved mental function).

Also remember that all of the primitive cultures Weston Price visited that had superb health (before the white man came with his white flour and sugar) ate many animal products. Personally, I have yet to see a truly healthy vegetarian. Many of them look pasty white and are mentally spacey with low endurance. As I mentioned before, I was a vegetarian for more than a decade and I did not get where I wanted to with my health. It wasn't easy to start eating animal foods again for mental and moral reasons. But we are on this planet to thrive, and if eating animal foods gets us there, then that's what was meant to be.

In her impressive book, *Nourishing Traditions*, Sally Fallon gives recipes for homemade formula that, although not as good as mother's milk, is much better than any store-bought formula. There is some time and effort involved in making formula from scratch, but isn't your baby worth it? Some of the ingredients may be unfamiliar, but they can be obtained from a good health food store or mail-order sources. (*Nourishing Traditions* can be ordered from The Weston A. Price Foundation at (202) 333-HEAL – I highly recommend it.)

Milk-Based Formula (makes 36 ounces)

2 cups	organic, certified clean, raw milk or organic pasteurized, nonhomogenized milk cultured with piima (see "1" below) or kefir grains (see "2" below), preferably from pasture-fed Jersey or Guernsey cows
1/4 cup	homemade liquid whey (see "3" below)
4 tbsp	lactose (see "4" below)
1 tsp	bifodobacterium infantis (see "5" below)
2 tbsp	good quality cream (not ultrapasteurized: pasteurized is OK and raw is best)
1 tsp	cod liver oil
1 tsp	unrefined sunflower oil (see "6" below)
1 tsp	extra virgin olive oil
2 tsp	coconut oil
2 tsp	brewer's yeast
2 tsp	gelatin (see "7" below)
1 7/8 cups	filtered water
1 100-mg	tablet acerola, crushed (see "8" below)

Add gelatin to water and heat gently until gelatin is dissolved. Place all ingredients in a very clean glass or stainless steel container and mix well (Note: If milk is from Holstein cows, add an additional 1 to 2 tablespoons cream). To serve, pour 6 to 8 ounces into a very clean glass bottle, attach nipple, and set in a pan of

The Truth About Children's Health

simmering water. Heat until warm but not hot to the touch, shake bottle well, and feed baby. (Never, never heat formula in a microwave oven!)

Goat Milk Formula Variation:

Although goat milk is rich in fat, it must be used with caution in infant feeding as it lacks folic acid and is low in vitamin B-12, both of which are essential to the growth and development of the infant. Inclusion of brewer's yeast to provide folic acid is essential. To compensate for low levels of vitamin B-12, add 2 teaspoons frozen organic raw chicken liver, finely grated, to the batch of formula. Be sure to begin egg-yolk feeding at four months.

About the ingredients:

1. Piima Milk is made as follows:

1 quart fresh whole milk, nonhomogenized

1 tbsp starter culture: 1 cup good quality cream, 1 envelope piima powder

Start with the best quality cream you can find, such as the thick old-fashioned cream available at health food stores and gourmet food shops. Raw cream is best, but pasteurized cream will do. Do not use ultrapasteurized cream – it doesn't contain enough nutrients to support your culture. Find a place in your house where the temperature is a fairly constant 72 to 75 degrees F, such as a closet or cupboard with a light bulb or a shelf over a refrigerator or near a heating vent. Place the cream in an impeccably clean glass jar. Stir in the piima powder and cover tightly. Leave in a spot that is 72 to 75 degrees F for about 24 hours until it thickens slightly. Transfer to refrigerator, where it will become firm. The culture will keep well chilled for several months. Always test it with your nose before using. If it smells bad, throw it out and start again. Do not use ultrapasteurized or homogenized milk. Place milk in a clean glass container. Add the starter, stir or shake well, cover tightly and place in a spot where the temperature is a stable 72 to 75 degrees F for 20 to 24 hours. Cultured milk does not thicken as does yogurt, but remains rather liquid. Chill well. Use in the preparation of cream cheese and whey, grain dishes and baby formula. Using piima is a good way to add enzymes and restore nutrients to pasteurized milk. Try to find milk from a dairy that allows its cows (or goats) to pasture-feed.

2. Kefir Grains can be obtained from G.E.M. Cultures, (707) 964-2922.

3. Homemade Liquid Whey: (makes about 1 cup whey and 2 1/2 cups cheese)

1 quart best-quality whole natural yogurt. You can use commercial yogurt if it is of the very best quality, containing no sweeteners or fillers. Place the yogurt in a strainer lined with cheese cloth or a clean linen dish towel, placed over a bowl. Cover with a plate and leave at room temperature for 12 to 24 hours, while the whey runs out. After the whey has run out into the bowl, you may tie up the cheese cloth or linen towel with the milk solids inside, being careful not to squeeze. Tie this little sack to a wooden spoon placed across the top of a bowl or pitcher so that more whey can drip out of the bag. When the bag stops dripping,

the cheese is ready. Store whey in a mason jar and cream cheese in a covered glass container. Refrigerated, the yogurt cheese will keep for about one month and the whey for about six months.

4. Lactose can be obtained from The Apothecary, (301) 530-0800.

5. Bifidobacterium Infantis (a beneficial bacteria) can be obtained from Life Start by Natren, (800) 992-3323.

6. Good-quality sunflower oil can be obtained from Omega Nutrition as the Arrowhead brand in health food stores or by mail order at (800) 661-3529.

7. Coconut Oil can be obtained from Omega Nutrition at (800) 661-3529, Carotec (800)522-4279, or Radiant Life (888) 593-8333.

8. Gelatin: Bernard Jensen Gelatin (made from beef) may be ordered from L & H Vitamins, (800) 221-1152 or P.K. Health Products, (619) 468-3543. (This is preferred to Knox gelatin since it's made from beef, not chicken.)

9. Acerola Tablets: Springreen (800) 544-8147. (Acerola has a very high vitamin C content.)

A meat-based formula is given below. This liver-based formula closely mimics the nutrient profile of mother's milk. In both the milk- and meat-based formulas, it's important to use truly "cold pressed" oils, otherwise they may lack vitamin E.

Meat-Based Formula:

3 3/4 cups	homemade chicken broth (see "1a" below)
2 ounces	organic liver, cut into small pieces
5 tbsp	lactose (see "4" above)
1 tsp	bifodobacterium infantis (see "5" above)
1/4 cup	homemade liquid whey (see "3" above)
1 tbsp	coconut oil (see "7" above)
2 tsp	coconut oil
1 tsp	cod liver oil
1 tsp	unrefined sunflower oil (see "6" above)
2 tsp	extra virgin olive oil
1 100-mg	tablet acerola, crushed (see "9" above)

Simmer liver gently in broth until the meat is cooked through. Liquefy using a hand-held blender or in a food processor. When the liver broth has cooled, stir in remaining ingredients. Store in a very clean glass or stainless steel container. To serve, stir formula well and pour 6 to 8 ounces in a very clean glass bottle. Attach a clean nipple and set in a pan of simmering water until formula is warm but not hot to the touch, shake well and feed to baby. (Again, never heat formula in a microwave oven!) It is very important to include the coconut oil in this formula as it is the recipe's *only* source or antimicrobial saturated fatty acids.

1a.   Chicken Broth:

>1   whole free-range chicken, or 2 to 3 pounds of bony chicken parts, such as necks, backs, breastbones and wings
>
>gizzards from one chicken (optional)
>
>feet from the chicken (optional)

4 quarts   cold filtered water

2 tbsp   raw apple cider vinegar

>1   large onion, coarsely chopped
>
>2   carrots, peeled and coarsely chopped
>
>3   celery stalks, coarsely chopped

1 bunch   parsley

If you are using a whole chicken, cut off the wings and remove the neck, fat glands and the gizzards from the cavity. By all means, use chicken feet if you can find them – they are full of gelatin (Jewish folklore considers the addition of chicken feet the secret to successful broth.) Even better, use a whole chicken, with the head on. These may be found in Oriental markets. Farm-raised, free-range chickens give the best results. Many battery-raised chickens will not produce stock that gels. Cut chicken parts into several pieces including the neck and wings. Place chicken or chicken pieces in a large stainless steel pot with water, vinegar and all vegetables except parsley. Let stand 30 minutes to 1 hour. Bring to a boil, and remove scum that rises to the top. Reduce heat, cover and simmer for six to 24 hours. The longer you cook the stock, the richer and more flavorful it will be. About 10 minutes before finishing the stock, add parsley. This will impart additional mineral ions to the broth. Remove whole chicken or pieces with a slotted spoon. If you are using a whole chicken, let cool and remove chicken meat from the carcass. Reserve for other uses such as chicken salads, enchiladas, and sandwiches. Strain the stock into a large bowl and put in refrigerator until the fat rises to the top and congeals. Skim off this fat and store the stock in covered containers in refrigerator or freezer. (72)

Let's compare the nutritional value of cow's milk vs. goat milk: goat's milk contains 13 percent more calcium, 25 percent more vitamin B-6, 47 percent more vitamin A, 134 percent more potassium, three times more niacin, four times more copper, 27 percent more antioxidant selenium. Cow's milk contains five times as much vitamin B-12 and 10 times as much folic acid.

Goat's milk contains less lactose, better for lactose-intolerant babies. It has more fat and this fat is easier to digest (owing to the fact that goat's milk does not contain agglutinin, so the fat globules don't cluster together). And goat's milk protein forms a softer curd that is easier and more rapidly digestible. Since most milk allergies are caused by milk protein intolerance, this is a major reason allergic reactions to goat's milk is less common. (73) Goat's milk has been shown to be less allergenic and babies fed goat's milk are less likely to develop colic and constipation.

However, goat's milk is low in iron, folic acid, and vitamins C and D and has a high solute load relative to cow's or mother's milk. Therefore, it should not be fed in the first month of life because it may cause metabolic acidosis. (74)

Given that goat's milk is deficient in some key and essential nutrients, if goat's milk is to be used as a substitute for human breast milk, it should be fortified with these nutrients. A baby on goat's milk formula should also receive a multi-vitamin with iron supplement prescribed by her doctor. In infants over one year of age, goat's milk can be readily used instead of cow's milk. Be sure to buy goat's milk that is certified free of antibiotics and bovine growth hormone (BGH). For more information about goat's milk call 805-565-1538 or 800-343-1185. (75)

Raw food is not only good for babies, but necessary for proper growth. Don't be afraid *not* to cook some of the ingredients in the above recipes. A quick and easy meal for baby is: 1 ounce fresh, wild-caught fish; 1 raw egg; 3 tablespoons raw cream; 1/4 cup fresh organic liver; 2 ounces raw milk; and 1/2 teaspoon raw honey. Blend in blender. If the child can eat solid food, feed as is. If an infant, strain through cloth or strainer, put in bottle and use nipple with large hole.

Food for Thought

Remember, all commercial formula is heat-treated (pasteurized), so again, the best alternative is to breastfeed your baby! If you're going back to work, you may consider pumping breast milk for later consumption. Expert Sue Gilber, M.S., recommends calling the experts in nursing, La Leche League, at (800)-LALECHE, or contacting a lactation consultant to learn more about how, why and the best way to pump breast milk.

It's wise to give all babies – whether breastfed or bottle-fed – a raw egg yolk a day (from free range chickens), starting at about 4 months old. Egg yolks supply the needed cholesterol for mental development, important sulfur-containing amino acids and omega-3 long-chain fatty acids found in mother's milk but that may be lacking in cow's milk. Doing so will help the child speak and take directions at an early age. Egg white, however, should not be given before the age of one year old since it contains difficult-to-digest proteins. (76)

When the time comes to add solid food to baby's diet, avoid cereal. Cereal grains should never be fed to infants. They are not equipped to handle cereals, especially wheat, before the age of one year since infants produce only tiny amounts of amylase, the enzyme needed to digest cereals. Some experts prohibit all grains before the age of two. Feeding babies cereals too early can lead to grain allergies later on.

The baby's first real food should be animal products, since his digestive system is better equipped to supply enzymes for digestion of proteins and fats than carbohydrates. (77) Grated, raw organic liver can be added to the child's diet at six months. It's rich in iron, a mineral which may be low in mother's milk. (African mothers chew liver before giving it to their baby as their first food.)

Bananas can be added at age six months. At 10 months, meats, fruits, and vegetables may be introduced, one at a time. If any adverse reactions take place, you'll be able to tell which one caused the problem. Potatoes, carrots, turnips, and other starchy vegetables can be given but should be mashed with butter. Orange-colored vegetables should be given in moderation since the baby's immature liver may have difficulty converting the carotenoids to vitamin A. If the baby's skin turns yellowish, discontinue the orange vegetables for a while.

A little buttermilk or yogurt can help with digestion. Remember, your growing child needs a lot of fat, much of it saturated, for optimal physical and mental development, so don't deprive him or her of animal foods.

A popular trend these days is to give babies fruit juices, especially apple juice. Mothers mistakenly think that this is a wholesome healthy beverage. However, the simple carbohydrates often spoil an infant's appetite for more nutritious foods, and the sugar-alcohol called sorbitol found in apple juice is difficult to digest. Studies have shown children struggle to thrive with diets high in apple juice. High-fructose foods are especially dangerous for growing children. All this sugar creates and acid environment in the body, and minerals needed for growth must be used instead to neutralize this acid. This can seriously hamper infant development. [78] (Recall that high-fructose corn syrup is just as bad if not worse than unhealthy table sugar.)

As for fat vs. fitness, babies should be chubby, with fat around their ankles, knees, elbows, and wrists. This fat ensures adequate nourishment to the growth plates at the ends of the bones. Babies with fat on them grow into sturdy children. Children, likewise, should be sturdy and strong, not slim. They too, need that fat to grow and develop properly.

The better you feed your baby in the beginning, the more likely he will desire nutritious foods as an adult and the better his body will be able to handle less-than-ideal foods later in life.

Baby Food

Most parents don't think twice about feeding their baby food from a jar. It has become a common occurrence and almost a tradition. Companies like Gerber's have made it very convenient for mothers to just pop open a jar and spoon it into trusting little mouths. But is it good enough for your baby? Does it have the right nutrition, and is it pure enough for the sensitive infant?

Susan B. Roberts, Ph.D., professor of nutrition at Tufts University School of Nutrition Science and Policy in Boston, says, "As a nutrition researcher, I have spent 20 years studying the importance of healthy food at all stages of life... Studies from my own laboratory and others around the world have taught me that the foods my daughter eats during the first months and years of life have long-lasting – and in some cases – permanent effects. Foods make an important difference in virtually everything – from mental and physical development to vitality, personality and health from childhood through old age." [79]

Melvin B. Heyman, M.D., and professor of pediatrics at the University of California in San Francisco, tells us that the foods babies eat can have a direct influence on disease, "One recent study reported that children who eat a diet with plenty of fruits and vegetables and very few high-nitrite foods – such as hot dogs, ham, bacon and sausage – have only one-seventh to one-tenth the incidence of leukemia seen in children with poor nutrition." (80)

Food for Thought

Children who consume many vegetables and few processed meats have a lower incidence of leukemia. Please don't take this to mean that your child should not eat animal foods and be a vegetarian. "Bad" foods Melvin Heyman, M.D., mentions have high nitrites because they are artificially treated with them. Good clean, organically raised bacon or sausage is fine in moderation. But don't buy nitrate-laden commercially prepared bacon and other processed meats from the regular supermarkets and feed it to your child.

The average baby eats 600 of those little jars of baby food (including baby food juices) in his or her first year of life. Some 1.78 billion jars are sold per year and three companies, Gerber, Heinz, and Beech-Nut, sell 96 percent of these. All three of these companies sell products in three stages: stage one for children up to six month of age; stage two for children from six to nine months and; stage three for children nine month and older. (81)

Aside from their actual nutritional content, there is a growing concern that these foods are contaminated with alarming levels of pesticides. The Environmental Working Group reports that in lab tests of eight brand-name baby foods made by the three companies that dominate the market, pesticides were found in seven of the eight foods. These pesticides (which not only kill bugs or fungus but also cause cancer, mutations, nervous system disorders, and hormonal disruptions in laboratory studies) have never been tested for safety in the way that babies are exposed to them. The federal government currently allows these levels. (82)

This study showed that infants are eating mixtures of many different pesticides in baby foods (and getting another dose of pesticides from drinking water or bug sprays and weed killers used around the home). This toxic load accumulates in the baby.

Results from testing done by the Food and Drug Administration on baby foods also found problems. The FDA tests baby foods for pesticides as part of its Total Diet Study (TDS). Under the TDS, the FDA purchases and tests 234 foods four times per year and tests them for pesticides and other contaminants. In 1993, the FDA reported finding dozens of pesticides in baby food purchased in grocery stores and tested in the TDS during the years 1985 through 1991. In the 227 samples tested during the seven-year period, the FDA found 12 pesticides in applesauce, 11 in pears, and seven in green beans, peaches, plums/prunes. The pesticides found most often were phosalone, dicloran, endosulfan, chlorpyriphos, and parathion. Perhaps more shocking, DDT was found in 26 of 27 baby beef dinners, 19 out of 27 chicken or turkey dinners, and 16 out of 27 pork dinner samples. No single company's products tested were significantly less contaminated than any other's. (83)

Food for Thought

Although the National Academy of Sciences reported in 1993 that current pesticide standards are out of date and allow too much pesticide in food and too little protection for infants, Congress is now considering weakening pesticide standards. Several bills (encouraged by special interest groups (i.e., the chemical companies) moving through Congress would allow many more – and more toxic – pesticides in all foods, including baby food. And to top it all off, a rider to EPA's appropriations bill would actually prohibit EPA from removing a number of carcinogenic pesticides from the market. The 104th Congress is moving to repeal several long-standing pesticide safety standards, in particular the Delaney clause, which bans cancer-causing pesticides that concentrate in processed food. This rollback of federal protections will allow more carcinogens and other pesticides not only in processed foods, but also in the raw foods that they're made from. If that is repealed, concentrations of pesticides in baby foods will almost certainly increase. (84)

Even the present standards for pesticide exposure are too high. Remember, an infant or child has a different physiology than an adult and is more sensitive since his or her organs of elimination and immune system are not fully developed and the metabolism is different. Therefore, young kids cannot throw off poisons as easily as an adult. But the existing regulations and standards are designed to protect an average person with an average diet from an average pesticide. Infants and children do not fit that mold. In spite of the evidence, the EPA evaluates the safety of most pesticides using protocols that require testing only sexually mature animals and these tests provide little or no information relevant to fetal, infant, and childhood exposure. Regulations would have to be tightened significantly to protect our youngsters.

And despite volumes of evidence supporting this from reputable sources, our government is going the other way. You know, I have mentioned many times that it's all about money. But sometimes as I evaluate the

---

obvious conclusions of all this research, I wonder if they're not trying to make us sick and kill us off on purpose. However, since these poisons become ubiquitous in our environment and food supply, they're going to sicken and kill the very people who are responsible for our toxic planet as well.

Store-bought baby foods are often overprocessed and contain unnecessary food additives. Although the label may say there's no added sugar, the manufacturer may still add fruit syrups and other sweeteners that can not only upset the baby's stomach but cause him to develop a sweet tooth that may last his whole lifetime, causing other nutritional problems along the way. High levels of nitrates have been found in many store-bought baby foods including beets, carrots, green beans, squash, turnips, spinach, and collard greens. (85)

Vital nutrients can be lost during production of commercial baby foods, so manufacturers may "fortify" their purees with vitamins and minerals. But these added synthetic vitamins and minerals are not nearly so good as the natural ones found in food. These foods are most often overprocessed, which may prolong shelf life, but does serious damage to the nutritional quality.

The best thing to do is to make your own baby foods. Use a blender to make a mush or puree from fresh and wholesome foods. These will taste better and contain more nutrition. Don't cook the ingredients too long since many vitamins are destroyed by heat. Make sure your child gets plenty of raw, uncooked foods. Of course, breastfeed your baby as long as possible – even up to two years of age.

Please note that the values in the tables below are mostly RDAs (Recommended Dietary Allowances) which are set to basically prevent starvation. Many doctors recommend higher amounts of many of these nutrients.

Foods Your Baby Needs

Fats

Many children are picky eaters. They often prefer heavier, fatty foods. Allow them these foods, making sure they are pure and organically grown or raised and raw as often as possible - raw butter, eggs, dairy, cold-pressed oils,. Children's bodies are telling them that they need that fat, and it's important they get it.

Daily Fat Requirements (Percent calories from fat)

Age	Amount
Under 6 months	50 percent
6-12 months	40 percent
1-2 years	35-40 percent
2-3 years	35-40 percent
3-6 years	35-40 percent
Adults	30-35 percent

Most people, especially children, benefit from the right kind of fat in the diet. Avoid all processed foods with hydrogenated fats and polyunsaturated oils. Use traditional vegetable oils like extra virgin olive oil and small amounts of unrefined fax seed oil. (The recent fad of canola oil is not beneficial and is explored in greater detail in Chapter XIII.) Coconut oil is good for baking, and using animal fats for frying is OK. Cooking like our grandparents did on the farm with lard and fatback is, believe it or not, much healthier than the way we do it now with hydrogenated margarines and imitation fats. Egg yolks and butter contain fats and nutrients essential for proper growth and maintenance. Eat as much raw, unheated fat as possible. The Eskimos do and they have the lowest incidences of heart disease in the world.

Food for Thought

Although the popular medical dogma has linked coronary heart disease and other problems with dietary fats, much research has shown this to simply not be true. The rise in coronary heart disease has increased as the consumption of margarine and other trans fatty acid fats have increased. Chemically made and synthetic products are never as good as the natural ones. More and more doctors are coming around to recommending diets high in the natural, beneficial animal fats like butter and wholesome oils like cold-pressed olive oil.

Fiber

Although it's important for adults to get enough fiber in their diets, it's not so important for babies and children. Babies lack the proper enzymes to process fiber and they don't need it at all in their diet. At about age two, the child should get minimal amounts of fiber, mostly from fruits and vegetables. About 3/4 to 1 1/2 cups of these a day is a good amount.

Daily Fiber Requirements

Age	Amount (grams)
Under 1	0
1-3 years	5-8
4-8 years	9-11
Adults	25-30

5 grams equals one teaspoon

Calories

Many Americans are obsessed with counting calories (a measure of the energy a food gives). However, as long as your child is eating healthily, this is a minor concern. Let your children eat freely of good quality foods, and their weight will take care of itself. Remember, a baby should be chubby and a toddler should be sturdy, not skinny.

Minerals

Minerals are involved in countless metabolic and enzymatic reactions in the human body. They're necessary to maintain and build strong bones, teeth, muscle, and tissue. The body needs a constant supply of these minerals since it cannot manufacture them on its own. Now, many nutritional experts suggest that many of today's degenerative diseases such as diabetes, heart disease, strokes, arteriosclerosis, and hypertension are caused by long-term nutritional deficiencies. Considering that recent studies have shown that 50 percent of children don't get enough iron, calcium, and zinc these diseases can start very early in life. [86]

Not only are minerals essential from a nutritional standpoint, but they also provide protection against pollutants as well. Since many minerals have similar physical and chemical properties, if there's a deficiency of one mineral, another mineral or substance which is similar but toxic may take it's place in biochemical reactions. Cadmium, silver, arsenic, and lithium – all toxic – can take the place of zinc, copper, phosphorus, and sodium respectively – all necessary for health. When the healthy minerals are present, they tend to neutralize the potentially harmful ones.

The best source of minerals is natural, wholesome food. Mineral supplements, although sometimes necessary, do not offer the mineral to the body in the form it can most easy absorb and use, and oftentimes contain toxic additives or ingredients. The best ways to ingest minerals are through mineral-rich water, fresh vegetable juices, nutrient-dense foods (raw), and meat and bone broths. Some traditional societies even add small amounts of fine clay or mud as a supplement. Clay compounds not only provide minerals but can also act as detoxifying agents. A good mineral powder is Azomite Mineral Powder.

Iron

Iron is the most important, and oftentimes lacking, mineral for your child. It's a vital part of hemoglobin (the protein in red blood cells that transports oxygen through the body) and many of the body's enzyme systems. Iron is essential for myelination of nerve cells in the brain and peripheral nervous system during the first two years of life. Not enough iron can cause permanent damage to motor and mental functions, leading to lower IQ and poor attention span along with aberrant social behavior.

A newborn's liver has a store of iron. Breastfed babies usually don't need additional iron until they're six months old. If the mother is feeding herself correctly with organ meats, egg yolks, and so on, additional iron is not necessary when breastfeeding. Bottle-fed babies are a different story. The homemade formulas recommended earlier are loaded with iron in a form the baby can use. All baby formulas on the market are fortified with iron, of course, but their other problems make that a small consolation.

If you're giving your baby (after four months old) an egg yolk a day, additional iron is probably not needed. Red meat also contains a lot of iron, and introducing it to your baby after 10 months (other than in the meat-based formula above) is advisable.

Vitamin C aids iron absorption, so fruits and vegetables are needed. Store-bought milk and dairy products decrease iron absorption by 30 percent to 50 percent. Cultured milk products do not have the same effect, however.

Food for Thought

An ancient Jewish tradition is to never combine milk and meat in the same meal. This is a good practice to follow since milk stops the absorption of the iron found in the meat. Sorry, no more cheeseburgers.

Even though it is virtually impossible to get too much iron from normal foods, you can get too much if taking iron supplements or multiple vitamin/mineral supplements. Avoid giving your child any iron supplements. Also, keep any adult supplements out of the reach of children, since ingestion of iron supplements causes many cases of poisoning in children.

Good dietary sources of iron are beef, lamb, eggs, sardines, spinach, and other dark green, leafy vegetables, wheat germ, dried apricots, peas, and beans.

Daily Iron Requirements

Age	Amount (mg)
Under 1 year	6-10
1-3 years	10
4-8 years	10
Adult	10-15

Calcium

A calcium deficiency can lead to teeth problems (and osteoporosis later in life) and many metabolic difficulties. Many nutrition experts may say that children don't get enough calcium.

Lower calcium levels are oftentimes caused by eating and consuming foods that leach calcium out of the body (more so than not consuming enough calcium). If a person consumes refined sugar (fruit juice sweetened with high-fructose corn syrup, cake frosting, etc.), soft drinks, coffee, and tea, the acidic reaction in the body caused by these products forces the body to neutralize the acid with calcium. That draws calcium out of the bones, muscles, and soft tissues and can contribute to osteoporosis, joint and muscle problems.

A child with a diet high in sugar or other acid-forming foods such as pasteurized milk will naturally need more calcium in the diet to offset the demineralization caused by these items. It's ironic that milk, especially the milk found in today's supermarkets, is acid-forming and actually leads to demineralization rather than mineralization of bones.

If the milk is raw and fresh, it actually has an alkaline effect on the body as evidenced by alkaline urine after ingestion of raw milk. After pasteurization, it becomes acid-forming. These days, dairy cows are being fed more protein because it increases milk production. The milk produced by these cows has more protein in it and thus has an even more acidic reaction in the body – even if it's raw. (87)

Consuming milk, unless it's raw and from pasture-fed cows, does children more harm than good. They will not get a good supply of calcium from it. It's better to feed children other more wholesome foods that are rich in calcium (in the form the child can utilize) and not so acid- forming to the body. Some good sources of calcium are fresh-squeezed orange juice, kale, collards, mustard greens, and other dark green leafy vegetables, yogurt (a cultured milk product), broccoli, sesame seeds (hulled), nuts, dulse, sunflower seeds, and kelp. (Dulse and kelp are "sea vegetables" that are very high in minerals. They can be found at health food stores.) Please note that modern "calcium-fortified" orange juice is second rate and not really a good source of calcium. This is because the product is pasteurized, and the heat renders the calcium biologically unavailable.

Daily Calcium Requirements

Age	Amount (mg)
Under 1 year	210-270
1-3 years	500
4-8 years	800
Adult	800-1,200

Zinc

Zinc is an important mineral for controlling cell division, growth and protein synthesis that occurs only during childhood. If a child doesn't get enough zinc during these times, he may be permanently stunted. It plays a part in more than 200 enzymatic reactions in the body and helps strengthen the immune system. Zinc is known as the "intelligence mineral" and is also necessary for a healthy reproductive system and collagen formation. It's involved in blood sugar control and protects against diabetes. If a person develops an inability to taste or smell and a loss of appetite, he or she is probably zinc-deficient. (88)

Zinc levels are diminished by oral contraceptives, so it's important for women to wait at least six months after discontinuing the pill before becoming pregnant.

Many pediatricians think that zinc deficiencies are a real health problem in children, especially considering the trend of eliminating or limiting the two best sources of zinc – red meat and egg yolks (for the mistaken fear of fat). And even the best sources of zinc supply only about 10 percent of the daily allowance for children in normal-size meals. Zinc deficiencies are even more common in vegetarians.

Even though adults may want to cut back on foods such as meat and eggs, children really need them for zinc and other minerals and fats. Don't stop your child from eating them, fearing there's too much fat or too many calories in these foods. The better nourished a child is, the less likely it is that that child will have a weight problem. It's junk food, soda, and sugar that cause children to get fat, not red meats, eggs, and other wholesome fatty foods.

The best dietary sources of zinc are beef, turkey, lamb, chicken (dark meat especially), egg yolk, yogurt, peas, pumpkin seeds, brewer's yeast, wheat germ, ginger, hard cheeses, and beans.

Daily Zinc Requirements

Age	Amount (mg)
Under 1 year	5
1-3 years	10
4-8 years	10
Adult	12-19

Iodine

Iodine is now believed to be necessary for proper mental development. It's necessary for proper thyroid gland function and the production of sex hormones as well as proper fat metabolism. Iodine deficiency has been linked to mental retardation and also to susceptibility to polio and breast cancer and coronary heart disease.

Signs of deficiency are cold hands and feet, poor memory, weight gain, constipation, depression, and headaches. Vitamin A is necessary for proper iodine utilization. Consumption of large amounts of inorganic iodine, such as that found in iodized salt or iodine-fortified bread, as well as organic iodine can cause thyroid problems similar to those due to iodine deficiency.

Good sources of iodine include kelp, dulse, fish broth, butter, pineapples, most seafoods, asparagus, artichokes, and dark green vegetables. Cabbage and spinach when eaten raw can block iodine absorption, however.

Daily Iodine Requirements

Age	Amount (mcg)
Under 1 year	40-50
1-3 years	70
4-8 years	90
Adult	150

Phosphorus

Phosphorus is needed for kidney function, cell growth, and bone growth. Too much phosphorus can lead to calcium loss and cravings for sugar and alcohol. The high levels of phosphoric acid in soft drinks can lead to excessive blood levels of phosphorus, thus encouraging these problems. Not enough phosphorus can lead to poor calcium absorption and osteoporosis. Good sources are animal products, whole grains, legumes, and nuts.

Daily Phosphorus Requirements

Age	Amount (mg)
Under 1 year	100-275
1-3 years	460
4-8 years	500
Adult	700

Magnesium

Magnesium is necessary for hard tooth enamel and resistance to tooth decay, bone formation, nerve transmission, and proper enzyme activity throughout the body. It is essential for calcium and potassium absorption and the metabolism of carbohydrates and minerals.

American soils are deficient in magnesium, the phytic acid found in whole grains (avoided by soaking grains overnight in water), the ingestion of raw spinach, and a high-carbohydrate diet can cause magnesium deficiencies. Magnesium deficiency can cause fatigue, epilepsy, and impaired brain function, chronic weight loss, obesity and coronary heart disease.

A strong craving for chocolate is a sign of magnesium deficiency. Good sources of magnesium are beef, chicken or fish broth, nuts, vegetables, and seafood.

Daily Maghnesium Requirements

Age	Amount (mg)
Under 1 year	30-75
1-3 years	80
4-8 years	130
Adult	310-400

Chromium

Chromium is needed for blood sugar regulation along with syntheses of fats, protein and cholesterol. Blood sugar problems can cause a host of mental problems. A high refined carbohydrate diet can lead to a chromium deficiency. Best sources are animal products, molasses, nuts, eggs, vegetables, and whole wheat.

Sodium

Sodium is essential to the proper functioning of the adrenal glands, and thus important for handling stress. It's vital for proper nerve functioning and muscle contraction. Deficiency may cause confusion, low blood sugar, weakness, lethargy, and heart palpitations. If a person consumes sodium from food, the chances of excessive sodium are diminished since these sources contain the necessary minerals for proper sodium metabolism. Meat broths and zucchini are good sources as is celery.

Amazingly, the consumption of large amounts of refined salt (the common table salt found in supermarkets) has been shown to cause sodium starvation. [89]

Potassium

Potassium and sodium work together to maintain the proper fluid balance in the cells. It's helpful in treating high blood pressure and is found in nuts, grains, and vegetables. Too much potassium can lead to a sodium deficiency, and too much sodium can cause a potassium deficiency.

Chloride

Chloride is necessary for the proper growth and functioning of the brain and efficient protein metabolism. Good sources are celery, coconut, and bone broths.

Copper

Copper is needed for the correct formation of bone, hemoglobin, and red blood cells. It's necessary for healthy nerves and collagen formation and is important for memory and brain function. It's believed that copper deficiency is widespread in America (due to poor soils) and that a copper deficiency along with a diet high in fructose can have disastrous effects on infants and growing children. Best sources of copper are nuts, molasses, oats, and particularly liver.

Manganese

Manganese is needed for a healthy immune system, nerves, blood sugar regulation, and healthy bones and is important for the formation of mother's milk. Trembling hands, seizures, and lack of coordination mark deficiencies. Good sources are nuts – especially pecans – seeds, butter, and whole grains. As already noted, too much manganese early in life can cause attention deficit and behavioral problems later in life – so no soy formula please!

Please note that some minerals are harmful (see Chapter II). Aluminum, for example, is believed to contribute to Alzheimer's Disease and is found in soy products, aluminum cookware, refined table salt, deodorants, antacids, and baking powder. Mercury is found in amalgam fillings. Lead, cadmium, and arsenic are also toxic. Vitamin A, carotenes, vitamin C, vitamin E, and selenium can protect against these heavy metals and help the body eliminate them.

Vitamins

Vitamins are cofactors in many biochemical reactions in the body. Not having enough of them available can cause many problems ranging from bleeding gums to rickets and beriberi. Fresh, wholesome organically raised fruits, vegetables and animal products are the best ways to ingest vitamins. And beware that most vitamin supplements are toxic.

Vitamin C

Vitamin C is crucial for bone development, tissue growth, and repair, and is a potent anti-oxidant. (Antioxidants slow the aging process by preventing damage to cells caused by free radical oxygen cells.) It's important for adrenal gland function, promotes healing of wounds, is good for the common cold, and can help fight cancer. Good sources of vitamin C are Kiwi fruit, oranges, cantaloupe, sweet peppers, broccoli, tomatoes, and strawberries.

Heat and alcohol, aspirin, oral contraceptives, and other drugs have been shown to destroy vitamin C and reduce vitamin C levels in the body.

Vitamin A

Vitamin A is an all-important nutrient that is a catalyst for numerous biochemical processes. Weston Price believed that protein, minerals, and many other vitamins cannot be utilized by the body without vitamin A from animal sources. It helps build strong bones and rich blood, is a potent antioxidant, and helps protect against cancer.

There is a "preformed vitamin A" (called retinol) that is present only in animal foods. There is also a "provitamin A" (carotene) that is found in all yellow, red, orange, and dark green fruits and vegetables.

Carotenes are converted to vitamin A – which is used by the body – in the upper intestine. However, not all people, especially children and infants (and diabetics or people with poor thyroid function) can make the conversion from carotene to retinol (vitamin A). And studies have shown that carotenes cannot be converted to vitamin A without fat in the diet. Price determined that the diets of healthy people in isolated areas had at least 10 times more vitamin A from animal sources than the typical American diet.

The best sources of vitamin A are butterfat, egg yolks, liver and other organ meats, seafood, and cod liver oil. Vitamin A from synthetic supplements can be toxic, and antibiotics, laxatives, fat substitutes, and drugs can interfere with vitamin A absorption.

Good sources of carotenes are broccoli, carrots, spinach, squash, sweet potatoes, cantaloupe, eggs, cheese, and dried apricots.

One of the most important things you can do for your child is to be sure he or she get enough vitamin A from animal sources.

Vitamin E

Vitamin E is necessary for tissue repair, healing, and circulation. It is a powerful antioxidant and helps prevent cancer and cardiovascular disease. If a person eats a lot of polyunsaturated oils, greater amounts of vitamin E are needed. Good sources are unrefined vegetable oils, butter, organ meats, grains, nuts, seeds, legumes, and dark green leafy vegetables.

Daily Requirements of Vitamins A, C, and E

Age	Vitamin A (Retinol Equivalents)	Vitamin C (mg)	Vitamin E (IU)
Under 1	375	30-35	6
1-3 years	400	40	9
4-8 years	500	45	15
Adult	800-1300	60-1,000	15-1,000

B vitamins

B vitamins promote healthy skin, eyes, hair, liver, nerves, muscle tone, and cardiovascular system. The best sources of B vitamins are whole grains and natural foods. Processing (as with white rice, white flour) removes the B vitamins from foods. Manufacturers will oftentimes add B vitamins and call the product "enriched," but these synthetic vitamins are not nearly so effective as the ones naturally found in whole grains.

B-1 (also called thiamin) deficiency causes beriberi and may be the root cause of anorexia and other eating disorders. Sugar consumption depletes the body's stores of B-1. B-2 (riboflavin) deficiency causes frequent cracks in the lips and corners of the mouth. A deficiency of B-3 (niacin) causes the disease called pellagra, which is characterized by dermatitis, dementia, tremors, and diarrhea. B-5 (pantothenic acid) plays a vital role in cell metabolism and cholesterol production and helps the body withstand stress. It's found in organ meats, egg yolks, and whole grains. B-6 (pyroidoxine) contributes to the proper functioning of more than 100 enzymes. It's found mostly in animal products. B-6 deficiencies may cause diabetes, nervous disorders, and coronary heart disease. A great source of B-6 is raw milk. Other sources are eggs, bananas, oatmeal, avocados, chicken, beef, fish, wheat germ, and prunes.

The lack of the B vitamin called folate or folic acid during pregnancy is known to cause neural tube defects such as spina bifida. If taken before conception and during pregnancy, folic acid will help prevent these problems. But is also important for the proper myelination of brain cells during the baby's first months of life. Folate is found in spinach, peaches, oranges, broccoli, and dark green lettuce.

B-12 is needed to maintain fertility, to promote normal growth and development, prevent anemia and nervous disorders. Interestingly, one common symptom of early B-12 deficiency is irrational anger. Forms of B-12 the body can use are found only in animal foods. Vegetable sources are not metabolized by the body and are thus ineffective. Good sources of B-12 are beef, chicken, fish, eggs, cheese, and whole, raw milk.

Daily B-Vitamin Requirements

Age	Folate(mcg)	B1(mg)	B2(mg)	B3(mg)	B5(mg)	B-6(mcg)	B-12(mcg)
Under 1	65-80	0.2-0.3	0.3-0.4	4-5	1.7-1.8	0.1-0.3	0.4-0.5
1-3 years	150	0.5	0.5	6	2.0	0.5	0.9
4-6 years	200	0.6	0.8	8	3.0	0.6	1.2
Adult	400-600	1.2	1.3	14-16	5.0	1.3-2.0	2.4-2.8

Vitamin D

Vitamin D is necessary for proper calcium and phosphorus absorption and thus is essential for strong bones, healthy teeth, and normal growth. Deficiencies can cause rickets and myopia. The body uses sunlight to manufacture vitamin D from cholesterol, so getting adequate exposure to the sun is vital for children. Foods high in vitamin D are butterfat, eggs, liver, fish oils, organ meats, and seafood, especially shrimp and crab.

What's the best way to ensure your children get all the vitamins and minerals they need? Make sure they eat an egg yolk a day and plenty of natural, fatty foods such as meat and butter. Compliment these with fresh fruits and vegetables, whole grains, and raw milk if you can, and they will grow to be healthy and strong. The RDA for Vitamin D is 5 mcg for children and adults.

As much as possible, the food you feed your children should be grown organically. Meats should be from free-range animals with no antibiotics or hormones added to their feed. Allow your children to choose their foods, as long as they are wholesome. The better nutrition your babies and children receive, the less likely they will be drawn to junk foods.

Contamination is not the only problem with baby foods. The ingredients themselves can cause health problems. A typical baby food may contain added sugar, food colorings, salt, preservatives, and is pasteurized. The foods in the baby foods themselves have not been organically grown and have, as already mentioned, contain pesticide residues. It's always best to buy organically raised foods and make your own baby food. That way you're sure of feeding your little loved ones fresh, nutritious, and clean food – so they can grow up strong, vital, and intelligent with few health problems.

Water

Lack of enough water in the body contributes to and is a cause of many diseases. Feyedoon Batmanghelidj, M.D., a leading expert on the value of water, says in his book *Your Body's Many Cries for Water* that dehydration can cause joint pain, back pain, angina pain, hypertension, asthma, allergies, high cholesterol, chronic fatigue, obesity, diabetes, migraine headaches, heartburn, colitis, and some emotional problems including depression. (90)

Bernard Jensen, D.C., N.D., Ph.D., an icon in the natural health care field, has this to say about water:

> When a newborn baby comes forth from the mother, it is 77 percent water. After a few years, the average child is about 59 percent water and the average adult may be around 60 percent water. We find out that even bones are about 20 percent water while blood is 83 percent water... The brain and muscle tissues are nearly the same – about 75 percent water... My experience in nearly 70 years in the healing arts verifies that ongoing dehydration is a serious problem. I have found that nearly all of my patients have some degree of bowel underactivity and constipation, which are signs of dehydration. I also find that symptoms such as dry, hard stools and infrequent bowel movements every two to five days are not uncommon... When we don't drink enough water, the lymph system, the kidneys, skin, lungs/bronchials, and bowel cannot carry off toxic wastes as they are meant to do. Digestion of foods and transportation of nutrients are impaired. At the cellular level, lack of water slows down all cell processes, including the making of proteins and development of

energy. Perspiration and temperature control becomes abnormal. All of these things make us more vulnerable to disease... We must understand there is no substitute for plain water. Coffee, tea, and milk are not acceptable substitutes because they act as diuretics, causing more water to be eliminated than is taken in. This increases dehydration. Alcoholic beverages are especially dehydrating... Diseases favored by dehydration include asthma, allergies, stomach ulcers, bulimia, Alzheimer's, hiatal hernia, arthritis, adult-onset diabetes, kidney problems, high-blood pressure, and morning sickness due to pregnancy... (91)

Most drinks – sodas, coffee, tea – contain caffeine, and caffeine is a diuretic (alcohol is too). That means it pushes water out of the body and dehydrates you. For every glass of caffeinated beverage you drink, you need to drink at least one or two glasses of water to replace the water you lose due to the diuretic action. This is a double-edged sword. Not only are you losing precious body water by drinking these beverages, the caffeine itself is a neurotoxin. It's vitally important you and your children give up these beverages..

One woman discovered an easy and painless way to give up her Coke:

My main source of water up to that time had been Coca-Cola. I loved Coke, and didn't think I could ever give it up, but I've managed to break myself of the habit rather painlessly. I decided that every time I felt the urge to drink a Coke, I would make myself drink a glass of water first, and then have my soda. What happens now is I go to the fridge, take out a can of Coke, and then go to the sink and drink a glass of water. About 75 percent of the time I don't even open the Coke, because my desire for it is gone. It was water my body wanted the whole time, but it didn't know how to tell me. (92)

This is a great strategy to wean yourself and your child off these unhealthy beverages. Let them have the soda, but before they do, have them drink a glass of water, raw milk or vegetable juice. You'll find they won't drink as much soda and eventually will give it up completely.

You lose water all night long simply from the act of breathing, and become slightly dehydrated as a result. You need to replenish this water to avoid dehydration. Adults should drink two glasses of water, raw milk or vegetable juice upon rising, and children less as determined by their size. Drink a glass of water, fresh vegetable juice or milk a half-hour before meals. That will ensure that your body does not have to withdraw water from other organs to produce digestive juices. You will have better digestion and experience a happier disposition.

You hear that the average adult should drink a minimum of six to eight glasses of pure water a day. But I don't think you should force yourself to drink – drink when you're thirsty. Water is a solvent and has the tendency to dissolve the mineral matrices in our body. Drinking raw milk or vegetable juices, replete with minerals, is better for you, your muscles, bones, and brain. When you do drink water, it's best to drink a good mineral water such as Perrier. If you're eating a largely raw diet, you will not need to drink as much. Dr. Batmanghelidj says:

It is more important for children to be properly hydrated than adults. Cells are comprised of approximately 75 percent water, so it is crucial that children receive enough water so they will grow properly. Their cells cannot grow without water. I would go so far to say that giving a child soda and not giving them water is the same as molding them for suffering from future problems with drug and alcohol addiction... The reason is that when you don't give children water and they only drink caffeinated drinks, the caffeine will promote the system into endorphin production. The more endorphin that is produced, the more the child gets high from the caffeine. The child eventually develops that program within their physiology, and must eventually drink more caffeine to produce that same false high. They will become much more predisposed to an alcohol problem as they seek to reproduce that feeling in latter years. I firmly believe this is why teenage alcoholism is such a widespread problem today – they are a generation of children brought up on caffeinated colas... (93)

It's important to ingest minerals and enough water-soluble vitamins if you increase your water intake. If you ever develop cramps, it's an indication that there are not enough minerals in your diet. I do not believe salt is the best source for minerals. You should get them from vegetable juices, milk and the food you eat. But in a pinch it will do. Batmanghelidj recommends 1/4 teaspoon of salt for every eight glasses of water you drink. If you don't have the salt, your body may not be able to retain the water and you will remain dehydrated.

Consuming enough minerals is vitally important, but don't get them from regular table salt. The regular salt in supermarkets is stripped of many of its minerals, especially the trace minerals that are important for proper cellular function. Table salt comes from the same batch as vacuum-refined industrial salt. It's treated with caustic soda or lime to remove magnesium salts. The removal of magnesium salts not only allows the salt to flow, but also frees them up to bring in more money on the chemical market. However, these magnesium salts fill important biological and therapeutic roles and are necessary for proper cellular functioning. Also to keep the salt flowing, alumino-silicate of sodium or yellow prussiate of soda are added. The salt may also be bleached. This chemically altered salt does not combine with human body fluid and may cause edema (water retention) and other severe health problems. (94) If you must use salt, the only salt you and your child should consume is Celtic Sea Salt.

Doctors say to avoid sodium (salt) in order to keep blood pressure down. But sodium is not the problem – we need sodium. If you eat the correct, balanced, untreated salt, blood pressure actually comes down. (Celery has a lot of the right kind of sodium.)

Making sure children are nourished correctly takes some understanding and effort. But if their little bodies are supplied with proper nutrition, they will be a lot brighter, better behaved, and healthier. It's worth the effort.

CHAPTER XI
The Truth About Vaccines

Here are some reports from parents who believe a vaccine affected their child:

"Terry was a beautiful baby... happy, healthy, strong baby from birth. When Terry was nine weeks old, his doctor gave him his first DPT shot and oral polio vaccinations. In the 48 hours after his vaccinations, Terry started to sleep more than usual and his mother couldn't wake him up to eat... his skin turned grey and mottled." Terry was put on a respirator and had to be fed through a tube in his nose because he was severely paralyzed. He loves to be picked up and held close but he can't hug you back. In 1996, the U.S. Court of Claims in Washington, D.C. officially acknowledged that Terry's paralysis was a result of the polio vaccine he received as a baby. (1)

Within ten hours of his first DPT shot, a mother reported that her son "had a red and swollen leg and was crying a strange cry. His temperature was 105 degrees. I called the doctor and he told me to give him Tylenol and put him in a tepid bath. As I was putting him in the bath, his eyes rolled back in his head and he quivered all over." From that moment on, her son continued to have seizures and high-pitched screaming. Today, he is hyperactive and physically and mentally handicapped.

After her fourth shot, an eighteen-month-old girl collapsed. Her mother said, "The day after her shot, her leg got really stiff, and she couldn't walk on it... The next night, she woke up screaming. It was a terrible, fearful kind of scream. My husband picked her up, and she got very silent and turned white with a purple-blue tinge around her mouth and went completely limp. We thought she was in the throes of Sudden Infant Death Syndrome." (1a)

Edward Jenner, a British physician, is often credited with starting vaccinations (or inoculations) in 1796 - but the history of vaccines goes back before that, probably originating in the Orient or by the Arabs. Jenner scraped cowpox pus into a cut on the arm of eight-year-old James Phipps. The boy came down with cowpox - a relatively mild disease - but later did not contract smallpox - a potentially fatal disease. There are reports the boy was sickly most of his life. He died at the age of 20 from tuberculosis (often a side effect of the smallpox vaccine). However, the same kind of inoculation failed to work with Jenner's own 18-month-old son, (who also died in his early 20s of tuberculosis), and bad reactions to inoculations in people during Jenner's day were widespread and serious. In fact, there was a serious outcry of public opinion against vaccines when they were first introduced because of their side effects and lack of effectiveness. (2,3)

Never the less, due to political and economic pressures, government mandates, bad science, and outright deception, vaccinations have become a mainstay of the traditional medical community's attempts to prevent and control infectious diseases. But as we shall see, there are serious questions as to whether vaccines help prevent disease at all. And, there are indications that they may actually contribute to a wide range of maladies that have increased dramatically over the past 60 years.

The theory of vaccines is that some disease germ is injected into a person that stimulates the body to produce antibodies, which are proteins that reportedly defend it from an invasion of harmful bacteria or viruses.

The National Academy of Sciences states that the incidence of disease and death caused by vaccines is "extraordinarily low." The Centers for Disease Control says that most vaccines are 90 percent effective at preventing their target diseases. UNICEF reports that vaccines save the lives of at least 1.5 million children every year.

The U.S. Government reports the following statistics purporting to show a correlation between vaccination use and the incidence of disease. (4)

Table 5

Government reported cases of various diseases 1970 - 1990

Reported Cases per 1000:	1970	1980	1990	1994
Diphtheria	435	3	4	2
Polio	33	9	7	0
Tetanus	148	95	64	51
Measles	47.4	29.1	27.8	1.0
Mumps	105	8.6	5.3	1.5
Pertussis	4.2	1.7	4.6	4.6

The global eradication of smallpox during the 1970s is attributed to worldwide vaccination campaigns. Many hail the pioneering work of Salk and Sabin for developing the polio vaccine in the 1950s. Some expect polio to be eradicated as well within the next few years.

However, as we shall see below, there are other researchers and scientists who believe that the decline in infectious diseases was not due to vaccination but other factors. Indeed, there is a brewing controversy over the safety, effectiveness, and even necessity of vaccines.

A document on vaccines by the World Health Organization prepared for parents gives general information concerning vaccines. The question is presented: "Are vaccines contrary to nature?" Their response:

> No, on the contrary, vaccines are simply utilizing the laws of nature. Science has gradually gained insight into some of the basic

mechanisms utilized by nature to prevent as well as cure infectious diseases. But whereas infectious agents often cause serious disease or even death before the body can mobilize its defense, the vaccines are designed to stimulate the natural defense mechanisms in the most efficient ways, with minimal harm to the body... (5)

But these trends and statistics do not necessarily prove a correlation, and not everyone believes vaccines are as effective as they are made out to be. They may even be harmful. William Campbell Douglass, M.D., says:

What the vaccinators don't tell you is that communicable diseases have been declining at a steady rate for 150 years and that there is no relationship between the various diseases and the onset of immunization. Without exception, the vaccine program for each of the childhood diseases was inaugurated after that particular disease had begun to disappear. Contrary to what you have been told, this included polio. What the vaccines have done is cause the various childhood diseases to become adulthood diseases - with far more serious implications, mumps in men and rubella in women for example. (6)

Are vaccines really hazardous to your health? Much research says so. Even the World Health Organization acknowledges potential dangers:

The vast majority of adverse effects following vaccination are minor, typically just a local reaction at the site of the injection... may occur in approximately 1-30 percent of the cases... On rare occasions, more serious adverse effects may occur, such as fever, aches or a widespread rash... Extremely rare cases of lasting damage or even death have occurred. Death in association with an injection of a vaccine has mostly resulted from individual hypersensitivity to one of the components included in the vaccine. The majority of such tragedies are in principle preventable; questions concerning possible allergies are routinely explored before any immunization, and persons with a history of severe hypersensitivity reactions should be referred to relevant medical expertise. (7)

Hardly any mother is aware of how many children have been killed or permanently injured due to vaccines. But the government does. They have records of thousands of children and babies who have been killed or permanently hurt by vaccines in a special database. And that's just the tip of the iceberg. The FDA acknowledges that 90 percent of doctors do not report vaccine reactions at all. FDA Commissioner David Kessler stated that only one in 10 adverse events following vaccinations are reported. (8) Even with this underreporting, every year there are more than 12,000 reports of adverse reaction to vaccines. These reports include hospital visits, irreversible injuries, and hundreds of deaths. If you consider only 10 percent are reported, then the true figure could be as high as 120,000 adverse events annually. (9) All this even though the Federal government set up the Vaccine Adverse Event Reporting System (VAERS) especially to document adverse reactions to vaccines. During one 20-month period 54,000 vaccine adverse events were reported to the VAERS which included 700 deaths.

More proof that the government acknowledges problems with vaccines: In 1986 the National Childhood Vaccine Injury Act (Public Law 99-660) was passed. It addresses the facts that vaccines do in fact cause injury and death. Part of this law requires doctors to inform parents of the potential risks of vaccines and to report any adverse reactions. But as we just saw, only about 10 percent of adverse reactions are ever reported. And I suspect the percentage of doctors informing parents of the potential risks of vaccines is even lower.

The National Childhood Vaccine Injury Act has a provision to give compensation to victims of vaccinations that have caused injury or death. As of January 2000, more than $1 billion has been paid out for hundreds of injuries and deaths caused by mandated vaccines, and thousands of cases are still pending. (10) Yet, this program currently dismisses 90 percent of all vaccine injury claims. The money for this fund is raised by taking a portion of the money the parents, insurance companies, or government funds spends on the vaccines and putting it into a congressional fund. The law awards up to $250,000 if a person dies or millions to cover lifelong medical bills, pain, and suffering caused by a vaccine the government requires by law.

Food for Thought

Lest you think the government is being generous in effectively insuring manufacturers against vaccine casualties, consider how easy the program makes it for manufacturers. The bottom line is that this government-run compensation program protects vaccine manufacturers from lawsuits. National Vaccine Information Center president Barbara Loe Fisher comments: "Imagine having the following business opportunity: You produce a product which the government guarantees to be free from liability and the marketplace is every child born. It certainly doesn't get much better than that... And the pharmaceutical industry currently has a monopoly on this 'business.' To date there has never been an independent, controlled study which proves that their vaccines are safe or even effective." (11)

There is very little control of the vaccine industry. The scientists and physicians in the pharmaceutical industry and government who are in charge of the mass vaccination system are policing themselves. There is no oversight mechanism in place to safeguard the public health.

Barbara Loe Fisher is president and cofounder of the National Vaccine Information Center (NVIC) – a consumer-led movement that monitors vaccine research, licensing, development, promotion, and policy making. She says:

It's a dream for the pharmaceutical industry involved in making vaccines, because there's no way anybody can say no. It's a stable, ready-made market, and the enactment of the compensation law in

The Truth About Children's Health

1986 has removed almost all liability for drug companies... You would think that, because vaccines are required to be used by everyone, they would be held to the very highest safety and efficacy standards, but that is not the case. What the NVIC has been pushing for is more consumer involvement in the public health decisions that are made in this country with regard to vaccination. We believe that health care consumers should have the right to choose the type of preventive health care that they want to use – including choosing whether to use one, ten or no vaccines... We are vaccinating in a vacuum of scientific knowledge. There have been no long-term studies set up, as has been done with heart disease and cancer, to evaluate all morbidity and mortality outcomes following vaccination in large populations of vaccinated and unvaccinated groups to see if we are paying a price for the control of infectious disease in childhood. Are we paying a larger price down the road, in terms of chronic illness?... Today in this country, a one-year-old child can be vaccinated with ten different viral and bacterial antigens on one day. That is an incredible assault on the immune system... (12)

A vaccine is made by first acquiring the disease germ (bacterium or live virus) and then processing in various ways to make it suitable for the intended use. Some of the processes include adding drugs, antibiotics, and toxic substances (e.g., formaldehyde, aluminum hydrochloride, streptomycin, neomycin, thimerosal [a mercury derivative]). The toxic effects of aluminum formaldehyde and mercury are well documented, and even microscopic doses of them can lead to permanent cellular damage. Remember, a vaccine is made of live viruses or bacteria, toxic substances, and diseased animal matter. Then, it's injected into children. Vaccines containing the carcinogenic toxins formaldehyde and thimerosal are being injected into infants as young as two months old whose immune systems are not fully developed. (13)

The CDC and the National Immunization Program post a Contraindications to Vaccine Chart on their website (www.cdc.gov/nip/recs/ contraindications_vacc.htm). The only official contraindication for most vaccines is if a child got a serious allergic reaction after a previous vaccine dose or exposure to a vaccine component. However, there are many health-care professionals who believe there are more reasons or situations not to give a child a vaccine. They include: the child being sick or having a cold; allergy to eggs; weak immune system; and simply being too young for a particular vaccine. The NVIC says a parent should ask the following questions before allowing their child to receive a vaccine: Is my child sick right now? Has my child had a bad reaction to a vaccination before? Does my child have a personal or family history of vaccine reactions, convulsions, neurological disorders, severe allergies, immune system disorders? Do I know if my child is at high risk of reacting? Do I have full information on the vaccine's side effects? Do I know how to identify a vaccine reaction? Do I know how to report a vaccine reaction? Do I know the vaccine manufacturere's name and lot number? (14)

DPT is a single vaccine combining diphtheria, tetanus, and pertussis vaccines into one shot. Formaldehyde is used to manufacture the vaccine and formaldehyde is known to cause cancer. The DPT vaccine also contains a preservative called thimerosal, which is a form of mercury combined with aluminum. Think of DPT as a triple threat: formaldehyde, mercury, and aluminum – all considered toxic.

Even the CDC recognizes there are more contraindications for the DPT vaccine including encephalophthy (coma, prolonged seizures, decreased level of consciousness) and progressive neurological disorder (infantile spasm and uncontrolled epilepsy). However, the CDC dismisses the following reasons not to give a baby a DPT shot: high temperature, fussiness after a previous DPT shot; family history of seizures; family history of SIDS; family history of adverse events following DPT shots, and; well controlled convulsions.

Food for Thought

Having a list of contraindications is to ensure that a person who has a high chance of being susceptible to a vaccine is determined so a serious adverse reaction can be avoided. Each box of vaccines comes with a package insert detailing the contraindications and doctors are supposed to find out if they apply to an individual before the vaccine is given. But how many doctors take the time to ask a parent if their child had an adverse reaction to their most recent vaccine, or if the child has any other characteristics that might indicate a vaccine should be avoided? As a parent, learn the contraindications and ask – even demand – to get them before letting your child get a vaccine. Do NOT assume the doctor knows everything... remember, he or she is very busy!

One of the most frightening and suspicious things about the whole vaccination issue is that vaccines have not been tested in any way for safety or effectiveness. The proof of safety comes from the state and local officials who are just following the advice of organizations who set the policies who in turn are influenced and educated by the companies who manufacture the vaccine. Nowhere in the literature is there any hint of a double-blind study performed with vaccines. The Advisory Committee on Immunization Practices (ACIP) makes immunization recommendations that the FDA follows in licensing vaccines. Their members are appointed by the Centers for Disease Control. The Chairman of the ACIP, Dr. John Modlin, said in February 1999: "...available data are insufficient to fully establish the safety and efficacy of Rotavirus vaccine in premature infants... To my knowledge we don't have data from a clinical trial specifically... Some bit of information from Seattle, as I recall, that had suggested that there was a slight increase in relative risk for hospitalization for premature infants...

The Truth About Children's Health

Obviously a situation where we have to make a judgment in the absence of data, and with a vaccine that has not yet been tested in the group..."

Modlin said that during an ACIP meeting held to determine if the Rotavirus vaccine (known to cause infant diarrhea) should be approved. Given this information, or declaration of the lack of information, the committee nonetheless voted nine to one for the Rotavirus to be given to premature infants. (15) This story does not stop there. It turns out that Modlin did indeed have data about the safety of the virus from being the Chairman of the Rotavirus working group of the Vaccines and Related Biological Products Advisory Committee (VRBPAC), which decides whether vaccines are licensed (Congressional Hearing). The data showed a risk of life-threatening bowel obstructions in clinical trials of Rotavirus before the February 1999 ACIP meeting. In these clinical trials, some babies suffered obstructed bowels a week after being vaccinated – some requiring intussusception surgery to remove a portion of the intestine. The committee called these reactions statistically insignificant. (16)

Once the vaccine was introduced (with 1.5 million doses given to infants), some bad things happened. One premature baby died and another five-month-old infant died from a bowel obstruction. In all there were 113 cases of life-threatening bowel obstructions reported because of the vaccine. Only then was the Rotavirus vaccine withdrawn from the market in October 1999. (17) In a March 1999 debate at the University of New Hampshire, Modlin defined his standard for scientific validity: "Has the information withstood the test of peer review? Has the information been published in a respected medical or scientific journal?... This is the standard that you should hold me to today... Has the information been published in a scientifically reputable Journal?" Nothing was published about the Rotavirus, and yet he voted for its approval. Modlin has subsequently been reappointed Chairman of the ACIP.

There were trials of the Rotavirus vaccine, though never published or reviewed, showing the vaccine to have a 49 percent efficacy rate, which is low. Also, the public has no access to the actual data concerning the side effects of the Rotavirus vaccine or for the chicken pox or hepatitis B vaccines. If all these are good for us, why don't they let us see the data?

Still, if you ask your doctor about vaccines, he or she will tell you that "everyone knows" you need them and "it is scientifically accepted" they work and are safe. But ask him or her for proof or studies to show that. Your doctor will more than likely try to evade your questions or get angry and tell you, "It's the law."

But if you ask someone for the data showing there are great risks associated with vaccines and they are really not that effective (if at all), they can turn up a library full, like I am here. Who are you more likely to trust... Someone who's an open book, or someone who defiantly objects to your questions? I'm perfectly willing to consider the establishment's side of the story, but they don't give it out! Why not? Show me the studies and tests showing safety and efficacy, and I'm all yours.

Another bit of history: In 1991 ACIP recommended that every newborn baby receive the hepatitis B vaccine in the hospital within hours of birth. Samuel L. Katz, M.D., was the ACIP Chairman at that time. He has stated that, "... there was no published peer-reviewed study" on the safety of the vaccine. Even though newborns have a negligible risk of getting hepatitis B unless the mother is infected, the vaccine was mandated for newborn babies. This was the first of its kind since no newborns were previously required to be immediately vaccinated. Not only that, but once again there was no proper safety study on the hepatitis B vaccine. Since its approval and use, there have been more than 36,000 adverse reactions and more than 440 deaths reported from it (VAERS records, which are accessible to the public through the Freedom of Information Act). So, let me get this straight. There's little chance of a newborn getting hepatitis B, and there were no safety studies done on the vaccine. Yet after they started vaccinating for it, 440 babies died? And 36,000 more had adverse reactions? (18) And the vaccine was originally developed to protect drug addicts who shared unsterilized needles or people who had multiple sex partners. (19) Does that sound like our babies?

Here's the extent to which the vaccine manufacturers and health officials will go to keep blame of harm off their products: There have been cases where a child had a post-vaccine reaction resulting in seizures, coma, or death, and then the parents were charged with causing it by excessively shaking the baby ("shaken baby syndrome"). It was the parents who killed their own baby or put it into a coma, not the vaccine – so the officials say. Talk about a raw deal. First their baby dies because of a vaccine reaction, and then they get accused of murder. I bet if the defense attorney would take the time to examine the baby's vaccination record, he would find the baby was recently vaccinated. Wouldn't that cause an uproar in the courtroom and in the press?

Encephalitis, (swelling of the brain) can be caused by a severe injury to the head, a severe burn, a high fever or from vaccines. Harris L. Coulter, Ph.D., a researcher and author of two books on vaccinations takes this a step further and says the childhood vaccination program is the principal cause of encephalitis in the U.S. today (and other industrialized countries). Coulter says that post-vaccinal encephalitis may be the greatest cause of developmental and learning disabilities in the country, and that "These manifestations of a vaccine reaction are identical to the symptoms of acute encephalitis from any other cause." (20) One of the most prevalent reactions to the measles vaccine – and other vaccines – is a kind of encephalitis.

Post-vaccinal encephalitis results in a loss and destruction of myelin on the brain stem and spinal cord (remember, myelin is the fatty protective sheath around nerves that acts like insulation around an electric wire. If it's not there, all sorts of short-circuits are possible and the nerves never fully develop).

The symptoms of, "Diarrhea, vomiting, flatulence, gastroenteritis, stomach aces, enuresis, constipation, loss of sphincter control, etc., are all found in encephalitis and are frequently reported after the DPT shot... When the baby reacts to a DPT shot wit a 'slight fever and fussiness' or drowsiness' for a few days, this may be, and often is, a case of encephalitis which is capable of causing quite sever neurologic consequences." But that's not all. Severe neurologic damage can occur in a child later, even if he or she showed no acute reaction to the vaccine. In fact, "encephalitis from all other causes [eg., fever, brain injury] is known to produce severe neurologic damage..." (21) So if vaccines cause encephalitis, how can they *not* cause severe neurologic damage?

Coulter believes that the long-term effects of vaccines are more widespread than anyone suspected. He says that these effects are more often than not "disguised" under different names: autism, dyslexia, learning disabilities, epilepsy, mental retardation, hyperactivity, minimal brain dysfunction. Those are the labels children are brandished with, when the cause of their problems originated with the nervous-system-attacking vaccine. These conditions then lead to violent crime, drug abuse, juvenile delinquency, and the seeming collapse of the public school system.

There have been studies showing that more violent crimes are committed by those with neurological damage than those without. And since encephalitis is neurological damage, children who have had it may exhibit cruel, abusive, and destructive behavior more often. Not just as children, but as adolescents and adults too. (22)

Hyperactivity and learning problems are another result of neurological damage and also predisposes a child to violent tendencies. An article in the *Journal of the American Medical Association* concluded that; "Adults with a history of attention-deficit hyperactivity disorder appear to be over represented in the ranks of felons." (23)

Other learning disabilities such as dyslexia are often found in convicted criminals. (24) And again, these violent tendencies may be a result of actual brain damage (from vaccine reactions?) and not necessarily from psychological or sociological problems.

Food for Thought

The number of hyperactive children has increased dramatically over the past few decades such that now one child in 20 is considered hyperactive. (25) Hyperactivity increases the likelihood of violent and criminal behavior. So it's not just your imagination that crime has increased in our society. Poisons injected into babies leads to hyperactive and learning impaired children which leads to unruly adolescents which leads to unlawful adults.

In attempts to cope with hyperactivity, a person may turn to alcohol or drugs. (26) What's more, encephalitis often causes a myriad of seizure disorders including epilepsy with episodes of convulsions, petit mal, grand mal, tics, tremors, and grimaces. (27) Movements can also be impaired resulting in paralysis, cerebral palsy, weakness of arms and legs, clumsiness, and spasticity. Later in life, chronic encephalitis can manifest as Parkinson's disease. (28) For over a century, scientists have noticed a link between epilepsy and violent tendencies, and studies have shown that the prevalence of epileptics in prisons is significantly higher than in the general population. (29)

It's an accepted fact (even by the vaccine manufacturers) that vaccines can cause convulsions. Isn't it interesting that the medical establishment is still hunting for the cause of epilepsy? Everyone wants to point to social and psychological reasons for the recent dramatic degeneration of our society. No one wants to consider that what we put into our and our children's bodies (the poisons present in vaccines among others) may be causing not just an increase in violence, alcoholism, and drug abuse, but an increase in learning and behavioral problems as well.

Another possible manifestation of encephalitis is that of abnormal sexual activity and desires. These may appear as hypersexuality (too much sex drive usually discharged by masturbation), pornography, a casual attitude towards sex, perversions, fetishes, confused sexuality, bisexualism, and homosexualism. (30) To see a display of many of these attitudes, all one has to do is watch the MTV channel on the television. This is what our children – the most vaccinated children in the history of mankind – relate to.

If a child shows signs of hyperactivity and aggressiveness (as in ADHD), he or she is often times given drugs (i.e., Ritalin, etc.) to control them. These hyperactive children in many cases may have some form of neurological disorder as mentioned above, and children with minimal brain dysfunction are more likely to start smoking, drinking, and using drugs as adolescents. (31) Could much of the problems with our children be attributed to vaccinations? A child is vaccinated at birth and throughout childhood. If the scientific studies on brain damage, encephalitis, and seizures are correct, the brain abnormalities resulting from vaccinations could then lead to hyperactivity, learning disabilities, and violent acts.

These lead to the child being prescribed drugs like Ritalin to control them. These drugs, harmful in their own right, then predispose the child to substance abuse and antisocial behaviors later in life. This is not to mention the increased susceptibility to other disorders such as cancer due to the poisoning effects of the vaccines.

Autism is a well-known syndrome suffered by approximately 118,000 children in U.S. schools and 400,000 Americans overall. (32) Experts estimate that autism rates have risen from around four per 10,000 in the early 1980s to between 12 and 20 per 10,000 in the 1990s. (33) In the state of California, autism has increased 273 percent over a 10-year period starting in 1989, with 1,685 new cases reported in 1999 alone. A national study based upon yearly reports to Congress from the U.S. Department of Education shows the incidence of autism is consistent with the data from California. (34) In Maryland, as another example, the autism rate has increased 500 percent.

Katz said that the adverse reactions to a vaccine are the same thing as the neurological complications from the disease itself. Since the introduction of the measles vaccine, the rate of autism has increased hundreds of percent. Autism has historically been called "postencephalitic syndrome" – and is essentially the same thing as measles encephalitis. Many parents report that their children were perfectly normal until the received the MMR (measles/mumps/rubella) vaccine. Then they became autistic. (35)

Robert Mendelsohn, M.D., says that the measles vaccine may cause the inability to coordinate muscle movements (ataxia), learning disabilities, paralysis, retardation, seizure disorders, aseptic meningitis, juvenile-onset diabetes, multiple sclerosis, Reye's syndrome, blood clotting disorders, and death. (36) An article in the *New England Journal of Medicine* said that giving vitamin A to children with measles reduces the likelihood of complications and their chances of dying. (37)

Regarding diabetes, the MMR vaccine has been heavily implicated in the causation of Type-I diabetes. (38) The rubella (German measles) component of the vaccine is believed to be the major suspect because rubella itself (along with mumps) is known to be a cause of diabetes. The action of the live MMR vaccine mimics that of the disease and it's believed that the rubella and mumps viruses infect pancreatic islet cells and severely reduce levels of secreted insulin. (39) Researchers believe that if measles or mumps can cause diabetes, the vaccine can too. (40)

The history of autism is particularly interesting and shows an amazing correlation to the introduction and increased use of the pertussis vaccine (and the MMR vaccine as we shall see a bit later, below). A well-known psychiatrists named Leo Kanner, while at Johns Hopkins, first described autism in 1943 in his article "Autistic Disturbances of Affective Content." He noted that the symptoms of aloneness and lack of social involvement started early and thus the syndrome was called "infantile autism." (41)

Autism is now characterized as a self-absorbed alienation where the child is detached, inaccessible and sometimes nervously hostile. It can start very early in the child's life, as Kanner initially observed. However, more recently, it has been observed that it can start later, during the age of two. This is now referred to as "late onset autism." It was virtually unheard of before the 1970s, but now such cases out number early onset autism cases 5 to one. (42)

The reported cases of autism have steadily increased over the years to the point of being at an epidemic level. "...The number of children aged 6 to 21 with autism in the U.S. schools rose steadily from 5,415 in 1991 – 1992 to 118,602 in 2001 – 2002." (43) And while the number of children with disabilities in general has increased 30% from 1991 – 2002, the number of cases of autism has increased a disproportionate 1700%. (44)

Two questions must be asked: Why did autism begin at all, and; why the steady increase in the number of cases of autism over the years?

Many researchers have made the link between autism and governmented mandated vaccinations – especially the pertussis vaccine. This vaccine, to combat whooping cough, was developed in the mid 1930s and it gradually achieved widespread mandated governmental use in the 1950s. Harris L. Coulter observed, "The increase prevalence of autism in the 1950s and 1960s precisely reflected the expansion of mandated vaccination programs during these same decades." (45)

And this trend occurred not only in the U.S. In Japan, France, Chile, Austria, Holland and England, the first cases of autism occurred after the introduction of the pertussis vaccine. (46)

Another reason to suspect the pertussis vaccine as being a causative agent in autism is because of the kinds of children it first affected. When autism first appeared, it did so in children of well-educated, intelligent, and affluent parents. Naturally, scientist tried to explain the outbreak of autism (unsuccessfully) as being a genetic trait. But there was something more telling going on. Since free vaccinations at public health clinics had not yet begun, only those who could afford private physicians and the new vaccinations they offered were having their children vaccinated. But as free and government mandated vaccines increased across the country, so has the incidences of autism. Not just in children of affluent parents, but in children of parents of every economic, social and ethnic class as well. (47)

Food for Thought

I realize that diagnosis and terminology have advanced since the 1940s. But for there to not even be a name for the symptoms of autism in the medical literature of that time is telling. Dr Yazbak says "Suggesting that a sudden and exponential increase in autistic disorders is not real, and results only from better diagnosis, amounts to denial." (48) And is it really a coincidence that the incidences of autism are in direct proportion to the number of mandated vaccinations given our children?

The agent in the vaccines believed to be largely responsible for inducing autism is mercury, which is in the thimerosal used to preserve more than 30 vaccines since the 1930s. Thimerosal is nearly 50 percent ethyl mercury. (49) Recall that the symptoms of mercury toxicity include depression, mood swings, withdrawal, tantrums, aggression, retardation and poor attention, problems with speech, hearing, movement, vision, sleeping, eating, and allergies. It's also been noted that thimerosal completely inhibits phagocytosis in blood, which is one of the body's most vital immune defenses. (50) Vaccinations are used to induce an immunization response, and yet one of its ingredients inhibits that very response! According to Lars Friberg, M.D., former head of toxicology at the World Health Organization, "There is no safe level of mercury and no one has actually shown there is a safe level, and I would say mercury is a very toxic substance." (51)

Thimerosal's potential danger has not gone unnoticed by the FDA. On July 1, 1999, the FDA sent a letter to vaccine manufacturers requesting plans for the removal of thimerosal from vaccines – or to justify the continued use of it. (52) On July 7, 2000, the American Academy of Pediatrics (AAP) and the U.S. Public Health Service issued a statement calling for the elimination or reduction of thimerosal in vaccines for children. The AAP also urged the FDA and manufacturers to quickly reduce the mercury content of vaccines. Why? Because of the mounting toxicity evidence, numerous babies building up harmful levels of ethyl mercury, and the fact that thimerosal exposure from the combination of vaccines in the first six months of life could exceed some government-recommended limits.

Walter A. Orenstein, M.D., head of the national immunization program at the federal Centers for Disease Control and Prevention, told concerned parents that..."Thimerosal will be out by the end of the year." Spokesman for the CDC Glen Nowak said that "Our goal is to [achieve] a thimerosal-free children's immunization schedule by early 2001." (53)

The FDA had previously ruled that thimerosal was safe.

One concerned mother, Lyn Redwood, RN, MSN, CRNP, reviewed her son's vaccine record and found that they contained thimerosal and he had received 187.5 mcg (micrograms) of mercury – all within the first six months of life. She said: "At each visit, two, four, and six, he received a total of 62.5 mcg of mercury. These levels exceeded EPA's allowable daily exposure of 0.1 mcg per kilogram at two months 125-fold." (54) The EPA allowable exposure of mercury for adults is only 0.1 mcg per kilogram per day. (55) Clearly, our children are underprotected.

Supposedly thimerosal has been removed from three or four childhood vaccines for influenza and one of four DTaP vaccines and has been replaced in vaccines for hepatitis B. (56) However, the vaccines given at the time of this writing still contain thimerosal, since doctors are still using up their stock of thimerosal-laden vaccines. No recalls have been issued.

Food for Thought

I went to the American Academy of Pediatrics web site on December 15, 2000, to see exactly what they had to say. The press release posted was dated July 14, 1999. In it they announced new recommendations regarding the reduction and/or elimination of thimerosal in many vaccines. Although they make this recommendation, they said, "There is no evidence that vaccines containing thimerosal result in adverse reactions, and government safety guidelines for mercury exposure are still well below a dangerous level. But since very high mercury exposure from fish and other sources has caused brain damage, it is crucial to ensure that mercury levels in vaccines are as low as possible." So mercury in fish can cause brain damage, but mercury in thimerosal doesn't? Mercury is a cumulative poison. That is, it accumulates in our tissues and builds up over time because it is not easily excreted. Repeated vaccinations of thimerosal (i.e., mercury) containing vaccines is just like eating mercury- contaminated fish repeatedly. The mercury is the same, and it accumulates in our tissues the same way.

For them to say what they did is out right chicanery. They're admitting there's a problem by recommending thimerosal be reduced, but at the same time deflecting any admission of negligence on their part by talking about mercury exposure from fish. Joel Alpert, M.D., president of AAAP, said in the article, "Parents shouldn't worry about the safety of vaccines. The current levels of thimerosal will not hurt children. Reducing those levels will make safe vaccines even safer." If it's so safe, why take it out? Because it isn't and he knows it and he's merely covering his and the AAP's behind. Can you imagine the AAP, the FDA, and other health agencies saying "Oh, well, we've been injecting this toxic metal, mercury, into your children for years. Now we've realized it can cause autism and other things, so we're taking it off the market. So sorry."

And you can tell where their priorities are. Although they agreed to make thimerosal-free vaccines, they are still dispensing the vaccines they had in stock that contain mercury. Heaven forbid the pharmaceutical companies lose any money by throwing out any known-to-be-toxic product. Does this sound like they care one little peep about your child's safety?

Thimerosal is not only used as a preservative in vaccines, but is also used during the production of vaccines. So even if the vaccine does not contain thimerosal as a preservative, it may contain trace amounts of it (less than 0.3 micrograms of mercury) because not all of it is removed during manufacturing. (57) And, even if EPA guidelines are followed, children and especially small children, can actually be inoculated with mercury levels over the recommended amounts. In fact, the smallest children receive approximately eight months of daily exposures of mercury in a single day if they receive all thimerosal-containing vaccines, and at two months of age, children of all weight categories receive more than 30 times the recommended daily maximum exposure if the Agency for Toxic Substances and Disease Registry guidelines are followed. (58) The EPA guideline is 0.1 micrograms per kilogram of child per day, the Public Health Service guideline is 0.3 micrograms per kilogram of child per day and the FDA guideline is 0.4 micrograms per kilogram of child per day. (59) There is also debate over which scientific data is used for establishing safety guidelines. Newer studies show that current guidelines are still too high.

Food for Thought

Even many over-the-counter drugs recommend different dosages for different sizes and ages. And though there are guidelines for the amount of mercury a child can be exposed to, are they ever followed or even considered? Dosages are not adjusted for the size of the child; an eight-pound infant receives the same amount of vaccine that a 40-pound five-year-old receives. Boyd Haley, Ph.D., confirms this oversight along with other things I've been saying: "A single vaccine given to a six-pound newborn is the equivalent of giving a 180-pound adult 30 vaccinations on the same day. Include in this the toxic effects of high levels of aluminum and formaldehyde contained in some vaccines, and the synergist toxicity could be increased to unknown levels. Further, it is very well known that infants do not produce significant levels of bile or have adult renal [kidney] capacity for several months after birth. Bilary transport is the major biochemical route by which mercury is removed from the body, and infants cannot do this very well. They also do not possess the renal capacity to remove aluminum. Additionally, mercury is a well-known inhibitor of kidney function." (60)

Is there even one pediatrician in the country who would tell a parent: "We can't give little Johnny any more shots today because we've already injected him with the EPA recommended safety limit guideline of 0.1 micrograms per kilogram body weight of mercury. Come back tomorrow."

Lifestyle can come into play as far as increased risk to thimerosal-containing vaccines. Mothers who eat more fish, which is known to concentrate mercury, can have babies who are more affected since mercury is transferred to their children both prenatally and in breast milk. (61)

The EPA estimates that 7 percent of women of childbearing age in the U.S. consume at least 0.1 micrograms/kg/day of mercury from fish (that's above the recommended safe limit). Still, a recent study suggests that intermittent large exposures to methylmercury pose more risk than small daily doses. Multiple vaccines on a single day can be considered an intermittent large exposure if all the vaccines contain thimerosal.

Food for Thought

It's not like our government is unaware of the problems associated with vaccines. We just don't hear about it in the media. The U.S. House of Representatives held a Government Reform Committee meeting on April 6, 2000, in Washington D.C. titled "Autism: Present Challenges, Future Needs - Why the Increased Rates?" The committee chairman was Representative Dan Burton, and portions of his opening statement are as follows:

"This morning we're here to talk about autism. As we learned in our August hearing, the rates of autism have escalated dramatically. What used to be considered a rare disorder has become a near epidemic. We've received hundreds of letters from parents across the country. They've shared with us their pain and their challenges. My staff tells me they cried from the heartbreak of many of these letters.

"I don't have to read a letter to experience the heartbreak. I see it in my own family. My grandson, Christian, was born healthy. He was beautiful and tall. We were already planning his NBA career. He was outgoing and talkative. He enjoyed company and going places. Then his mother took him for his routine immunizations and all of that changed. He was given what so many children were given – DTaP, OPV, Haemophilus, Hepatitis B and MMR - all at one office visit. That night Christian had a slight fever and he slept for long periods of time. When he was awake he would scream a horrible high-pitched scream. He would scream for hours. He began dragging his head on the furniture and banging it repeatedly. Over the week and a half after the vaccinations, Christian would stare into space and act like he was deaf. He would hit himself and others, which was something he had never done. He would shake his head from side to side as fast as he could. He lost all language.

"Unfortunately, what happened to Christian is not a rare isolated event. Shelly Reynolds will testify today. Her organization, Unlocking Autism, will be displaying thousands of pictures of autistic children... Forty-seven percent of the parents, who provided these pictures, felt that their child's autism was linked to immunizations.

"We frequently hear about children with chronic ear infections and children who became autistic after spiking a fever with their vaccinations.

"Liz Burt was one of the hundreds of parents who contacted us. Her five-year-old son, Matthew, has been classified autistic. He was developing normally. At age 15 months, following his MMR vaccine, he began to regress. Since the time of his vaccination, he's had chronic diarrhea. This is very prevalent in autistic children. He also didn't sleep on a regular basis for over three years. Liz took her son to numerous gastroenterologists in prominent medical facilities in the United States with no resolution. Finally, this past November, Liz took her son to London, to the Royal Free Hospital. A team of medical experts there examined Matthew. They felt that he was severely constipated. To the family, this seemed impossible since he had constant diarrhea. A X-ray indicated that Matthew had a fecal mass in his colon the size of a small cantaloupe. After the obstruction was cleared with laxatives, Matthew underwent an endoscopy and colonoscopy. The lesions in Matthew's bowel tested positive for the measles virus.

"Dr. Andrew Wakefield and Professor John O'Leary will be testifying today. Their research has uncovered a possible connection between inflammatory bowel disorder in children with autism who received the MMR vaccine and have measles virus in their small intestines. Since coming home from England and being treated for chronic Inflammatory Bowel Disorder, Matthew has finally begun to sleep through the night. I know it's a welcome relief for his family.

"Unfortunately Matthew's story is not that unusual in children with autism... Dr. Mary Megson of Richmond, Virginia, will testify about the correlation she has seen in children with autism and attention deficit disorder. She's seen a correlation between Vitamin A depletion and immune-suppression after receiving the MMR vaccine...

"There is probably a genetic component to autism. But genetics is not the only issue. Many children seem to have severe food sensitivities – particularly to gluten and casein – ingredients in the most common foods – dairy and wheat. Many of these children show signs of autism shortly after receiving their immunizations. Some of these children, as we will hear from Jeana Smith, have metal toxicities – aluminum and mercury. What is the source of these toxic substances?

"I'm very concerned about the increased number of childhood vaccines. I'm concerned about the ingredients that are put in these vaccines. I'm concerned about the way they're given. We've learned that most of the vaccines our children are given contain mercury, aluminum, and formaldehyde. Last year the Food and Drug Administration added up the amount of mercury our babies were being given to learn that in the first six months of life they received more mercury than is considered safe. Why is it that the FDA licenses vaccines that contain neurotoxins like mercury and aluminum?

"When asked about the increased rate in autism, many will immediately discount that there even is an increase. Even though the latest statistics from the Department of Education show increased rates in every state. Others will say the increase is due to better diagnostic skills. Others will say it is because the diagnostic category was expanded.

The Truth About Vaccines

"California has reported a 273 percent increase in children with autism since 1988... "Florida has reported a 571 percent increase in autism. Maryland has reported a 513 percent increase between 1993 and 1998. You can't attribute all of that to better diagnostic skills...

"If we want to find a cure, we must first look to the cause. We must do this now before our health and education systems are bankrupted, and before more of our nation's children are locked inside themselves with this disease. Families are forced to spend huge sums of money out-of-pocket, even when they have good insurance, because autism is often specifically excluded. California passed legislation recently to require insurance companies to cover autism. Parents spend $20,000 and $30,000 a year. What medical care is covered is often done so after extensive struggles with insurance providers...

"I think that as a top priority, we have to do much more research on the potential connections between vaccines and autism. We can't stick our heads in the sand and ignore this possibility. If we don't take action now, 10 years from now may be too late, not only for this generation of children, but for our taxpayer-funded health and education systems that will collapse from trying to care for these children..." (62)

As we've seen, a link between hyperactivity and learning disabilities in children can be made to vaccines as well. The incidences of ADHD were already discussed in a previous chapter, but just to remind you: It became prevalent in the 1950s and by 1963 was being called minimal brain dysfunction; and the symptoms called by various names have been on the rise ever since. Nationwide, the number of children classified with learning disabilities and placed in special education programs increased 191 percent between 1977 and 1994. (63) Even with an increase in detection and reporting, that number is very high.

In her book *Endangered Minds*, Jane M. Healy, Ph.D., notes that teachers have observed that many of their students are not as bright with shorter attention spans compared with the students they had in the 1960s. Beginning in 1964 until the early 1980s, the average SAT scores (tests given to high-school students prior to graduation) in both English and math steadily declined. If that's not bad enough, Healy also shows that since the early 1960s, the tests themselves have actually been made easier. Publishers of the tests, school administrators, and teachers are all under pressure to have students look good and to show that the education system is working. (64) When in fact, children are becoming dumber and learning impaired.

The pertussis vaccine is not the only one implicated in the startling rise in autism. R. Edward Yazbak, M.D., says that the MMR (measles, mumps, rubella) vaccine, when given to women before and after conception presupposes them to having children with autism. (65) The CDC and vaccine manufacturers caution that the MMR vaccine should not be given to pregnant women. In one study by

Yazbak, 18 mothers had received a live virus vaccine just before or after conception. Seventeen of the 18 women had children with early onset autism. The report goes on to say... "Several mothers who were in good health and had normal children report that after they were re-vaccinated with MMR or rubella vaccines they experienced health problems; they had miscarriages or delivered prematurely; they still remained rubella-susceptible; their children developed autism and other disabilities." (66)

In another study by Dr. Yazbak, 60 mothers had been revaccinated with the MMR vaccine after childbirth. Forty-five of these women now have children diagnosed with autism; another 10 have children with ADHD and four women have children with other serious health problems. (67) Yazbak, a well recognized expert in immunology, began his research when one of his grandsons, who was perfectly normal, became autistic at 15 months immediately after he received his first MMR shot. His autism worsened drastically after his second MMR shot. This boy's mother had received 4 MMR shots before conception, and Dr. Yazbak believes by her receiving these shots, her son became more susceptible to autism. Yazbak believes it's imperative to scientifically explore the relationship between vaccines and autism. "It is now up to them to prove that vaccines do not predispose to autism. Independent, large-scale studies should be promptly initiated," he said. (68)

The American Medical Association, The American Academy of Pediatrics, the CDC, the FDA, the U.S. Department of Health and Human Services, pharmaceutical companies and the U.S. Congress all maintain the position that there is absolutely no autism-vaccination connection and that the onset of autism around the time of an MMR or pertussis (DPT) vaccine is purely coincidence. (69)

Food for Thought

Imagine what would happen if a herb or vitamin caused a person to become hopelessly deranged – even if the connection of the product to the person's derangement was not scientifically established. And even in spite of the evidence of vaccines being a causative factor in the development of autism, the correlation is explained away by organized medicine as merely coincidental. Sounds very similar to the tobacco industry denying that smoking caused cancer and cardiovascular problems. There was no hard, scientific evidence to support this connection. That is, there were no scientific double-blind studies conducted under strict scientific protocols showing that this was in fact the case. That's what these industry and governmental spokespeople mean when they say there's no "scientific evidence." They are right in saying this since there have been no scientific studies conducted under accepted scientific protocol. All the evidence is merely "anecdotal," meaning it is hearsay and not statistically proven. That's correct. But just as in the case of the tobacco industry, there are a growing number of people making the connection between their children's illnesses, injuries

---

and deaths to the vaccines their children were subjected to. And I predict that within the next 10 years you'll see class-action lawsuits filed against the pharmaceutical companies who make these vaccines. There have already been many lawsuits filed (and won) by individual parents claiming vaccines caused harm to their child. You just haven't heard about them because the mass media doesn't report them, and the parents must file the suit in accordance with the National Childhood Vaccine Injury Act, which buffers the pharmaceutical industry from exposure. And the government – we taxpayers – pay the settlements!

Are vaccines effective in preventing the disease they are designed to prevent? The first measles vaccine was given in the U.S. in 1963. But the death rate (reflective of the number of measles cases overall) had already declined almost 98 percent from its recorded high in 1900. A survey of 30 states in 1978 showed that of all the children who got measles, half of them had received the measles vaccine. Other research documents the amazing fact that someone who receives the measles vaccine is actually 15 times more likely to get the disease than someone who is not vaccinated for it. (70) There are similar statistics for other diseases that show that they too were on the decline before a vaccine was developed for them, and that the vaccine actually does little, nothing, or actually contributes to the incidences of the disease it is meant to prevent.

The pertussis vaccine is implicated in diabetes. Since the 1970s the vaccine has been known to cause over-production of insulin by the pancreas in test animals leading to exhaustion and destruction of the "islets of Langerhans" cells. This then prevents the cells from producing enough insulin, thus causing hypoglycemia and latter diabetes. (71) As early as 1949 it was noted that the vaccine could cause low blood sugar in children. In 1977, Gordon Stewart wrote, "More than any other vaccine in common use, pertussis vaccine is known pharmacologically to provoke... hypoglycemia due to increased production of insulin." (72)

J. Barthelow Classen, M.D., a former researcher at the National Institutes of Health, has done extensive studies, which support the vaccine-diabetes connection. He showed that DPT injections in lab rats caused them to have a significantly higher rate of diabetes than those not injected. (73) He also reported that in Finland there was a marked increase in the incidence of Type I diabetes following changes and increases in the childhood vaccination schedule. Dr. Classen concluded: "The net effect was the addition of three new vaccines to the 0 to four-year-old age group and a 147 percent increase in the incidence of IDDM [insulin dependent diabetes mellitus], the addition of one new vaccine to the five- to nine-year-olds and a rise in the incidence of diabetes of 40 percent, and no new vaccines added to the 10 to 14-year-olds and a rise in the incidence of IDDM by only 8 percent between the intervals 1970 - 1976 and 1990 - 1992. The rise in IDDM in the different age groups correlated with the number of vaccines given." Also, in New Zealand, the incidences of diabetes went up from 11.2 cases per 100,000 children per year to 18.2 per 100,000 children per year following a massive campaign from 1988 to 1991 to vaccinate babies six weeks of age or older with hepatitis B vaccine. That's a 60 percent increase. (74)

Children born since 1990 are the most vaccinated generation in American history and probably the world. The nation's public health "experts" currently recommend 36 vaccinations by the age of five and many people have been vaccinated their entire lives with the recommended regimen plus tetanus boosters and periodic hepititis A & B inoculations. Never before has children's health been so in question, with numerous maladies now at epidemic proportions.

Food for Thought

Statistical analysis holds that if something changes by more than 5 percent, it's seen to be a "significant" change. If there's a change of less than 5 percent, it's seen to be "insignificant." Many of the surveys concerning vaccines and diseases that manifest after inoculations show changes well above this 5 percent mark. This indicates a possible "causational relationship" worthy of further investigation using accepted scientifically sound protocols. But testing costs money.

More than $1 billion is appropriated by Congress to federal health agencies every year to develop, purchase, and promote mass vaccinations of American children. However, none of that money (that means absolutely $0) is used to fund independent vaccine researchers to investigate vaccine-related health problems such as diabetes and autism. The government relies solely on scientific data supplied by drug companies (who make and sell the vaccines) to approve and license the vaccines for mandated mass-vaccination programs. There is no corroboration of data with independent research. It's the fox guarding the chicken coop. The National Vaccine Information Center (NVIC) says there is a serious conflict of interest in allowing the same health officials who are responsible for researching, developing, regulating, making national policies, and promoting vaccines to also be in control of monitoring vaccine reactions and health problems associated with vaccines. We need checks and balances. Barbara Loe Fisher, president of NVIC says, "Health officials in federal agencies have no accountability to anyone when it comes to setting priorities for how our tax dollars are used when it comes to vaccine research. They can choose to do whatever they want to do with the money they get from Congress. And they choose to ignore the mounting evidence that vaccines are playing a role in the current epidemic of chronic disease, such as diabetes, in our society. Instead, our tax money is used to create more vaccines to add to the mandatory vaccination schedule for our children. There have never been and there are no plans to fund large independent studies to back-up the scientific validity of the government's current vaccine policies and independently confirm they are safe." (75)

The Truth About Vaccines

Pertussis, also called whooping cough, was first described by French physician Guillaune Baillou in 1578 during an epidemic in Paris, France. There have been many other pertussis epidemics since, and most of the victims were children. Symptoms include a severe, short, dry cough, vomiting, runny nose, and later a high fever and possibly convulsions. It usually affects children between the ages of 2 and 6 years, but infants and older children are also vulnerable. (76)

Many people believe that the incidences of pertussis declined because of vaccinations. However, in America, England, and Sweden, the death rate from the disease declined by 90 percent in the 1940s before mass vaccinations. (77) Further, a study published in 1994 showed that at least 80 percent of children under the age of 5-years-old who got pertussis had been vaccinated for that disease. (78)

Some reactions to the pertussis vaccine include vomiting, diarrhea, a hard swelling at the site of the injection, fever, runny nose, bronchial congestion, ear infections and possibly SIDS. However, the most distinctive symptom to the pertussis vaccine (which is part of the DPT shot) is a loud, high pitched screaming. One mother described her child's screaming after a DPT shot: "It was a blood-curdling scream like someone was stabbing him, and he never, never cried like that. Then he became unresponsive. His arms dropped to his side, and he became flaccid. About an hour later, the same thing happened again. His arms dropped to his side, he let out this terrible scream and became flaccid." (79)

Robert Mendelsohn, M.D., the pioneer in the fight against vaccinations, has this to say about the whooping cough vaccine:

> Whooping cough (pertussis) vaccine is one of the most controversial immunizations, even after all these decades of use. It is included automatically in the "triple shot" given almost all babies, the other two being diphtheria and tetanus. Yet it is the least effective of the three and the most dangerous. Most of the bad reactions, including high fever and convulsions, come from the whooping cough element, and the official recommendation is that the shot usually not be given to anyone older than six. The incidence of whooping cough in this country has certainly declined, but the disease is not that rare. Doubts persist as to whether the pertussis vaccine itself has had very much to do with the decline in the disease and whether the vaccine, if introduced today, would pass FDA standards. If you're concerned about giving the whooping cough vaccine to your child, ask your doctor if he really feels that your child should be immunized with the triple shot, or whether he believes that the duo of diphtheria and tetanus immunization is enough. (80)

Sudden Infant Death Syndrome (SIDS) usually happens when the infant stops breathing, most often during sleep. The medical community does not know exactly why it occurs, but the popular explanation is that the central nervous system is somehow affected so that the involuntary act of breathing is suppressed.

Mendelsohn has his own opinion. He says,

> What caused the malfunction in the central nervous system? My suspicion, which is shared by others in my profession, is that the nearly 10,000 SIDS deaths that occur in the United States each year are related to one or more of the vaccines that are routinely given children. The pertussis vaccine is the most likely villain, but it could also be one or more of the others. (81)

Mendelsohn says that breast feeding can help children avoid SIDS (along with other ailments such as allergies, respiratory disease, gastroenteritis, hypocalcemia, obesity, and multiple sclerosis).

Food for Thought

All this bad news about the pertussis vaccine may be new to you, but it isn't to the medical community. As early as 1948 researchers from Harvard Medical School reported about children who had suffered brain damage after getting a pertussis shot. And product insert sheets from a vaccine manufacturer, the Public Health Services Immunization Practices Advisory Committee (ACIP) and the American Academy of Pediatrics all advise against further pertussis shots if a child exhibits high pitched screams or abnormal crying. (82) Isn't it comforting to know that all those experts know there are hazards with the vaccine, but the general public doesn't?

DPT shots (which include diptheria, pertussis, and tetanus), are typically administered at two months, four months, and six months. (There is a newer version of this vaccine is called DTaP, but we will call it the DPT in this discussion). A study at the UCLA School fo Medicine examined 145 SIDS victims and found a high percentage of them died soon after receiving their DPT shots: 6 died within 24 hours; 17 within one week; and, 27 within 28 days. (83) Another study reported in Neurology, the author reported that close to 70 percent of children who reportedly died of SIDS had received the DPT vaccine. The deaths were clustered around the time when the shots were given (i.e. 2 and 4 months). (84)

There have been 579 deaths adjudicated through the Federal Count of claims against vaccines since the National Vaccine Injury Compensation Program began in 1986. Two hundred twenty-seven of these were misdiagnosed as SIDS. (85) (There is also evidence that the mattress a baby sleeps on may contribute to SIDS. Please see the Special SIDS Section near the end of the book.)

The DPT vaccine is one of the worst for causing problems. Barbara Loe Fisher of the NVIC says,

> We have been most involved in trying to inform the public about the hospitalizations, injuries, and deaths that have been associated with vaccines, particularly the DPT and DPTH vaccines. The DPT vaccine – the whole cell pertussis, or whooping cough, vaccine – is

the most reactive vaccine used in the U.S. It's still on the market, even though the FDA finally licensed a less toxic, acellular pertussis vaccine, after 15 years of pressure from NVIC and parents. Although the DTaP vaccine causes fewer reactions, it still contains pertussis toxin that is somewhat bioactive, and so has the potential of causing injury. Even though studies have shown that the DTaP vaccine is associated with far fewer severe reactions than the whole cell pertussis, or DPT, vaccine, the FDA won't take the whole cell vaccine off the market. In the compensation program that was set up under the National Childhood Vaccine Injury Act of 1986, most of the nearly 1,000 awards that have been made are for DPT vaccine injuries. There's no question that it is the most reactive vaccine that we use. (86)

So far we've addressed the problems that result from properly made vaccines. But just like in preparing anything, mistakes can be made and problems can arise in the manufacture of vaccines. Not every batch of each vaccine is as safe as the next one and some batches are more potent than others. An improperly prepared vaccine that gets past safety testing is called a "hot lot."

You would think that upon discovering a "hot lot," public health officials would recall that batch of vaccines. But history shows that this is not the case. The state of Michigan, in 1975, knowingly allowed a "hot lot" of DPT vaccine be given to several hundred children to see just how potent it actually was. The result? Several children suffered seizures, paralysis, and brain damage. When the parents tried to sue the state of Michigan for negligence, the case was dismissed because of the "doctrine of sovereign immunity." This protects the state from claims against it when damages are a result of services only the government can provide. (87) That's our justice system for you.

Even more tragically, in 1990 and 1991 in Los Angeles, approximately 1,500 minority infants were given an experimental measles vaccine. Parents were not told that it was experimental nor were they warned about immediate or long-term risks. (88)

"Hot lot" or not, children are vulnerable to reactions to any vaccine. Most children show some kind of reaction, be it as minor as a red soreness around the site of the injection. But not all children are strong enough to handle a shot, and some react more violently than others. Some so severely they are left brain damaged or dead.

Diphtheria is an upper respiratory disease causing a sore throat, fever of 100 to 104, and swelling of the lymph nodes in the neck, possible heart muscle inflammation and paralysis of the breathing muscles, which can be fatal. Robert Mendelsohn, M.D., in his book *How to Raise a Healthy Child in Spite of your Doctor* gives us some interesting insight into the diphtheria vaccine:

"...there is ample evidence that the incidence of diphtheria was already diminishing before a vaccine became available [as it is with all vaccines]... only 5 cases were reported in the United States in 1980... Today your child has about as much chance of contracting diphtheria as he does of being bitten by a cobra. Yet millions of children are immunized against it with repeated injections at 2, 4, 6 and 18 months and then given a booster shot when they enter school. This despite evidence over more than a dozen years from rare outbreaks of the disease that children who have been immunized fare no better than those who have not... Episodes such as these shatter the argument that immunization can be credited with eliminating diphtheria or any of the other once common childhood diseases... In view of the rarity of the disease... the questionable effectiveness of the vaccine, the multimillion-dollar annual cost of administering it, and the ever-present potential for harmful, long-term effects from this or any other vaccine, I consider continued mass immunization against diphtheria indefensible. (89)

Polio, sometimes referred to as Infantile Paralysis, is a disease of the Central Nervous System (CNS) that plagued American children in the 1940s and 1950s. The greatest incidences of the disease are in children between the ages of 5 and 10 years. Early symptoms include fatigue, headache, fever, vomiting, constipation, stiffness of the neck, diarrhea, and pain in the extremities. The symptoms depend on the site of involvement of the disease in the CNS. Permanent paralysis, including fatal respiratory paralysis, may occur. However, only a small percentage of people who have the polio virus ever exhibit definitive symptoms of the disease at all. (90)

The American epidemiologist, Jonas Edward Salk, developed a vaccine for polio. He used inactivated or "killed" poliomyelitis viruses of three known types and the first use of this vaccine in the U.S. occurred in 1954. Later, another "live" vaccine was developed by Albert Sabin and was first licensed for use in 1961. (91)

These vaccines are credited for halting the polio epidemic. However, Dr Mendelsohn reports that there is "...no credible scientific evidence exists that the vaccine caused polio to disappear." (92) In fact, polio epidemics ended in Europe around the same time as in the U.S., where the vaccines were not nearly as extensively used.

What's worse is that the polio vaccine itself can cause the very disease it's meant to prevent. Even Jonas Salk stated that most of the polio cases in the U.S. since the 1970s were caused by the live virus vaccine. (93)

Besides the vaccine, is there anything else that could cause polio, or the symptoms associated with it? During one of the worst outbreaks of polio in 1948, Dr. Benjamin Sandler of North Carolina publicized findings from his research on polio showing that the disease actually resulted from the over-consumption of sugar and refined starches such as white flour products and corn meal. He showed that as sugar consumption in the U.S. increased over the years, so did the incidences of polio. In addition, countries with high amounts of sugar consumption also had high rates of polio; low consumption countries had few cases of polio. The Asheville, North Carolina, Times newspaper published an article on August 4, 1948, that discussed Dr. Sandler's theory and his dietary recommendations to eliminate sweet and starchy foods. He said:

"I am willing to state without reserve that such a diet, strictly observed, can build up in 24 hours time a resistance in the human body sufficiently strong to combat the disease successfully. The answer lies simply in maintaining a normal blood sugar." (94)

By the way, his dietary recommendations are consistent with those I make in this book: no sugary foods like soft drinks, candy, fruit juices, ice cream, cakes, pies, candies, etc; no cereals, breads, rolls, pancakes, etc; more protein from natural sources like eggs, fish, beef, chicken; raw milk; raw cheese. (This diet is not just good for preventing polio, but for avoiding all diseases.)

Dr. Sandler also showed that polio outbreaks occurred during the summer months when the consumption of sugary drinks and ice cream was the highest. In 1948, polio was at epidemic levels in North Carolina and its residents were desperate. So following the newspaper article and other newspaper and radio coverage, they started following his advice and sugar consumption decreased by 90 percent. The result? The number of polio victims also decreased a full 90 percent. This improvement didn't last long, however, because the manufacturers of soft drinks and ice cream made some announcements of their own discrediting Dr. Sandler's findings. By 1950, the sales of pop and ice cream were back to normal, and so were the high incidences of polio. (95)

Food for Thought

Here's another way to get the incidences of a disease down to make vaccinations look effective: change the definition of the disease! That's what happened with polio. In 1962, Dr. Bernard Greenberg, head of the Department of Biostatistcs at the University of North Carolina School of Public Health, testified in front of Congress that this was in fact the case. He said that between 1957 and 1958, polio actually increased 50 percent, and from 1958 to 1959, it increased 80 percent (after the polio vaccine was administered). But the disease was redefined. In 1955. Instead of having to exhibit paralytic symptoms for 24 hours per the old definition, the patient needed to exhibit symptoms for a full 60 days under the new definition. Dr. Greenberg said, "This change in definition meant that in 1955 we started reporting a new disease..." (96) And in order for polio to be considered an epidemic, 20 people per 100,000 people per year had to exhibit the symptoms under the old definition and 35 people per 100,000 people per year under the new definition. Before the vaccine, cases of aseptic meningitis (similar to polio itself) were often reported as polio. After the vaccine, these cases were counted as a separate disease. No wonder the incidences of polio dropped after the vaccine! It was harder to get it, according to their new definitions! Ever wonder why there are so many names for so many seemingly similar diseases? Most of an M.D.'s work is trying to diagnose the disease – to give it a name. Getting the right name seems to be important for people and it puts them at ease. At least they know what it is! But many times even the M.D.s are stumped. How many times have you heard of someone going to the doctor, getting all the tests, and the doctors still don't know what to call his illness. Boy, then that person is really in for trouble! After the polio vaccine was introduced in 1955, there were 273 cases of polio reported in Los Angeles County and 50 cases of aseptic meningitis. In 1961 there were 161 cases of polio and 65 cases of aseptic meningitis. By 1966, there were only 5 cases of polio but 256 cases of aseptic meningitis reported. (97) Numbers like that sure make it appear like the vaccine is working. But the governmental report that reported these numbers even stated, "Most cases reported prior to July 1, 1958 as non-paralytic poliomyelitis are now reported as viral or aseptic meningitis." (98) (Again, the symptoms of aseptic meningitis are virtually identical to those of the "old polio.")

Mankind sure is clever. Don't worry folks, the U.S. is not the only clever one. The same renaming charade happened in Great Britain. "After vaccination was introduced, cases of aseptic meningitis were more often reported as a separate disease from polio, but such cases were counted as polio before the vaccine was introduced. The Ministry of Health [the Great Britain version of the FDA] admitted that the vaccine status of the individual is a guiding factor in diagnosis. If a person who is vaccinated contracts the disease, the disease is simply recorded under a different name." (99)

Again, in 1995, the federal government arbitrarily rewrote the definition of encephalophy (brain dysfunction) that had been used in medicine for decades. This was done in the Table of Compensable Events used to determine what injuries, under the 1986 National Vaccine Injury Act, were eligible for compensation. Compensation for encephalophy from the DPT vaccine, with this new definition, has become virtually impossible to claim. In addition, they removed seizures from the table, although the fact that the pertussis vaccine causes them is uncontested, and a warning that seizures may result from the vaccine is even on the manufacturer's package insert! Barbara Loe Fisher comments on the changes: "The federal compensation system that we were told would be 'simple justice for children,' has become a cruel joke, a sad commentary on a national health policy that forces children to take the risk and then leaves many families to cope with the catastrophic consequences on their own when the risk turn out to be 100 percent." (100)

Doctors and members of the traditional medical community, either knowingly or unknowingly deny the existence of vaccine reactions. But it goes further than that. Rarely is a vaccine listed as the cause of death. Instead, the coroner uses the subterfuge of complicated medical language to falsify the death certificate. When in truth the death was caused by a vaccine, they say it was due to bronchial bilateral pneumonia, infantile paralysis, SIDS, lymphatic leukemia, tubercular meningitis or a number of other names to ensure the real reason is not listed and thus discovered.

George Bernard Shaw was privy to these shenanigans. He wrote, "During the last considerable epidemic at the turn of the century, I was a member of the Health Committee of London Borough Council, and I learned how the credit of vaccination is kept up statistically by diagnosing all the revaccinated cases (of smallpox) as pustular eczema, varioloid or what not – except smallpox." (101)

Before we go on with this discussion, I want to remind you that there is strong evidence that the incidences of infectious diseases were already declining when the vaccines were introduced; vaccines have actually been shown to increase the incidences of that particular disease; and that the classification and diagnosis of many diseases have been changed to help reflect the "benefit to our society" of the vaccines. What could actually be happening is that the incidence of acute "infectious" diseases is really not being curbed by vaccines at all and that chronic diseases like diabetes and asthma are also increasing. The worst of both worlds.

In 1997, two highly respected magazines, *The Economist* and *Science News*, had featured articles posing the question of whether the decrease in infectious diseases in childhood through the mass use of vaccines has been replaced with an increase in chronic diseases such as diabetes and asthma. Citing data from England and New Zealand, the *Science News* article entitled "The Dark Side of Immunizations," showed that vaccinated children have a higher incidence of asthma and diabetes than do unvaccinated children. The article cites data from England and New Zealand supporting this. (102)

The Economist article entitled "Plagued by Cures" says that exposure to infections in childhood may prevent chronic disease later in life and that "intervening in infections may have undesirable effects on the hosts – that is, on people – as well as on the pathogens themselves." The article says that one study showed that children who had not had measles were significantly more likely to suffer from asthma, eczema, and hay fever. One theory for this is that recovery from naturally occurring childhood diseases is important so that the immune system can respond and be strengthened by viral and bacterial attacks. Depriving the immune system to naturally develop this way may cause the immune system to "eventually attack itself, which is what happens in autoimmune diseases like asthma and diabetes." (103)

Another study by New Zealand researchers reported in the November 1997 *Epidemiology* analyzed 1,265 people born in 1977. Twenty-three of these did not get any childhood vaccinations and none of them suffered asthma. Of the 1,242 who got polio and DPT shots, more than 23 percent later had episodes of asthma. (104)

Food for Thought

Some people do refuse vaccines and their numbers are increasing. The American Medical News reported on February 9, 2004 that 93 percent of pediatricians and 60 percent of family physicians reported a parent refusing a vaccine for their child. (105) Many parents are now home schooling their children to avoid subjecting them to vaccinations. Even some military personnel have refused to take the anthrax vaccine though doing so could ruin their careers. But for the most part, people follow the advice of their physician. People faithfully go get their injections and subject their children to them to avoid coming down with a disease or the dreaded strain of flu making the rounds that year. But are flu shots effective, safe, and necessary?

In 1999 there were about 85 million doses of flu shots given (billions and billions of dollars worth). There are over 200 common types of influenza viruses documented (the "flu" is influenza – an infection of the respiratory tract). Which one will appear in any given year is unknown, so doctors literally guess at which strain will might come around each year. And even if they guess right, there's always a chance that the virus will mutate into a new kind. Often times, the flu shot leaves the person sicker than the disease itself, and there's still the chance of paralysis, seizures, allergic reactions, and death. (106)

In 1976 there were 565 cases of Guillian-Barre paralysis associated with the swine flu vaccine along with 30 unexplained deaths of elderly persons. Dr. John Seal of the National Institute of Allergy and Infections Disease says, "We have to go on the basis that any and all flu vaccines are capable of causing Guillian-Barre." (Guillian-Barre Syndrome is the inflammatory destruction of the nerve sheath causing rapid paralysis.) (107)

It's hard for me to rationalize how injecting poisons into someone can be healthy. Call me an extremist. Healthy things promote health. Poison and death (vaccines) promote sickness and misery.

Are vaccines absolutely required by law? Most doctors and school authorities tell parents that state laws and school regulations require their children to receive mandated vaccines. However, most states provide waivers allowing parents to decline the mandated vaccines on personal, religious, or philosophical grounds. Contact your State or County Health Department and your State Board of Education and request a copy of the immunization laws in your area. Know what you are up against and learn if there's any way out of having your child vaccinated. Probably a better approach is to get a written statement from a medical doctor stating that the vaccine (or vaccines) would be harmful to the child's health. If you can find a sympathetic doctor, this would probably work. If neither of these methods works, contact the National Vaccine Information Center in Vienna Virginia for help (703) 938-DPT3 or www.909shot.com.

If you try to fight the system, be prepared for resistance. Some parents have been charged with child abuse for not having their children vaccinated and on rare occasions parents have lost custody of their child. That's why getting a doctor's statement instead of a waiver would probably be the safest and surest way to go.

The logic behind denying someone the right to refuse a vaccine is also flawed. If vaccines provide true immunity, as the health officials and manufacturers would have you believe, then the people who are vaccinated should be safe. If parents choose not to vaccinate their child, then that child would be the only one at risk, not endangering those who received the vaccine. So getting a vaccine to protect society is not relevant with these mass-inoculation policies.

In examining 70 years of medical literature, it's apparent that scientists and doctors have long noted how vaccines can cause injury and death in lab animals and humans. It's known and documented that substances such as mercury, aluminum, and formaldehyde are used in their manufacture. Some vaccines are even cultured from aborted human fetuses and potentially contaminated human and animal tissue cultures. And there's no guarantee they won't injure or kill. But why don't the authorities and doctors tell this to the people being vaccinated?

The deception goes further. Barbara Loe Fisher reports,

> Then, after the National Childhood Vaccine Injury Act was passed in 1986, when the Departments of Health and Justice worked together to rewrite the law and withhold federal compensation from three quarters of all children with vaccine associated injuries applying for help; when contraindications were narrowed and sick children started being vaccinated in emergency rooms; when each new vaccine produced was recommended for mandatory use; and when government and industry subsequently joined together to launch a mass media campaign to achieve a 100 percent vaccination rate by denying vaccine risks exist or suggesting that, if risks do exist, they are only experienced by children who are genetically compromised, there was a further erosion or trust.

And how does our government react? Fisher continues:

> ...despite evidence supplied by the Institute of Medicine in their published reports on vaccine adverse events in 1991 and 1994, U.S. government officials continue to promote the idea that children who die or are brain injured following vaccination have an underlying genetic disorder and that (a) either the vaccine simply triggered the inevitable; or (b) these children were predestined to die or become brain damaged even if no vaccine had ever been given. Without any empirical evidence whatsoever in most individual cases of vaccine associated death and brain damage, health officials repeat the seduc-

tive and dangerous mantra to pediatricians and parents alike when referring to children with vaccine associated health problems – underlying genetic disorder.

And so, when parents take the state mandated vaccine risk and it turns out that the risk for their child is 100 percent, everyone has been carefully preconditioned to accept the idea that the vaccine is not responsible. The doctor is not responsible. The vaccine manufacturer is not responsible. The government is not responsible. The genetically defective child is responsible.

How convenient. No need for questions to be asked. No need to report deaths and injuries following vaccination. No need to pull vaccine lots associated with high numbers of deaths and injuries off the market. No need to commit dollars or time to conduct scientific studies to find out exactly what vaccines do in the human body at the cellular and molecular biology level. No need to develop pathological profiles for vaccine injury and death or develop a genetic marker to separate out high risk children and save their lives. No need to be concerned about the immune and neurological dysfunction of these genetically defective individuals who have been legally required to sacrifice their lives on the battlefield of our nations' War on Disease... And of the haunting question remains: just how many are being sacrificed? How many of the mentally retarded, epileptic, autistic, learning disabled, hyperactive, diabetic, asthmatic children in the inner cities and the suburbs and the big and small towns of America are part of that sacrifice? (108)

Food for Thought

George Bernard Shaw, one of the great minds of the 20th century, wrote, "All great truths begin as blasphemies." This may be helpful to keep in mind as you read this sidebar...

Not only are vaccines risky, but the understanding of how they work and of immunology in general is incomplete. The concepts of immunology are filled with assumptions and stretches of the imagination. Barbara Loe Fisher comments about the lack of understanding the medical community has when it comes to the immune system: "I remember standing in a lab at the FDA... talking with Dr. Chuck Manclark, who... conducted pertussis vaccine research for many years at the Bureau of Biologics... In one conversation he pointed out to me that the problem with developing a safe and effective pertussis vaccine was that medical science still doesn't really understand precisely how the pertussis bacterium acts on the human body during the course of the natural disease and so it was difficult to develop a vaccine with the right components in it... If you add this basic gap in understanding to science's limited general understanding of precisely how the human immune system functions and how it interacts with the neurological system, a frontier that is being explored by the new neuroimmunologists and molecular biologists, you have a window for possible past miscalculation of the biological effects over time of repeatedly manipulating the human immune system with single and multiple antigens." (109)

How then, can anyone be sure that the vaccine that's being injected into babies, children, or adults will work if the science and understanding behind vaccines and the human immune system is incomplete? And how can the manufacturers of new vaccines be so sure about them that they not only recommend them but force children to take them?

Let's take a look at the history and science behind immunology to see where it all came from, what the original theories were and why sickness and disease don't always follow the rules it has invented.

In the mid 1800s there was a debate going in the scientific community – the outcome of which would set the modern medical paradigm for the cause and prevention of disease. The principal players in the debate were Louis Pasteur and Claude Bernard. Pasteur (1822-1895) believed that disease came from preexisting microorganisms that invade the human body. He also believed that bacteria are not normally found within the body. The tissues of normal, healthy animals, he said, should be totally bacteriologically sterile. He contended that bacteria caused cells to decompose, or putrefy, thus leading to disease.

Of course, science has proven Pasteur wrong on that. Bacteriologists have since found that all animals need healthy bacteria in their bodies in order to live. In fact, animals delivered in aseptic (germ-free) conditions, kept in sterile cages, and fed sterile food and water do not live more than a few days. It would seem that this "contamination" by outside bacteria is essential for healthy life. (110)

Pasteur was a French chemist who became famous for inventing a heat process that saved wine from being overtaken by mold and extended it's shelf life. This was during a time in Europe when mold was so seriously affecting the vineyards that the industry was on the brink of financial failure. His heat process, or "pasteurization," gained him instant fame, and he derived his livelihood from the sale of wines and beer. He was neither a doctor or biochemist, but was given an honorary doctorate degree which made him appear to be more than he really was. (111)

Pasteur was a prolific writer and had a vocal and flamboyant personality. He promoted his views with zest and conviction and made it his mission to preach his ideas to the world. This attitude and energy did much to get him and his ideas recognized which further advanced his career and theories. The bottom line is he was not just a scientist, but a good salesman. And, his original theories that the blood and everything else of a truly healthy person should not have one single microorganism in it have not only been proven wrong, but conveniently ignored and forgotten. The scientific community still considers him a hero.

Claude Bernard (1813-1878), on the other hand, not only had a different personality – being quite and reserved – but different beliefs on the origin of disease as well. Bernard, believed that disease was not caused by outside invaders. He believed that "the microbe is nothing, the terrain is everything." Others, most notably Antoine Bechamp (1816-1908), a medical doctor, chemist and biochemist, contended that no outside germ was necessary for a healthy person to become sick. Bechamp was quoted to have said, "Disease is born of us and in us." (112)

In the Pottenger's Cats study (see Chapter XII), the healthy cats – fed the healthy diet – were generally kept in close proximity to the sick and diseased cats. The diseased cats had all sorts of diseases that one would normally classify as "contagious.'" But the healthy cats never got sick – they never came down with the "contagious" diseases. Either the healthy cats (who were never immunized) had a strong enough immune system to fend off those nasty germs from the sick cats, or something else was happening.

Dr. Weston Price observed that members of remote tribal villages, who were very healthy before the white man came, would start coming down with tuberculosis (among other diseases) after white flour and sugar were introduced into their diets. Tuberculosis is thought to be a contagious disease. But Price never got it and the tribes-people that stayed on their original natural diet never got it either, despite constant contact with people (and their germs) who did have it. Price said the reason these people got tuberculosis was because of deficiencies they developed from eating refined sugar and flour, not because of a contagious germ. Dr. Paul Carton corroborates this with his observations of patients in his clinic in France. He said, "In tuberculosis the soil is practically everything. One becomes tuberculous by enfeebling one's organism, and the only means of getting rid of the bacillus… is the heightening of the spontaneous resisting power. In a word, Koch's bacillus is not much more than a saprophyte, a moss, a parasite which fastens upon failing organisms and seals the fate of those already falling into ruin." (113)

Germs alone can no more produce a disease than a seed alone can produce a tree. They both need food, water, and a place to live. When these conditions are present, germs become active. When a lot of food is available, as in undigested food or abundant excretion of waste from the cells as they attempt to cleanse themselves from toxicity, these germs will multiply. Herbert M. Shelton, N.D., D.N.Sc. said, "The germs feed on the excretions. They are scavengers. They were never anything else and will never be anything else. They break up and consume the discharge from the tissues. This is the function ascribed to germs everywhere in nature outside the body and is their real and only function in disease... The medical profession has coued itself into hysteria over the germ theory and is using it to exploit an all too credulous public." (114)

Bechamp said that there is what he called "little bodies" or "microzymas," that exist in all living cells of animal and plant life. They change form depending on the condition of the host organism (this changing form is called pleomorphism) and actually help the body get rid of dead and useless matter. He said that no outside germ was necessary for a healthy person to become sick. The German scientist Dr. Robert Koch also believed that germs couldn't cause disease. If that were the case, then germs must be found in every case of the disease and never found apart from the disease. But in the real world, this is not observed. (115)

Another well-respected German scientist, Guenther Enderlein, also believed in pleomorphism. He contended that bacteria could go through many forms during a life cycle – similar to a caterpillar "morphing" into a butterfly or a tadpole into a frog. (Every living creature I can think of goes through different developmental stages where their appearance changes as they grow. A seed becomes a tree, an egg becomes a fish, an embryo becomes a man. Why would bacteria be any different?) In his book *Bakterien Cyclogenie*, Enderlein explained that when a person is healthy, the bacteria live in a harmonious relationship with it and actually help the immune system. If there are factors such as poor nutrition, dehydration, stress, alcohol, nicotine or drug use, the internal environment of the body changes and becomes toxic, the pH of the blood becomes imbalanced (it becomes acidic), and then the bacteria change form into a disease indicating (not causing) form. (116) It seems, then, that the health of the person determines the kind of germ present, and not the other way around!

As you can see, many researchers believe that germs do not cause disease. If true, the very foundations upon which vaccinations are built are terribly flawed. Remember, 90 percent of the people with the polio virus show no signs of the disease even under epidemic conditions. Why? Remember the events in North Carolina? When the consumption of sugar and ice cream went down, so did the incidences of polio.

This also explains why some germs may emit toxins into our bodies, which do in fact have an unhealthy effect on us. But the germs only emit toxic byproducts if the environment they are in is first toxic. It is not the other way around, namely, the bacteria causing the body's toxicity. Sir Richard Douglas Powell was a leading bacteriologist in the early 20th century. He observed that if tetanus and gas gangrene germs are washed clean and freed from their environment, they are quite harmless. Shelton comments, "It would seem that they [the germs] depend for their toxicity and supposed specificity upon a toxic environment, and if this is so, the chemistry of their environment really determines toxicity." [117] Other researchers agree. Nancy Appleton, in her book *Rethinking Pasteur's Germ Theory*, recounts the work of Dr. Arthur Kendall, Dean of Northwestern University Research Laboratory in Chicago, Illinois, and Royal Raymond Rife. She says their conclusions were, "The human body is chemical in nature. The bacteria that exist normally in the body feed on these chemicals. If the chemicals change as a result of a toxic environment – an unbalanced body chemistry – these same bacteria, or some of them, will also undergo a chemical change." And Dr. Kendall said, "We have often produced all the symptoms of a disease chemically in experimental animals without the inoculation of any virus or bacteria into their tissues." [118]

Louis Pasteur is credited with developing the modern germ theory. He believed that all diseases resulted when microorganisms invaded the body and that healthy tissues had no microbes present. He did however, admit that the health of the individual was important in the formation and severity of a disease, but no one ever publicized this fact. [119] Very fortunate and convenient for the soon-to-be pharmaceutical industry. Even Rudolph Virchow, the famous German pathologist and founder of cellular medicine, stated: "If I could live my life over again, I would devote it to proving that germs seek their natural habitat – 'diseased' tissue – rather than being the cause of the 'diseased' tissue." And George White, M.D., states that "If germ theory were founded on facts, there would be no living being to read what's written." [115] (i.e., they would completely overtake an organism once they gained a foothold.)

Florence Nightingale (1820-1910), the famous English nurse, held a similar view. "Is it not living in a continual mistake, to look upon diseases as we do now, as separate entities, which must exist, like cats and dogs, instead of looking upon them as conditions like a dirty or clean condition, and just as much under our own control; or rather as the reactions... against the conditions in which we have placed ourselves?... The specific disease doctrine is the grand refuge or weak, uncultured, unstable minds, such as now rule in the medical profession. There are no specific diseases; there are specific disease conditions." [120]

As an environmental engineer, I inspected my share of wastewater treatment plants. As you might imagine, they have a characteristic smell. The smell is mostly one of bacteria. You see, the way to treat wastewater is to take a thing called an aerator and blow the wastewater up into the air in a mist. This is so the bacteria have plenty of oxygen to carry on respiration so they can eat the waste in the water (i.e., the carbon source). There's plenty of food in this dirty water for these bacteria. All those little germs need is enough air and they multiply like rabbits. The goal of a wastewater treatment operator is to make sure there's enough bacteria in the water so the waste will get eaten up. Many wastewater treatment plants I inspected were ones that got waste from regular houses, businesses, and hospitals, laden with every kind of germ imaginable. I never met a sick wastewater treatment operator and I never got sick inspecting a plant, even though we all breathed the air filled with every kind of bacteria and virus during inspections. And isn't it ironic that the very thing we're trying to avoid (germs) is the same thing that actually cleans our water and makes it safe to drink (among other treatment procedures)?

When they start up a wastewater treatment plant, all they do is take the dirty water and blow it up into the air. They don't need to put the bacteria in it. The bacteria are plentiful in the air we breathe, and are considered ubiquitous. It's estimated that we breathe in an average of 14,000 germs an hour. (121) They are everywhere. They'll find the waste, show up, eat it, and have a party.

If you've put impurities into your body, they have to come out or your body can't function correctly. Your body knows what it's doing, so it starts cleaning house. It throws out the garbage and you have a discharge. Then the bacteria show up and start eating and multiplying. The bacteria did not cause the disease – they just showed up, or changed form, because their food (our waste) was available. Just like the bacteria at the wastewater treatment plant. The food, or soil for the disease, comes first. Then the germs arrive or existing germs change form into the "pathological" strain. That's why Walter R. Hadwen, M.D., "one of the most experienced men in tuberculosis," said, "Nobody has ever found a tubercle bacillus in the earliest stages of tuberculosis." (122)

As the poisons and waste come out in an accelerated way, you don't feel well because now there are poisons in your bloodstream. And often, you'll get a fever because the body speeds up its metabolism to get rid of the waste as quickly as it can. It is the excess waste and toxins in our system that cause disease, not the microscopic germs that are everywhere just looking for their next meal.

My mom was a nurse for 30 years – exposed to all sorts of germs. I can't remember her getting sick. Has your doctor been sick lately? If germs caused diseases, with all the sick people he or she sees, he or she should have been dead by now.

Have you ever noticed the flu season is always around the holidays? You would think there would be more bacteria around during the warm summer months than the cold winter months since they multiply better in warm temperatures. But as the days get shorter, so does our exposure to healthy sunlight. Concomitantly we get less exercise, eat fewer fresh foods, and consume more "party" food than our system can handle. Our internal environment becomes fouled and overloaded and the body tries to rectify this by accelerating its waste disposal. Runny nose, fever, diarrhea, feeling bad, and so on, arise simply from the body trying to clean itself up, not as a reaction to germs. You'll find that as you clean up your diet and consume more life-giving foods, you won't come down with a cold or flu. I haven't had either in close to 20 years.

I also worked as a county health inspector inspecting restaurants to make sure they were clean and safe to eat in. During our training at the state capital, I asked the head of the certification board just what it was about bacteria that caused illnesses. He said he didn't know. I doubt many microbiologists can tell you logical, scientifically proven reasons either.

Think about it. A bacteria is an organism that takes in food (carbon), oxygen (from the air) and water, and gives off carbon dioxide – just like us. (This is aerobic bacteria. There are also anaerobic bacteria that function when there's no oxygen available.) Just what do they do that causes such havoc? And why are some OK and some not – when they all do basically the same thing from a biochemical point of view?

If a doctor took a cell culture of your throat right now, I guarantee he'd find streptococcus germs present. But you don't have strep throat do you? (I hope not. If so, cut out the sugar and other bad foods and you'll get better.) Even the textbooks on bacteriology admit that diphtheria, typhoid, tuberculosis, pneumonia, or any other disease germ may be present in an individual without he or she having the disease these germs supposedly cause.

You may ask, "What about when my whole family got sick? Isn't that because of a contagious germ that got passed around?" Doubtful. You were probably all eating a similar diet and leading a similar lifestyle with similar beliefs. The residents of whole cities and societies lead similar lifestyles, and thus their bodies react similarly to toxic overload. The bubonic plague first appeared when sugar became popular, tribes-people got tuberculosis when they left their natural diet, and Pottenger's cats succumbed to various "contagious" diseases when fed a deficient diet. What I'm saying is, that 99.999999 percent of the time we bring sickness on ourselves (ignorantly or otherwise) by doing things the body doesn't like and can't handle. Most disease states are weaknesses brought on by improper lifestyle and/or toxic contamination and poisoning. The germs only appear in abundance after the body is weakened and toxic.

The Truth About Vaccines

In a CDC publication titled "10 Things You Need To Know About Immunizations," the point was made that "Immunizations must begin at birth and most vaccinations completed by age two... Children under five are especially susceptible to disease because their immune systems have not built up the necessary defenses to fight infection." (123) My question to this is: if the children's systems are not developed enough to fight infection, why are we subjecting them (via vaccines) to the very bacteria and viruses that (supposedly) cause the infection? This flies in the face of logic, does it not? Even if the germ theory were correct, should we not be protecting them against these agents, with better sanitary conditions, etc., and keeping them away from germs instead of pumping these agents into them with vaccines? As we saw in Chapter I, the biology and physiology of a child is still immature and cannot handle assaults on it like fully developed adults' system can. Yet, we subject them to vaccines that not only have the very thing that modern medicine tells us causes the disease (the bacteria or virus), but are also loaded with impurities and toxins that any healthy body has a difficult time coping with (i.e., mercury, formaldehyde, aluminum, etc.) Why would you give an already weak and undeveloped organism – a baby or child – something (a bacteria or virus) that is believed to make a healthy child sick? I don't get it.

The theories of immunology are just that – theories. In my medical school classes, the immunology students were called the "black magicians" because everyone realized they really don't know how immunity works! T-cells, B-cells, phagocytes, lymphocytes, and all those mechanisms that are supposed to somehow remember the germ that was injected into you years ago and come to your rescue when you're exposed to it again. They try to explain it scientifically – but it defies logic.

It's my belief that all these different cells and "immunity" mechanisms are nothing but the body's waste-disposal system. If germs don't cause disease, then what is there to build immunity against? All we need is to have the body be efficient at getting rid of the wastes (from outside as well as inside sources), and we'll be just fine.

The whole idea behind immunology is to prevent epidemics. Vaccines, the theory goes, protect us from bacteria and viruses that might cause disease in otherwise healthy individuals. These healthy individuals are just that – healthy and strong with no symptoms of the disease (diphtheria, measles, or whatever). Going along with this theory, the germ then has the power to make a healthy person sick. In order to do this, it has to be more powerful in its actions than the defenses and biological systems of the healthy and strong individual. If it were not, the individual would not be affected by it. And once the person is affected, the person becomes weaker. If the person is now weaker, would he or she not have less power to eradicate or "kill" the germ? If a germ can cause disease in a healthy person, then the germ should be able to continue to cause disease in the just-stricken sick person. (And the germ would be there. But we've seen that often times the germ is not even present at the very beginnings of the disease.) The germs would be more powerful and proliferate at a faster and faster rate – with less and less resistance from the body – until they completely overtook the individual and rendered him or her totally powerless - i.e., dead. That's why Dr. White could say, "If germ theory were founded on facts, there would be no living being to read what's written."

This is what logically would happen if germs caused disease. They would infect a healthy person and the infection would grow until the person was totally overcome. But immunology says that if we have the necessary defenses built up from prior exposure, we can fend off these germs – our immune system would gobble them up. We will give a healthy person some germs so that he or she can build a resistance to it. If a healthy organism – strong and uncompromised – doesn't have the necessary biological strength to render an invader harmless, then how can a diseased, sick, and weakened organism have the biological strength to do it? That's like saying we're going to open the gates of the castle to let in the enemy (to make us stronger in order to fight them better). The enemy kills and maims some of us. But somehow, that makes the rest of our army stronger. So now that we're stronger from having some of us killed and maimed, we're better able to defend against the enemy who has come in our open gates and is still killing and maiming us and multiplying before our very eyes! That's the logic of immunity.

There are two ways of looking at what would happen in a logical world. One: if the body doesn't have the defenses against that particular germ, then it doesn't have the defenses. So one little germ, one little virus or bacteria, can get into us and take over and make us sick. No defense against that germ means absolutely zero resistance and that germ would multiply and cause us sickness until we were totally overcome and dead. Two: let's say that one diphtheria germ won't hurt you. You have enough "immunity" built up to defend against it and render it harmless. But how about a hundred germs or a thousand germs? Still, with just these few, you don't get sick. But let's say that once you get "infected" with one million diphtheria germs, you get sick. Effectively, your defenses are overwhelmed. Then the germs begin to multiply and you get even sicker. Diseases just don't start at their peak, they progressively get worse. More and more bacteria mean more and more disease. If your defenses were so overwhelmed at just one million bacteria, and then you got weaker and sicker, how are they going to defend against a billion or a trillion at the peak of the disease?

Logically, they can't. And that's why modern medicine gives us drugs and antibiotics - to kill these germs so they don't keep you sick and kill you. But if germs multiply unchecked and we need drugs to kill them, then everyone who was ever infected who did not get drugs would have died. (And you know that's not true.) Not one person would overcome the disease because the germs would keep them sick and eventually kill them. Why have so many people died of pneumonia, malaria, and other diseases? Could it be that they were toxic and had deficiencies so the body did not have the tools to throw off the poisons effectively?

On one hand medicine tells us we need antibiotics and drugs to kill the germs because if the germs go unchecked, the germs will kill us. How many times have you heard the virtues of antibiotics touted and how many millions of lives they have saved? They (supposedly) saved these lives because they stopped the inevitable onslaught and destructive and deadly nature of germs. They stopped the weakening downward spiral these germs cause. We need drugs to stop the deadly nature of the germs because once they make us sick they may kill us or render us debilitated. Where would we be without them?

But immunology, on the other hand, says we can become resistant to these germs by being exposed to them and "building up" immunity. Why do the germs in the vaccines not cause the same downward spiral into death that we need to stop with drugs and antibiotics? After all, they are the very same germs (or facsimiles) in the vaccine as those that caused this down-ward spiral we need drugs to stop. Why, when we're exposed to that nasty diphtheria germ in the atmosphere or by drinking out of the same glass as a sick person, does our immune system not respond in the same way as when we're vaccinated?

According to immunology, exposure creates immunity. But, also according to immunology, the only way you can get the disease is by being exposed. Which is it? If the laws of physics, chemistry, biology, and simple logic are followed, it cannot mean both.

As you can see, modern medicine and the pharmaceutical companies have the best of both worlds. They have convinced us that we need drugs to stop germs so they don't continue to multiply and kill us. And then, they've convinced us we need vaccines to have these very same "killer" germs injected into us so we can have immunity so they never bother us! But as you see, the logic is flawed. And I was trained to believe that logic is the cornerstone to science – and medicine.

In a lot of articles and studies I've read, especially concerning vac-cines, the point is raised that there is no scientific evidence proving they or other environmental agents cause health problems. Just because a high number of children become autistic following vaccines doesn't prove a thing scientifically. This is what's called "anecdotal" evidence, or hearsay, which is not accepted as conclusive evidence capable of proving a theory.

I would like to extend this argument to the subject of germs and how they "cause" disease, and I challenge anyone to show me definitive "scientific" proof using accepted and verified scientific testing protocols that germs do, in fact, cause disease. All the evidence for this theory is strictly anecdotal and coincidental. The germ is there when the disease is present (and that not even all the time). So everyone believes that the germs caused the disease. But there's no hard evidence. We all assume it's fact, because "everyone knows" it's true. They have plenty of theories about how it's done – the DNA from a virus taking over the DNA of a healthy cell and so on – but no one has ever actually tested it "scientifically." Oh, wait! Hold on! Someone has!

A series of experiments were undertaken between 1914 and 1918 in Toronto, Canada, where numerous volunteers subjected themselves to germs to see if they would become ill. First, they drank water with 50,000 diphtheria germs. No reaction. Then 150,000. Still no reaction. One million, and then literally millions of diphtheria germs were swabbed over the tonsils, under the tongue and in the nostrils. Still no illnesses resulted.

They did the same with typhoid germs, meningitis germs, pneumonia germs, and tuberculosis germs, by themselves and in various combinations. The volunteers were observed for several months, and no illnesses were reported. Five years later they were checked on again. In no case did any of them come down with diphtheria, meningitis, pneumonia or tuberculosis. This study was reported in Physical Culture for May 1919. (124)

In the June, 1916 issue of the London Lancet Medical Journal of Canada, another similar experiment was documented where a medical doctor and six others were subjected to diphtheria, pneumonia, and typhoid in doses ranging from 50,000 to 1.5 million germs. After two and a half years, no disease.

In 1918 and 1919, about 30 volunteers in the U.S. Navy had blood and secretions from influenza patients' upper respiratory passages sprayed and swabbed in their noses and throats. The Public Health Report summed up the results saying "In no instance was an attack of influenza produced in any one of the subjects." (125) Similar experiments were conducted in San Francisco and Philadelphia resulting in no diseases. (126)

Dr. Thomas Powell challenged his medical colleagues to produce even a single disease in him because of germs. He was subjected to cholera germs, bubonic plague germs, diphtheria germs, and others over the course of many years. His contemporaries did their best to make him sick by inoculating him and having him eat foods laden with these germs. But not once did he become ill.

Why did these experiments fail to produce diseases in their subjects? Simple. Germs do not cause disease!

(If you discount these experiments because they took place many years ago and science wasn't advanced enough to be reliable back then, may I remind you that the germ theory itself originated in the 1860s.)

We've all heard the proclamations by the medical community and the mass media that smallpox was eradicated thanks to vaccinations (although now we're hearing it's making a comeback). But remember how they changed the definition of polio? Something similar happened with smallpox. Daniel Marchini, M.D., comments: "Since (the advent of vaccines), entire whole populations and generations have been vaccinated against smallpox, and cases of fatal encephalitis and motor and mental handicaps have multiplied... Suddenly the World Health Organization announced (in 1978) that smallpox had disappeared and the edict to vaccinate against it in France was set aside (in 1979)... In the following years cases of smallpox were officially reported. In truth, the illness had not disappeared, but the damage produced by the vaccine was of such importance and the legal reparations so costly (for law suits against the French State, since the vaccination was obligatory), that it became urgent to suppress this catastrophic vaccination and remove the State's accountability... Even though WHO recognized before 1978... that smallpox had not been beaten by vaccinations... the public and medical domains still believe that it was vaccination that beat smallpox." (127)

It appears the powers-that-be don't let the truth stand in their way of making billions from vaccines.

Don't confuse germs with toxins. Toxins are known poisons that interrupt cellular processes and have been shown, through scientific testing, to cause biochemical reactions to short-circuit. Take a pesticide, for example. A common way for a pesticide to kill is to flood the synapses between the nerves with neurotransmitters causing convulsions and death. The poison causes a change in the cellular process, which can lead to sickness and even death. Or like the mercury in a vaccine, which is a known neurological poison.

In a healthy, untoxic person, a germ is just living, breathing, and eating debris and giving off normal cellular wastes which are easily disposed.

On the other hand, if a person does not follow a healthy lifestyle and consumes things that are toxic (caffeine, sugar, food additives, alcohol, tar and nicotine, heavy metals, etc.), their internal environment will also be toxic. The bacteria that come to scavenge are now consuming toxins as well, and not only excrete these toxins as their cellular waste, but also adapt to their environment by changing form (pleomorphize). That's why Dr. Tilden said, "The disease condition present determines the morphology of the germ and not vice versa." (128)

Many cultures all over the world consume bacteria-rich foods on purpose believing they gain stamina and endurance from them. The Hunzas in Pakistan, Eskimos, Masai and Samburo tribes of Africa and others regularly consume foods that according to the germ theory would be considered pathogenic. And yet, these peoples are hearty and healthy. In fact, the Hunzas are one of the longest lived people on earth. By modern medicine's standards they should have died from pathogenic infections centuries ago!

Consider more recent research that undermines the germ theory - that being that many microorganisms are actually now being used to treat cancer. Salmonella has been used by researchers at Yale University to reverse cancer. Cancer is also being treated with "pathogens" by other notable research facilities: Duke University is using a measles virus; Stanford is using the common cold virus; Harvard is using a herpes virus and; the Mayo Clinic is using a measles virus.

Microbiologists believe that mitochondria, the bacteria-like looking organelle inside a cell that produces energy, are the vestige of bacteria that adapted through evolution to have a symbiotic relationship with the cell. Could it be that microorganisms are not our enemy at all, but are in fact beneficial to us and work symbiotically (living harmoniously and beneficially together) with us, helping us cleanse and purify our internal environment much the way microorganisms work in a wastewater treatment plant? Some researchers go so far as to say the doctors of the future will actually be injecting us with microorganisms to help us regain health!

If you're raised your whole life believing something a certain way, sometimes it's hard to realize or consider another point of view. I realize thinking that germs don't cause disease is a real stretch for most people. But again, whether they do so or not doesn't seem to matter simply because a healthy body does not get sick – even if it's exposed to disease "germs." And being healthy does not appear to be dependent on vaccinations. In fact, they just as often (or more) cause more severe and lasting problems than they are supposed to prevent.

One of the main objectives of this book is to empower you and your child. Knowledge and understanding of our bodies and the environment goes far in this regard. To live in a state of fear and worry does not, especially when it is unwarranted. Healthy beings need not fear germs because either germs will not effect a strong immune system or, they simply don't cause disease. Take your pick. The solution to not having to fear them is the same – be healthy!

And remember, many companies make a heck of a lot of money from people living in fear. They will naturally tend to emphasize the fear factor because it means more money in their wallet. The more knowledge and understanding you acquire, the less vulnerable you will be to their deceptions and the less fearful you will be.

Do me a favor... for just a moment or two, imagine how you would feel if you knew and all the experts agreed that germs did not cause disease. Would that be freeing, or frightening? On one hand, you would no longer have to fear being sneezed on or "catching" a cold or flu or more serious disease. On the other hand, if you did get sick, you would know it's your own doing and that you did something outside the laws of nature to cause it.

Could you handle that responsibility? Could you deny yourself and your child that pizza, Twinkie, and soda if not "catching" the measles, mumps, smallpox, and other illnesses depended on it?

Again, I quote George Bernard Shaw: "...intelligent people do not have their children vaccinated... The result is not... the extermination of the human race by smallpox; on the contrary more people are now killed by vaccination than by smallpox." (129)

The Truth About Children's Health

CHAPTER XII
"The Ancestry Factor"

It's highly evident that the health of our children (as well as adults) is not what it should be. The incidences of degenerative diseases such as cancer and diabetes have increased dramatically over the past 50 years. Disorders such as ADHD that were once rarities are now commonplace. Violent crimes by children and adolescents are happening with greater and greater frequency.

With all our medical knowledge it seems paradoxical that this should be happening. Our health and the health of our children should be getting better. But obesity, asthma, and diabetes are occurring in epidemic proportions, many children have learning disabilities, and their morals seem to be unraveling. It appears that instead of evolving to some higher state of being, we are actually degenerating into a sick, miserable and highly stressed society. The omnipresent question is why?

As we have already explored, there are many contributing factors to this dilemma. Pesticides, lead, sugar, water pollution, chemicals, food additives, TV... The list seems endless. Each one is a straw added onto our backs. As they get piled higher and higher, it gets harder and harder to function normally – physically, mentally, emotionally, and spiritually.

One of the most disturbing trends is that diseases are happening to people at a younger and younger age. First, cancer was rare and only the aged would get it. Now it almost seems commonplace for people to be getting cancer and dying from it in their thirties and younger – even children are getting it. Autopsies of teenagers are showing significant amounts of atherosclerosis - their arteries are that of what is expected in an elderly person. One estimate is that by the year 2020, people living in industrialized countries will not be able to successfully reproduce – we'll all be infertile! (1)

Although the effects of environmental stresses on people are the best evidence we can use, much knowledge is gained by performing experiments on animals. There's been enough scientific evidence to show that experiments on lab animals can be successfully interpreted to be used as guidelines for humans.

An intriguing experiment was conducted on numerous generations of cats between the years of 1932 and 1942. It was not performed under the same scientific protocol as experiments are today, but it was quite advanced for its time. The important thing to realize is that the experiment showed a trend that can be extrapolated to apply to any living system. I see it as a law of nature. If I put a cat's paw over a flame, it will get burned. If I put my own hand over the flame, I too will get burned. (Singeing cat's paws was not the experiment – I use this only to illustrate my point!) I know there could be many objections to my thesis in this chapter - from "cats are not people" to highly sophisticated arguments using quantum physics to prove that any experiment is affected by the consciousness of the observer. I know, I know – but let's be realistic. What you are about to learn concerning the cats in this 10-year experiment *may be* the same thing or at least similar to what's happening to us as a species. All signs point to it as far as I can tell. In fact, it was this evidence and its concomitant realization that led me to write this book. Some people can rationalize anything away. Whether you accept or reject my ideas here is up to you. But I think that if you observe what is happening in our society, you may agree it's plausible. If you do, you'll see that there is a need to change the direction of our vessel. Because right now, it's headed into the perfect storm.

Back to the study: Francis Pottenger Jr., M.D., performed the experiment on more than 900 cats to determine why the cats he was using in some of his other experiments were poor operative risks. An excerpt from the introduction (written by Elaine Pottenger) of his classic work titled *Pottenger's Cats - A Study In Nutrition*, is fitting...

In his effort to maximize the preoperative health of his laboratory animals, Francis fed them a diet of market grade raw milk, cod liver oil and cooked meat scraps... This diet was considered to be rich in all the important nutritive substances by the experts of the day... Therefore, Francis was perplexed as to why his cats were poor operative risks. In seeking an explanation, he began noticing that the cats showed signs of deficiency. All showed a decrease in their reproductive capacity and many of the kittens born in the laboratory had skeletal deformities and organ malfunctions. (2)

Pottenger divided the cats into numerous groups and fed them different diets. The result of his study showed that the cats on deficient diets developed: heart problems; nearsightedness and farsightedness; under activity of the thyroid or inflammation of the thyroid gland; infections of the kidney, of the liver, of the testes, of the ovaries and of the bladder; arthritis and inflammation of the joints; inflammation of the nervous system with paralysis and meningitis... [The] cats show much more irritability. Some females are even dangerous to handle because of their proclivity for biting and scratching... The males, on the other hand, are more docile, often to the point of being nonaggressive and their sex interest is slack or perverted. In essence, there is evidence of a role reversal with the female cats becoming the aggressors and the male cats becoming passive as well as evidence of increasing abnormal activities between the same sexes. Such sexual deviations are not observed among the raw food cats. (3)

[Note: the "raw food cats" were fed exclusively raw, uncooked food, which was seen to be sufficient (i.e., not deficient) for these cats.]

The cats fed deficient diets resulted in heterogeneous reproduction and physical degeneration, *increasing with each generation*. Kittens of third generation cats failed to survive six months. Vermin and parasites abounded. Skin diseases and allergies increased from an incidence of 5 percent in normal cats to over 90 percent in the third-generation. Bones became soft and pliable; calcium and phosphorus content diminished. The cats suffered from adverse personality changes. Females became more aggressive while males became docile. The cats suffered from hypothyroidism and most of the degenerative diseases encountered in human medicine. *They died out completely by the fourth generation...* (4) By the time the third deficient generation is born, the cats are so physiologically bankrupt that none survive beyond the sixth month of life, thereby terminating the strain... A study of the microscopic sections of the lungs of the second- and third- generation deficient cats show abnormal respiratory tissues. The lungs show hyperemia, some edema and partial atelectasis, (incomplete expansion of the lungs at birth) while the most deficient show bronchitis and pneumonitis... At autopsy, cooked meat-fed females frequently present ovarian atrophy and uterine congestion, and the males often show failure in the development of active spermatogenesis. Abortion in pregnant females is common, running about 25 percent in the first deficient generation to about 70 percent in the second generation. Deliveries are generally difficult with many females dying in labor. The mortality rate of the kittens also is high as the kittens are either born dead or are born too frail to nurse. Following delivery, a few mother cats steadily decline in health only to die from some obscure physiological exhaustion in about three months. Other cats show increasing difficulty with their pregnancies and in many instances fail to become pregnant. (5)

The mother cats that were fed the deficient diets eventually showed no inclination to care for their offspring. They could not nurse their kittens because their mammary glands were not developed enough for lactation.

As you can see, there are many similarities to the health of the cats fed deficient diets and the state of our own health:

- Heart problems, vision problems, kidney, liver, testicle, ovary, bladder problems, arthritis, nervous disorders – all are reaching epidemic proportions in our society.

- "Irritability" – we and our children are becoming more violent. We are constantly stressed. Violence is in demand in the cinema and on TV.

- "Sexual deviation" – a deviation from normal biological sexual behavior. Perversion on the Internet and seemingly everywhere else.

- "Skin diseases and allergies" – who doesn't seem to have allergies these days? Now they are advertising allergy medicine that can be taken by children as young as four years old.

- "Bone became soft and pliable" – soft and pliable bones are called osteoporosis - rampant among the elderly and even teenagers are showing signs of it. Hip replacements are commonplace.

- "Personality changes" – how many times have you seen on TV reports of someone committing a crime no one thought he or she was capable of committing? Our children are becoming more distant and reserved and difficult to reach.

- "Abnormal respiratory tissues" – asthma is increasing at an alarming rate and is at epidemic proportions – especially in our young.

- "Ovarian atrophy and uterine congestion" – blocked fallopian tubes causing infertility.

- "Failure in the development of active spermatogenesis" – males sperm counts are plummeting.

- "Abortion in pregnant females is common" – by this, Dr. Pottenger meant miscarriages. They are increasing in women, especially those who have been exposed to toxic chemicals.

- "No inclination to care for their offspring" – have a baby, put it in day care, and go back to work. Fewer parents seem to care enough about their children to raise them themselves.

Food for Thought

There are a couple points here I'd like to comment on. The "sexual deviation" definition is by no means a judgment. It is neither right or wrong. However, it is a deviation from the normal biological processes that nature has in place to propagate the species. In that sense, it is a "deviation." I'm speaking from a strictly biological point of view. I personally could not care less what sexual preference someone has. That's up to them. But there may be biological and physiological reasons for the propensity towards it – as there appeared to be in the cats.

As for the lack of inclination of diseased cats to care for their offspring, I see it as a ramification of biological and physiological deficiencies that affect organisms to act in certain ways. If someone is healthy and whole, he or she will likely be loving and caring. If someone is out of sorts and in any kind of diseased or degenerative state, he or she is likely to be less loving and caring. Are you more likely to lose your temper when you're in a good mood and feeling well, or when you're stressed out and feeling poorly? If your body itself is under some sort of physiological stress – from chemicals, pesticides, diet, and so on – you'll be more likely to be irritable and selfish. The uncaring atmosphere of our society is, in my opinion, in large part due to subtle biological stresses we are all experiencing from environmental factors that are difficult to avoid and have accumulated in us over the past three generations.

In a way all these aberrations are not our fault. We are victims of our environment (although we as a society created it). It's not a question of willpower to overcome these inadequacies and transgressions. If I'm missing an arm, all the willpower in the world won't give me the power to clap my hands. If my biological system is missing a key nutrient or is hampered by a pollutant that interferes with normal biological function, how can I be at my best? How can I be giving and loving and caring when my own body is crying out in pain and needing attention? How can a child read and write correctly and have a normal attention span if his brain has not developed correctly? If the child's brain were fixed, he would be able to function normally.

What will become of us? In the cat study, the cats on the deficient diet eventually got so diseased and nonfunctional that they could no longer reproduce. These groups of cats essentially became extinct. I call this law of nature "The Ancestry Factor": *An organism under undue stress or nourished inadequately will pass on its weaknesses and degeneration to its offspring, making that generation weaker and more susceptible to disease earlier in life. This will continue through the generations until reproduction is no longer possible.*

The high infertility rate we are experiencing in our society parallel's those in the cat study. Each generation is becoming less and less efficient at reproducing and carrying on normal reproductive activities. Fertility drugs are prescribed to the tune of a billion dollars a year. Viagra and other pharmaceutical solutions to impotency abound. We look to science and think it will solve all our problems. We trust with religious fervor that our intellect and technology will make everything better. But can it? Is it more powerful than nature and the laws of physics themselves?

Throughout this book I have attempted to detail the changes that have occurred in our society over the last century. From the exodus from the small farms to the cities during the industrial revolution to the introduction of pesticides (spawned out of chemical warfare during World War I) to the use of lead and its eventual ban in paint to the escalation in the consumption of sugar, soft drinks, food additives, and nutrient deficient foods and the use of drugs such as Ritalin by our children. All of these things have occurred so quickly that we really haven't taken the time to examine closely enough what their long-term, and sometimes even short-term effects might be. We are a proud, sometimes egotistical society that believes that we are not subject to physical law — that even though a pesticide will kill a bug, it won't do us any harm. We myopically believe that food additives are metabolized and have no effect on us. That drinking caffeinated beverages, alcohol, and eating tons of sugar a year are magically rendered harmless.

We are also trusting. We trust that the government will tell us if and when something is bad. The FDA, EPA, and international organizations such as the WHO, are our watchdogs. If they say something is OK, then it must be so. We have the best universities and research facilities in the world, don't we? Filled with the brightest minds, the smartest researchers and professors. They'll tell us when something is not right. So we go on eating, drinking, consuming harmful foods and drinks, and we continue to subject ourselves to unhealthy environments at work and at home – much out of simple ignorance, some out of egotistical denial, some out of greed, and some out of laziness. The ramifications of this ignorance, denial, greed, and laziness are disastrous. Your child may develop a brain tumor, leukemia, attention deficit disorder, diabetes, or asthma. He or she may struggle with learning, struggle with others, struggle with their temper, struggle with reality itself. All because he or she have been subjected to agents and conditions not natural to the human body.

In the Pottenger's Cats study, the diets that were shown to be deficient were ones that included predominantly cooked meat and cooked milk or condensed milk. The diets shown to be healthy were all raw. No cooked meat and no pasteurized milk. It's easy to come to the conclusion then that a raw-food diet is healthy and a cooked-food diet is deficient. Although an all raw-food diet can be very healthy, it is not the only point of this discussion, however. There are very few people who will go on an all raw-food diet. And although cooking does destroy some vital vitamins and nutrients, it also renders some harmful substances in food harmless or makes some food easier for the human digestive tract to handle.

In exploring the scientific literature further, an another reason the cats became sick on the cooked-food diet emerges. It's now known that an essential amino acid of cats is taurine (recall that "essential" means the nutrient must be procured from an outside source – i.e., the body cannot manufacture it on its own). (6) Cooking destroys taurine. Since this is now known, cat foods are fortified with taurine. That's why we still have cats around today. Since commercial cat food is cooked and processed, if cooking were the only reason their diets were deficient, then cats would have become sick and died out long ago.

The point here is that the cats' diet was *deficient*. The reason why it was deficient is not as important as the fact that the cats developed diseases and died out on that deficient diet. And even though cats are not people, aren't they subject to the same laws of nature people are?

A typical toxicology study will look at the lethal dose of a substance given to lab animals. In many studies, the LD_{50} is used to set a benchmark for a harmful substance. The LD_{50} is the lethal dose of that substance which causes 50 percent of the test animals to die. As we have seen in exploring numerous studies, many decisions are made on whether a substance can be used or how much of a substance can be used or allowed in our environment based on these kinds of toxicological studies. The point here is that these substances, whatever they may be, do harm.

Similar to the harm that was done to the cats on the deficient diet. The deficient diet is really just another harmful substance. It causes stress, does not allow the organism to operate normally, and results in sickness and disease.

In the cat study, the diseases the cats contracted increased with each generation and affected the cats *earlier in their life cycle*. That is, the first generation on the deficient diet developed degenerative diseases late in life. The next generation developed the same degenerative diseases in middle age. The third generation developed these diseases when they were still young so much so that they had trouble reproducing.

The same scenario is happening with us. If we use 1940 as the watershed year when pesticides, food additives, and chemicals were becoming omnipresent in our environment, then we are now beginning the third generation under these conditions. Each human generation is considered to be 30 years. So the first generation under these conditions was from 1940 to 1970; the second, from 1970 to 2000. The third generation will play out around the year 2030. This is not far from the estimate by some researchers already cited that humans in industrialized nations will be unable to reproduce by the year 2020. The same thing that happened to the cats – extinction after the third generation – could be happening to humans.

Not only were numerous manmade substances such as chemicals, pesticides, and fertilizers becoming common around 1940, the soil we grow our crops in had also become deficient which also leads to disease.

In 1936 the U.S. Senate published Document 264, which stated that American soils had become exhausted and were deficient in many minerals. Therefore, the plants grown on these soils and the animals and humans eating these mineral-deficient crops are often times mineral deficient as well. The document states: "Laboratory tests prove that the fruits, the vegetables, the grain, the eggs, and even the milk and meat of today are not what they were a few generations ago – which, undoubtedly explains why our forefathers thrived on a selection of foods that would starve us!"

Since minerals are such an important part of our diet – as important as vitamins – these mineral deficiencies can lead to disease. Just as the cats' diet was deficient, the human diet has been deficient as well.

A more recent study (1992) compared the mineral content of today's soils with soils 100 years ago from around the world. The findings showed that today's soils contained far less minerals than those of a century ago. The percentage of less minerals were African soils – 74 percent less minerals; Asian soils – 76 percent less; European soils – 72 percent less; South American soils – 76 percent less, U.S. and Canadian soils – 85 percent less. (7) The World Health Organization reports that in 2000, American soils were 95 percent deficient compared with soils of 100 years ago. (8)

The use of chemical fertilizers does little to replace the minerals lost due to their uptake by plants. As the plants take up the minerals they need to grow, the soil becomes deficient in those minerals. Repeating crops without replenishing those minerals results in deficient soils. A typical fertilizer provides only three minerals. Old-fashioned farming methods used natural fertilizers, which contained most if not all the necessary minerals to support healthy, mineral-rich plants. So the soils were replenished and the plants grew replete with an abundance of minerals. Even then, however, the soils could become deficient. "Bottom land" – land near a river in the flood plain – was prized because when the floods came, minerals were washed down onto the land and replenished the soils, thus making it mineral-rich again.

The progressive depletion of the soils was one of the reasons for western expansion of the U.S. in the 1800s. A farmer would plant for several seasons and deplete the soils. The food would become less nutritious and his family would take ill. They would move to virgin land, grow crops on this new rich soil, and become healthy again.

Food for Thought

I have a friend who's about 65 years old. Although he's not really health- conscious, he's generally healthy and has amazing endurance and stamina. He can work eight hours, go home, eat dinner, and then deliver papers on his paper route until 4 a.m. A few hours' of sleep, and then back to work. He can do this for a week or so at a time with no real problem. I've remarked to him that if I (over 20 years younger) had to do that, I'd probably be dead by the end of the week – even though I'm quite conscious of maintaining a healthy lifestyle. My theory on why he can do it, and I could not, is that he has a stronger constitution than I. He grew up on a farm during a time when the soils were richer, and they didn't use chemical fertilizers or pesticides. He ate what they grew or slaughtered, had cleaner water and air, and a less stressful lifestyle. Although his grandchildren are having all sorts of health problems, he remains strong and healthy as an ox. He's a first-generation cat. I'm a second-generation cat and am weaker and more prone to breaking down.

Isn't this what we're seeing in our society? Older people, although still susceptible to diseases, get the diseases late in life. Their constitution is stronger than the generations raised on deficient foods and in toxic environments. Now we're seeing middle-aged people – the first generation raised totally on commercially grown food and one that has been exposed to modern toxic chemicals – getting cancer earlier in life; becoming depressed; having difficulty having children; not caring for their young as vigilantly; contracting diabetes, cancer, allergies and so on in epidemic proportions; becoming fatter, lazier, less able to cope with life. And the offspring of that generation have all sorts of learning disabilities, attention deficit disorders, asthma, allergies, childhood cancers, hyperactivity problems and tendencies towards violence. This generation will – if the trend continues – give rise to a very sick and demented generation. The one after that will not be able to reproduce.

Harold Buttram, M.D., agrees with my assessment. In a personal communication he said, "Yes, many of today's children are in comparable stages of 3rd and even 4th generation Pottenger cats, and the numbers are steadily growing. I believe we will pull through as a society, but I fear our children will pay a fearful price before people come to their senses and the trend begins to reverse itself." (9)

We are coming to a fork in the evolutionary tree. Those who continue to live as is now prevalent in our society will whither in numbers, cease to reproduce and become extinct. Those who heed the warning signs and live within the laws of nature will become stronger with each generation, grow in number and give rise to a new, more enlightened and more harmonious humanity.

Can we produce more nutritious food? Does it really matter what the soil is like or what kind of farming methods are used? The answer to both is a resounding "yes." A study by Firman E. Baer way back in 1949 compared commercially grown produce from different soils around the country. They found that the richer the soil, the more nutrition the crops had. In fact, some crops had from three to 100 times more as nutrition as others. Many other essential trace elements are completely absent in some produce whereas trace minerals are abundant in others. Simply put, richer soils mean more nutritious food. Table 6 shows the results of the study. (10)

Table 6

Mineral content of food grown on rich soil vs. poor soil

Vegetable	P	Mg	Na	Mn	Cu	Ca	K	B	Fe	Co
Snap beans										
Rich Soils	0.36	40.5	60	99.7	8.6	73	60	227	69	0.26
Poor Soils	0.22	15.5	14.8	29.1	0.9	10	2	10	3	0
Cabbage										
Rich Soils	0.38	60.0	43.6	148.3	20.4	42	13	94	48	0.15
Poor Soils	0.18	17.5	13.6	33.7	0.8	7	2	20	0.4	0
Lettuce										
Rich Soils	0.43	71.0	49.3	176.5	12.2	37	169	516	60	0.19
Poor Soils	0.16	4.5	4.5	58.8	0	3	1	1	0	0
Spinach										
Rich Soils	0.52	96	203.9	237	69.5	88	117	1584	32	0.25
Poor Soils	0.27	47.5	46.9	84.6	0	12	1	49	0.3	0.2

P, Mg, Na, Ca and K are millequivalents per 100 grams dry weight.
Mn, Cu, B, Fe and Co are parts per million dry matter
P = Phosphorus, Mg = Magnesium, Na = Sodium, Ca = Calcium, K = Potassium
Mn = Manganese, Cu = Copper, B = Boron, Fe = Iron, Co = Cobalt

As previously noted, commercial farming methods typically use fertilizers with only three nutrients: nitrogen, phosphorus, and potassium (NPK). Organic farming methods often times use fertilizers that contain many more nutrients, including the trace elements that science is finding are vital to optimal health.

Consequently, the organically grown food will have more nutrients and be better for you, not to mention they are devoid of harmful pesticides.

A more recent study in 1993 compared organically grown food versus commercial supermarket foods for basic element levels. The conclusion was that "...the average elemental concentration in organic foods on a fresh weight basis was found to be about twice that of commercial foods." [11] For example, organically grown sweet corn had 1,000 percent more calcium, 2,200 percent more iodine and 300 percent more magnesium. Organically grown wheat had 360 percent more potassium, 160 percent more copper, and 80 percent more zinc.

The 10 percent to 20 percent more you pay for organic food translates to usually more than a 50 percent gain in nutritional value. So, per unit nutrient, you actually pay less for organically raised food than commercially raised food. Not only that, you don't have to contend with pesticides and herbicides that may "soak up" some of the nutrition or be outright poisonous in themselves.

Is it possible to reverse the trend of degeneration that deficient foods and toxins in our environment cause? Pottenger tried to return some of the degenerating cats back to health. He found that it took four generations on raw meat and milk to bring the kittens of second-degeneration cats back to normal. He wrote, "Improvement in resistance to disease is noted in the second generation regenerating cat, but allergic manifestations persist into the third generation. In the third generation, skeletal and soft tissue changes are still noticeable, but to a lesser degree; and by the fourth generation, most of the severe deficiency signs and symptoms disappear – but seldom completely." [12]

As you can see, the degeneration/regeneration occurs not just in the generation that is fed a certain diet. The deficiencies seem to accumulate through the generations, impacting the next generation more severely. Likewise, it takes several generations for degenerated organisms to return to good health. But it is possible. There is hope.

Food for Thought

An interesting correlation can be made between the state of our health and the actions of our government. As with theater, government is a reflection of society – its wants and needs. A trend in our government over the last 50 years or so is towards more and more programs aimed at helping people. There's welfare, Medicare, Medicaid, Social Security, food stamps, educational programs for the learning impaired, housing assistance programs, handicapped parking and building codes for handicapped accessibility, and so forth. More and more, people are asking for and even demanding that the government step in and help them. In no way do I denounce these actions. They are – considering the conditions – quite necessary. But *why* are they necessary? Is it because we are just now becoming compassionate toward those less fortunate? Or is it because now there are so many of us in one way or another impaired or needing assistance that it's becoming a driving force in determining governmental policies?

I get newsletters from a number of doctors and health practitioners. One doctor told of a friend he has who's a stockbroker. This stockbroker invests in a number of medical and drug companies who manufacture products or drugs for kidney disease. He does this because he says kidney disease is out of control and there's no cure in sight. One of the companies is an adult diaper manufacturer – more than 10 million American adults wear diapers. His portfolio of kidney drug, dialysis and diaper stocks is going through the roof. A sad statement on the state of our health.

So, the government must keep up with the demands of the people. Since more and more people are getting sicker and less able to care for themselves, you'll see more and more government programs aimed at helping them. The more the government must act to create these programs, the bigger government must become. A more socialistic state will result. The more people have to depend on the government, the less autonomous they and society become. As government expands to meet the needs of the many, more money is needed to support this growth and taxes will inevitably rise. To collect these taxes, more programs and policies will be needed. "Big Brother" will not arise strictly out of computer technology, but from a simple need – the need for the people to be taken care of.

The bottom line is this: If we don't reverse the trend of degeneration, our health and the health of our children will continue to decline. The degeneration cannot be stopped by more medicine and more technology. Rather, we must care for our bodies, minds, and spirits in accordance with the laws of nature. Then our children will grow up strong, healthy, and happy. They will learn easily, be gentle and loving, and enjoy life. It's the only way to save our children (and ourselves) from getting sick and going crazy.

CHAPTER XIII
Alternative Health Landmines

Throughout this book, I've steered you toward health food stores to obtain many of the items I recommend. But just because you see something in a healthfood store doesn't automatically mean it's healthy for you or your child. There are many products sold and promoted as being healthy that, in my opinion, are far from good for you. That is especially true now, since many mainstream companies are entering the alternative health industry with the sole intent of exploiting it and making more money. I present this information to give you other perspectives that you may not have seen before. I urge you to evaluate it along with any and all other information, and then use your own common sense. Always decide for yourself what's right for you.

The position I take on most issues is, "The closer to nature, the closer to health." All of our knowledge will never compare with the wisdom of nature itself. The more we tamper with things, the further from nature we get, and the more chances there are for mistakes. If we can consume a food directly from nature – such as a fruit, vegetable or animal – it will be much better for us than something that can only be consumed after extensive processing (such as soy products) or genetic engineering (such as canola oil). We should remember how humans ate thousands or even millions of years ago. That's closer to the truth of what the body really needs.

Soy

There's no better illustration of something bad turned on its head and made to look good than soy. The contention that soy and soy derived foods are healthy is pure lunacy. If you read the chapter discussing formula and baby foods, you already know a lot of the problems associated with soy. To even eat a soybean, we must process it extensively with high heat, caustic soda, solvents, and so on. Does that sound to you like something "edible?"

I know a lot of people who read this book are already health-conscious, and many of you may think soy is manna from heaven. "Look at all the good things soy has to offer – the phytochemicals, (isoflavones), protein, unsaturated fat, and essential fatty acids," you may cry. But just because something contains a lot of good things doesn't make it good for you. On paper, one of the most nutritious plants in nature is tobacco. It's loaded with vitamins, minerals, and so on. Problem is, it also contains a substance called nicotine, which is deadly. Should we eat tobacco just because it's a storehouse of nutrients? The overall effect of tobacco in the human body is a negative one. The same with soy.

It's my opinion that if we err, we should do so on the side of caution, using nature as the standard. If something is on the borderline and there are questions as to its safety and viability, it's more prudent to exclude it from our experience. Throughout history, there have been societies, civilizations, and long-lived peoples who have survived and thrived without ever seeing a soybean. Is it possible to achieve superior health without it? Of course it is. Simply use the foods that have nourished mankind for millions of years – before science and agricultural practices started "creating" new foods to turn a profit.

Do you want to know the real reason soy is touted as a health food and is being embraced by mainstream media and medical doctors? You know what it is: money.

Ask any farmer what he plants on barren land where nothing else will grow. His answer? The soybean plant. It's also easy to cultivate and cheap to raise. This gives the farmer and the food processing giants another way to make money from an otherwise unexploited resource. Originally, soy was grown not as a food for human consumption, but as a way to fix nitrogen in the soil. And for centuries, soy was only consumed in its nontoxic fermented form (such as soy sauce, tempeh, and miso), even in Asia. It wasn't until recently that processing made soy edible (if you can call it that). To expound on these points, I would like to quote an excellent article by Tim O'Shea, a chiropractor and clinical nutritionist:

> ...In spite of claims to the contrary, no bean is a complete protein because all beans lack two essential amino acid – cysteine and methionine – which we must get from other sources in our diet. A diet in which soy is the only protein source will cause an abundance of health problems from the ensuing protein deficiency... Soy is among the most highly commercially processed of food sources, and after processing it still retains many undesirable substances.

The point is, soybeans are not a natural food like other vegetables. First of all, soybeans contain high amounts of digestive enzyme inhibitors, blocking the function of the pancreatic enzyme trypsin in particular. These enzyme inhibitors are not removed by cooking. They interfere not only with the digestion of the soybeans, but also with the digestion of other foods that happen to be present in the tract.

The second main "antinutrient" soybeans contain is phytic acid. Present to some degree in all types of beans, phytic acid blocks the uptake of important minerals, such as iron, magnesium, calcium, and especially zinc. Soybeans have the highest phytic acid levels of any legume, and as such have an extraordinary ability to cause mineral deficiencies. Third World countries with diets high in grains and soy have the most profound deficiencies of these minerals. (1)

This is especially bad for infants. The soy in infant formulas robs zinc from the baby's system. And since zinc controls iron uptake, abnormally high iron levels may occur if zinc is not present and liver damage can result. Zinc is crucial for growth and brain and nervous system development (remember, it's sometimes called the "intelligence mineral"), as well as protein digestion. It is also necessary for immune system development and normal insulin function.

Another component of soy that is problematic is hemagglutinin – an agent that causes red blood cells to clot. When red cells clump together, the oxygen supply to the entire body is diminished. Those who already have a history of heart problems should be especially wary of soy.

Aluminum, another toxin found in some processed soy products, is said to be 10 times higher in infant soy formulas than in milk-based formulas – and 100 times higher than in unprocessed milk. Aluminum can damage the newly forming kidneys of an infant who drinks soy formula. Worse yet, it directly damages the infant brain because the blood-brain barrier has not yet formed.

Soy products may also be a causative factor in cancer. O'Shea states:

> Processed soy can also contain a known carcinogen called lysinoalanine. It is a by-product of a processing step called alkaline soaking, which is done to attempt to eliminate enzyme inhibitors. Even though the beans are thoroughly rinsed, the lysinoalanine by-product can remain from the interaction of the soybeans with the alkaline solution.

It's ironic that the same manufacturing processes used to render soy edible are the very processes which render soy inedible from a health standpoint. The beneficial soy enzymes, minerals, fiber, vitamins and nutrients are lost, rendering the end products – soybean oil and soy protein isolate and concentrate - totally devitalized commercial foods. (2)

If wholesomeness is what you're looking for, don't turn to soy. Producing it sounds like some kind of chemical manufacturing process:

The first step in soy processing is high-temperature cooking to try and get rid of the phytic acid. High temperatures denature the natural enzymes of the soybean. Without enzymes, any plant becomes a devitalized food, very difficult to digest in the human digestive tract. Consider that enzymes, vitamins, and minerals are three legs of the tripod of metabolic activity. Take away any one and the other two cannot function properly.

After cooking, soy oil is removed by one of two paths: pressing or solvent extraction. Soybean oil is rarely cold-pressed, as many claim, but is usually subjected to heat, which produces destructive free radicals. An easier method of oil extraction is by the use of solvents. Several are used in soybean oil processing. Hexane, a petroleum distillate, is the standard chemical used. Traces of this toxic solvent may be left behind in the finished products, both in the oil and in the protein isolate.

The next step in the refining process is degumming, the removal of residual fiber, or gum, from the oil. The problem is that valuable trace minerals like calcium, copper, magnesium, and iron, as well as chlorophyll, are removed as well.

Next, the refined oil is mixed with sodium hydroxide (which is what drain cleaners are made of) at a temperature of 167 degrees F. The purpose of this step is to remove any remaining free fatty acids.

To remove extra pigments and make the oil completely clear, bleaching is accomplished by more high heat followed by filtering. Other free radicals called peroxides are thus introduced.

Alternative Health Landmines

Deodorizing is then thought to be necessary to destroy any natural aromatics. This process uses extreme heat, up to 518 degrees F, which destroys whatever vitality and antioxidants the oils might have left. The oil is thus rendered absolutely tasteless, colorless, and odorless. It is now devoid of any useful vitamin, mineral, enzyme or nutrients content whatsoever. And even though it has undergone extreme high temperatures at several steps, as long as no external heat was added during the actual pressing step, the oil can still be sold as "cold-pressed."

As if no further biological indignity could have been levied against the lifeless processed oil, researchers in the 1930s at Dupont figured out a way to harden the oil into a perfectly engineered non-food: margarine. They found out that if they subjected the refined oil to yet another round of high temperatures – up to 410 degrees F – and also forced hydrogen gas in the presence of an aluminum catalyst through the oil, they could produce a substance with the desired spreadability and shelf-life. That's what hydrogenated margarine means. And at least 80 percent of the margarine made in the U.S. comes from refined soybean oil. (3)

Most soybeans on the market these days have been genetically modified (see more on this below) and have had a gene inserted that makes them resistant to herbicides. With this the soybeans can withstand more herbicides being sprayed near them to kill weeds. Less weeding equals more profit. But what about the buildup of herbicides within the soybean plant itself? Won't the plants exposed to all these herbicides become unsafe for human consumption? No one knows because no one has ever tested them!

To underscore how much the role of money plays into the contention that soy is healthy, O'Shea tells us more unsettling facts:

> The soy protein fad also has an uneasy background – it stems from the soy oil manufacturing process. With six million tons of soy beans being made into oil every year, there was a lot of product waste. After the oil was removed, what was left? Soy protein – the perfect remedy for the American obsession with obesity and cholesterol. Suddenly everyone was dining on soy burgers to meet their protein requirements. They are unaware that they are eating the residue of the oil-refining process. Soy protein isolate is just as toxic and foreign to the human body as processed soybean oil.

> Soy protein isolate is big business. We must appreciate the brilliance of taking a waste product from an already extremely processed food source and getting the majority of the population to think of it as a natural food. (4)

Soy is supposedly great for women approaching menopause, so the advertisers claim, because it supplies a "natural" estrogen, or phytoestrogen, which may prevent osteoporosis and other problems. These estrogen-like compounds come from the isoflavones in soy.

Most isoflavones come from genetically modified soy and are definitely not natural. And the amount that soy isoflavones increase estrogen levels in the body may well be pathological (but it's never been studied). But it *is* known that high

The Truth About Children's Health

levels of estrogen compounds may cause sex organ malformation, tumors and menstrual disruption. So do you think it's good for infants who eat soy to have phytoestrogen blood levels from 13,000 to 22,000 times higher than normal? I don't.

The soybean is America's third largest crop and supplies more than 60 percent of the world's soybean demand – that's a crop value of close to $20 billion per year. And if we take into account the retail market value of the dozens of *finished* soy food products sold in supermarkets, the total value approaches $100 billion per year.

Yes, you can find soy in burgers, margarine, cooking oil, and soy milk. But soy is hidden in a lot of other foods where it's not even listed on the label. Soy can be in items like chocolate, soup, French fries, and potato chips. Other names used to disguise soy are "vegetable flavoring," "natural flavoring," "vegetable shortening," " hydrolyzed protein," and "textured vegetable protein." These disclosures, which are all the FDA requires, are terms that indicate that the product contains hydrogenated soybean oil or protein isolate (probably from genetically modified plants). Yet you might never know it.

Soy products are not adequate for human protein requirements. They are devitalized, nonfoods with many toxic substances and little to no nutrient content. What can we do? Stay informed. Make choices for you and your children that are not determined by product ads and hype. Let's try to keep ourselves and our children away from the foods that contain processed soy products.

The only soy product that is not detrimental to your health is traditional soy sauce that's been "naturally brewed." Modern processing methods produce large amounts of the kind of unnatural glutamic acid that is found in MSG, which was discussed in Chapters VI and IX. Buy only the kind of soy sauce that says "Naturally Brewed" on the label. Commercially available tempeh and miso, although probably not "naturally brewed," are marginally acceptable also.

Vegetarianism

Over the past 30 years or so it's been more and more popular to be a vegetarian. Proponents cite moral as well as health reasons. Although it may be possible to be a healthy vegetarian, you must be very careful and vigilant to ensure adequate nutrition. In his article *Vegetarianism: An Anthropological/Nutritional Evaluation*, H. Leon Abrams, a noted anthropologist, says, "No culture in the history of mankind has been based on a 100 percent vegetarian diet, and although one can theoretically, in the light of contemporary nutritional scientific knowledge, obtain all the nutrients needed to provide good health, the technology to ensure such has not been developed and such a vegetarian diet is extremely risky." (5)

That is especially true for children. As already discussed, children need a high fat diet or else their nervous system and brain will not develop normally. They need iron in adequate amounts and vitamin B-12, which is absent or lacking in nonanimal foods. Children need to eat meat or animal products every day once they stop breast feeding and start eating solid food.

Abrams goes on to talk about the "macrobiotic diet," which primarily consists of cooked grains and no animal products: "... Research and clinical observation found that babies who eat no animal protein fail to grow at a normal rate; this study found that infants on 'vegan' diets, except for early breast feeding, did not grow nor develop as normally as babies on diets containing animal products or vegetarian diets supplemented with cow's milk.... The results of such diet can be scurvy, anemia, hypoproteinemia, hypocalcemia, emaciation and even death." (6) He also reported that the Hindus of India, although not 100 percent vegetarian, come the closest of any culture. He said that "... the greater percentage of the population, who subsist almost entirely on vegetable foods, suffer from kwashiorkor, other forms of malnutrition, and have the shortest life span in the world." (Kwashiorkor is a severe protein deficiency that is marked by severe tissue wasting and retarded growth.)

Food for Thought

Some of you reading this may be hard-core vegetarians. As I've said, I was a vegetarian for about 10 years, but started eating animal products again about five years ago. I changed because of scientific evidence and personal observation. I simply wasn't getting where I wanted to healthwise on a strictly vegetarian diet. The findings of researchers examining the diets of primitive cultures and long-lived and healthy peoples were also instrumental in changing my mind. Consider that for the 3 million to 4 million years mankind has been on this planet, 99 percent of the time he was a hunter/gatherer. That means he ate large amounts of animal food. It wasn't until 10,000 years ago that people finally started cultivating plants – only because they had in large part exhausted the supply of wild game. Interestingly, this stationary agricultural activity spawned political organizations (societies) and religions. And some of the religions imposed dietary restrictions – such as not eating meat – out of population growth pressures and for other pragmatic reasons. The Hindus, for example, once consumed beef. But because of the increased population and the fact that cows were valuable for their milk, dung (as fuel for cooking), and as draft animals, they were banned as food and became religious icons. (7) Clearly, mankind has been, and should now be, an omnivore, consuming a wide variety of foods, including meat. (For a more detailed discussion on this, see *The Cambridge World History of Food, Volume Two*, Cambridge University Press, 2000.)

My personal observation also showed that the vegetarian people I knew were frankly not very healthy and always struggling with one problem or another. I think part of the problem with most vegetarians is that they eat

---

a high percentage of cooked foods – rice, especially. Cooking robs the foods of vital nutrients. Rice, unless soaked overnight, contains enzyme and growth inhibitors which interfere with normal metabolism.

When I was a vegetarian, I ate a lot of uncooked foods, mostly nuts and seeds, and not too many cooked grains. I didn't get sick, but I wasn't healing either. Now that I eat animal foods, I try to consume some of them in their uncooked form. I eat only organic raw milk cheese, take unheated glandular supplements (i.e., liver, kidney, heart, etc.), and am now experimenting with raw meat dishes. Every long-lived culture consumed unheated animal products to some degree – cultured milk, organ meats, eggs, butter, and so on. It's a stretch for us to think of eating meat raw, but I now believe eating some animal products in their natural state is vital to optimal health.

If we examine the history of primitive man, Dr. Abrams tells us that "Ancient cave-man was a flesh eating animal . Perhaps he ate a few wild fruits and plants which he found in the area, but for the most part he preferred meat... man depended almost entirely, if not completely, on meat for his subsistence... He probably ate most of his meat raw, and that which was cooked was most likely rare." [8] And if you think that that might be fine for a cave-man, but not for us, consider that "man hasn't changed physiologically from ancient cave-man, and not at all from the men of 10,000 or more years ago." [9]

Did this diet of mostly raw animal food suit early man? "...the skeletal remains which we have, show that he was very healthy. He had to be in order to survive..." [10]

Sally Fallon clues us in on more of the history and culture behind raw food: "Almost all traditional societies incorporate raw, enzyme-rich foods into their cuisines – not only vegetable foods but also raw animal proteins and fats in the form or raw dairy foods, raw muscle and organ meats, and raw fish. These diets also traditionally include a certain amount of cultured or fermented foods, which have an enzyme content that is actually enhanced by the fermenting and culturing process. The Eskimo diet, for example, is composed in large portion of raw fish that has been allowed to 'autolate or predigest,' that is, become putrefied or semi-rancid; to this predigested food they ascribe their stamina." [11] This shows that the germs in their semi-rancid food did nothing to harm them, and in fact made them stronger – more evidence that germs do us no harm.

One more point worth noting is that pre-industrial cultures that consumed cooked meat usually included fermented vegetables such as sauerkraut, pickled cucumbers, beets or carrots with their meals. This increases the enzyme content of the meal making it easier to digest. So if you eat a steak, chop or hot dog, don't hold the 'kraut!

Aajonus Vonderplanitz is a nutritionist who has been eating a diet of predominately raw meat and animal products for nearly 20 years. He claims to have healed himself of numerous ailments, including cancer, and has reported success within three months time with 236 out of 240 cancer cases (the cancer was checked) that he put on his diet. (12) His findings are further validation that raw animal products are necessary for good health. In fact, he says that "experience has shown me that over time raw animal products produce the calmest, most balanced human nature with excellent mental clarity." (13) Vonderplanitz also cites the Eskimo, saying, "By several accounts of world travelers and explorers they considered the Eskimo the happiest of all races... the Eskimo ate 99% raw animal products and lived free of degenerative disease before white men introduced cooking cauldrons, breads and refined sugar to them... Their first case of dental decay was 50 years after [these] were introduced. The dental caries only existed among those who ate some or all of white man's food. Cancer never occurred among primitive Eskimo." (14) I recommend you check out his book *We Want to Live*, to learn more about his theories and practices.

Some vegetarians will cite physiological reasons for their choice, saying that the human body is not equipped to handle animal foods. Science disagrees. Again I quote Dr. Abrams:

> Actually, the digestive mechanism of man is adapted to a mixed meat and vegetable diet. Human teeth consist of three types: canines or piercing teeth of the meat-eating animals, and the molars or grinders of grain-and-nut-eating animals. With respect to structure, human teeth are conclusive proof that the human body is adapted to a mixed animal and plant diet. Man has specific digestive ferments for meat proteins and other special digestive juices for carbohydrates. His stomach and intestinal tract are equipped to handle both. (15)

Speaking of teeth, how strong and resistant to decay they are is a measure of how strong your bones are and how healthy you are in general. Healthy people (and animals) will simply not have cavities. And although tooth decay has been known throughout human history, it was extremely rare through the Paleolithic period, which spanned some 3 to 4 million years. It wasn't until mankind started agriculture (abandoning hunting because of lack of game) and consumed a diet high in carbohydrates (i.e., grains), did tooth decay become a major problem. Skeletal remains of ancient societies showed increases in tooth decay between 75 percent and 85 percent around the time agriculture became predominant and the diets became largely vegetarian. (16) Weston Price also found a dramatic increase in tooth decay of people of primitive cultures who abandoned their traditional diets and started consuming more agricultural products such as white flour.

Of particular concern for vegetarians is obtaining adequate amounts of vitamin B-12. This vitamin, also called cyanocobalamin, is critical for healthy blood and a properly functioning nervous system. Since vegetarian sources cannot supply adequate amounts of B-12, deficiencies in vegetarians are the rule instead of exception. And once one becomes a vegetarian, this deficiency may not become apparent for a while since the body stores a supply of B-12 that can last from two to five years.

Deficiencies can cause pernicious anemia, panic attacks, impaired eyesight, schizophrenia, hallucinations, weakness, loss of balance, numbness in the hands and feet, and irregular menstruation including sparse flow or no flow. (17,18) An article in the *British Medical Journal* reported that a deficiency of vitamin B-12 brought on devastating mental and emotional symptoms such as difficulty in thinking and remembering, mood disorders, confusion, agitated depression, paranoia, delusions, visual and auditory hallucinations, maniacal behavior, and epilepsy. (19) Another study found that an extremely high percentage of inmates in psychiatric wards suffer from low blood levels of B-12. (20)

Vegetarian women are not only making themselves vulnerable to a vitamin B-12 deficiency, but their children as well. Many may eat sea vegetables, tempeh, miso, and tamari that theoretically contain adequate amounts of vitamin B-12, thinking they are supplying the body's vitamin B-12 requirement. However, tests reveal that individuals who ingested such products showed no increase in vitamin B-12 blood levels leading to a B-12 deficiency in their baby. Dutch biochemists demonstrated that ingested seaweed products did not correct vitamin B-12 deficiencies in infants. Neither did spirulina, a micro algae. Why? Vitamin B-12 is only well absorbed from animal sources. The Dutch searchers reported that infants of many vegetarian women have abnormal red blood cells, delayed motor skills, and slow growth, compared with control group babies. What are the best sources of vitamin B-12? You won't find them growing on trees. They're liver, sardines, mackerel, herring, salmon, lamb, Swiss cheese, eggs, haddock, beef, blue cheese, halibut, scallops, cottage cheese, chicken, and milk.

As you can see, children and infants are especially vulnerable to the inadequacies of a strictly vegetarian diet. A research team made up of scientist from the University of Cincinnati, Harvard School of Public Health, Vanderbilt and Brandies Universities reported that strict vegetarian women who breastfeed their infants may be subjecting them to possible long-term brain damage. (21)

As I mentioned before, examining the diets of primitive cultures and our ancestors is interesting and enlightening. Native Americans were healthy and robust (before the white man came). They were not vegetarians. Recalls John Lame Deer, a full-blooded Sioux born 80 years ago on the Rosebud Reservation in South Dakota,

> We always had plenty of food for everybody, squaw bread, beef, the kind of dried meat we called *papa*, and *wasna*, or pemmican, which was meat pounded together with berries and kidney fat...

wasna kept a man going for a whole day... In the old days we used to eat the guts of the buffalo, making a contest of it, two fellows getting hold of a long piece of intestines from opposite ends, starting chewing toward the middle, seeing who can get there first; that's eating. Those buffalo guts, full of half-fermented, half-digested grass and herbs, you didn't need any pills and vitamins when you swallowed those. (22)

A couple of other points about vegetarianism. Vegetarian men have a slightly higher annual all-cause-death rate than nonvegetarian men (0.93 percent vs. 0.89 percent), and vegetarian women have a significantly higher annual all-cause-death rate than nonvegetarian women (0.86 percent vs. 0.54 percent). Vegetarianism is not better for your heart, either. The International Atherosclerosis Project found that vegetarians had just as much atherosclerosis as meat eaters. (23)

As far as children are concerned, I believe they are headed for trouble if some high-fat animal food is not included in their diets. If you're worried about cholesterol, please realize that it is vital to the proper functioning and development of the brain. Low cholesterol levels are believed to contribute to aggressive and violent behavior, depression, and suicidal tendencies. Cholesterol is needed for the proper functioning of serotonin (the "feel-good" neurotransmitter) receptors in the brain; is a precursor to hormones; is an antioxidant; is necessary for healthy cell membranes and is a precursor to vitamin D (needed for healthy bones and nervous system, insulin production, immune system function, proper growth, and mineral metabolism). Nature knows best, so it's no surprise that mother's milk is very high in cholesterol, and 50 percent of its calories come from fat (much of it saturated fat). That should be evidence enough that growing infants and children need a high-fat diet.

A popular item vegetarians consume is alfalfa sprouts. Although other kinds of sprouts are generally nutritious, alfalfa sprouts contain a substance called cadaverine that can be toxic. Tests indicate that alfalfa sprouts can inhibit the immune system and can contribute to inflammatory arthritis and lupus. (24)

My advice? Eat animal products! And above all, have your kids eat them regularly. There's a reason why they love hot dogs so much! (But please get them the best at the health food store.)

Canola Oil

In recent years many nutritionists have claimed that canola oil is a good, healthy oil, especially for the heart. They make these claims based on the accepted medical dogma which says that polyunsaturated and unsaturated fats and oils are healthy, and saturated fats like those found in animal products are unhealthy and lead to cardiovascular and heart problems as well as cancer.

At the turn of the 20th century, most fat in the diet was either in the saturated or monounsaturated form, coming primarily from lard, butter, coconut oil, and olive oil. Heart disease was rare, as was cancer. Today, heart disease is the leading killer and cancer is an epidemic – and as much as 30 percent of the calories in our diet comes from polyunsaturated oils. This is in large part due to the abundance of margarine in our diets along with vegetable oils derived from soy, corn, safflower, and rape seeds (canola oil).

Primitive, healthy populations in temperate and tropical regions consume about 4 percent of their calories in the polyunsaturated form – far less than the 30 percent in Western diets. (These come from legumes, grains, nuts, green vegetables, fish, olive oil, and animal fats.) Studies have shown that polyunsaturated oils actually increase cancer and heart disease, damage the liver, reproductive organs and lungs, cause digestive disorders, depress learning ability, and impair growth and weight gain. (25) Why? Polyunsaturated oils become rancid easily when subjected to heat, oxygen, and moisture (when cooking or processing). When an oil is rancid, it has many "free radicals" that attack cell membranes and red blood cells, damage DNA/RNA and cause mutations in tissues, blood vessels, and skin.

Free radicals cause skin to wrinkle, organs to develop tumors, and blood vessels to develop plaque. Not only have numerous studies shown that high consumption of polyunsaturated oils causes heart disease and cancer, but also contribute to premature aging, arthritis, Parkinson's disease, Lou Gehrig's disease, Alzheimer's, cataracts, and autoimmune disorders.

Most of the polyunsaturates in commercial vegetable oils are in the form of omega-6 linoleic acid. Too much omega-6 in the diet can cause blood clots to form, high blood pressure, depressed immune function, sterility, cancer, weight gain, inflammation, and irritation of the digestive tract. Too little omega-3 linolenic acid in the diet can cause asthma, heart disease, and learning problems. The healthy ratio of omega-6 to omega-3 fatty acids in the diet is about one to one. However, our modern diet contains far too much omega-6 and not enough omega-3, due largely to the prevalent use of polyunsaturated vegetable oils. Canola oil has twice as much omega-6 as omega-3, making it unbalanced oil. Even worse, during the processing of canola oil, much of the omega-3 fatty acids are transformed into trans-fatty acids, similar to those found in margarine and known to be dangerous. (26)

Mold develops very quickly in baked goods made with canola oil. Canola oil also contains a very long-chain fatty acid called erucic acid, which is associated with fibrotic heart lesions. Even though canola oil is bred to contain little erucic acid, it is likely still present. And even though canola oil is touted as being good for the heart, a recent study has shown that it may actually cause a deficiency in vitamin E, which is needed for a healthy cardiovascular system. (27)

While we're on the topic of fats and oils, it's important to realize that hydrogenated fats (like margarine – made from rancid vegetable oils) and partially hydrogenated vegetable oils have a very deleterious effect on the human body. They have been associated with cancer, diabetes, obesity, low-birth-weight babies, birth defects, sterility, atherosclerosis, immune system dysfunction, lactation difficulties, sexual dysfunction, and increased blood cholesterol. The next time you pick up a product in the supermarket, read the label. Many foods contain "partially hydrogenated vegetable oil." It's a testimony to the advertisers that they could brainwash generations of people into thinking that natural fats, such as those in animal products, are bad and manmade products from rancid and over-processed oils are good.

On the other hand, good old-fashioned butter contains short- and medium-chain fatty acids that are easily metabolized by the body and have antimicrobial and antitumor qualities. Butter also contains virtually the only dietary source of butyric acid, which has antitumor as well as antifungal properties.

Food for Thought

The quest for health is not an easy one, especially these days with so many differences in opinion, misinformation, and the huge financial implications. We must be vigilant and always question whether recommendations, no matter what their source, are really correct and really makes sense. No matter how advanced we become technologically, we will never have the wisdom of nature itself and we should always use it as our rule of thumb. Soy products, vegetarianism, and canola oil are three things that nature didn't intend for us and best be avoided if you want a healthy and happy child.

The Truth About Children's Health

CHAPTER XIV
How to Prevent and Reverse Disease

> Disclaimer: The ideas and suggestions contained in this book are not intended as a substitute for the appropriate care of a licensed health care practitioner. Qualified medical assistance should always be sought before beginning any treatments. The following is intended for educational purposes only. Suggestions are not made to treat a specific condition. They are made to help you and your child achieve a healthier lifestyle that will promote proper biological function.

The following are suggestions and strategies to help you and your child deal with many of the health problems discussed this book. An important thing to keep in mind is that you don't need to be perfect in your implementation of these suggestions. The human body is designed to take a fair amount of abuse and thrive in less than ideal conditions. If you've been functioning without benefit of the knowledge you've just gained in these pages, then you yourself are evidence of that! So don't obsess over these. The anguish and frustration that may result from trying to do everything and do it perfectly in some cases would be worse than not doing anything at all. Your mental health and peace of mind are just as important as eliminating the problem. Do the best you can, and realize that it's a long journey. A change here, a change there – and in time you'll be surprised at how far you've come. You may eliminate a specific problem in a few hours or a day, or it may take years. But realize that you are doing something great and something of true value. Not just for you and your children, but for society and future generations.

The first place to start helping your child is, perhaps surprisingly, by helping yourself. If you've ever flown in an airplane, the flight attendants give directions on what to do in case the airplane loses air pressure. You're instructed to put the oxygen mask on yourself first, and then attend to your child. The same priority applies in the case of the health and well being of your child. You, the parent, must be in good health – physically, mentally, and emotionally – to best help your child. Most of the recommendations made here, especially dietary, should be followed by the parents as well as the child. That way, you will both be working toward a brighter, healthier, and more harmonious tomorrow. You'll be facing the challenges together, and you as the parent will be better able to understand and feel what your child might be going through which will give you more compassion and patience. When you're in good health, you'll be better able to serve your child and his or her progress will be accelerated. And you'll get healthier and happier in the process.

Many treatments and changes in lifestyle can turn a seemingly hopeless child into one who is manageable and bright. Diet is of utmost importance and will be discussed first.

There's no sense in using your time, effort, and money on other treatments if you keep sabotaging yourself by consuming things that fan the fire of disease. The dietary guidelines presented below are simply the basic fundamentals we've lost sight of that have nourished and healed the body for millions of years. Implementing these suggestions in your diet and that of your children will go a long way to helping your child become healthy, happy, and smart.

Changes to our foods were initially made during the industrial revolution to preserve those foods to get them to market. With such changes, we discovered these foods didn't taste or look that good. So we added flavor enhancers, artificial flavors, preservatives, dyes, and colorings. All to make us think we were getting the real thing. The problem is, altered foods are not just deficient in their nutrient content, but also polluted by the additives.

In our quest to produce more food with less labor, we developed pesticides, herbicides, and chemical fertilizers. They further degraded the food supply and added to air and water pollution. We want to avoid foods with any of these in them as much as possible. They interfere with normal cellular processes and are also less nutritious. Anything not found in nature is suspect. Use this as your rule of thumb: "The closer to nature, the closer to health."

I realize it may be very difficult to get your youngsters or teenagers to change their dietary habits. If the media and their friends have influenced them, it can be especially tough. Take it slow, introduce one new thing at a time, and avoid pressuring them to change. Leading by example is always the best. And, your own health will improve along the way.

Don't be afraid to get creative with your encouragement. A friend of mine was having an especially tough time with her learning-impaired child. This child was slow in school and was in special education classes. She struggled to get him to do his homework, complete chores around the house, and to eat properly. After trying to discipline him, which just made him belligerent, she came up with what she called the "Pass System." She made a list of things she wanted her child to do and assigned each one a value. Taking out the garbage, for example, got him three passes. Making his bed, got two passes, doing homework on time got five passes and so on.

Then she made a list of all the things the child liked to do: watch TV, go to a movie, play video games and so on. Each activity got a value too. Watching TV for a half-hour required two passes, video games for an hour took three passes – you get the idea. She sat her child down and explained to him this new "game." In no time, the kid was not only doing the chores on the list, but also doing other things such as sweeping the floors, vacuuming, and cleaning out the garage and then asking how many passes he would get! It was amazing. Why such a turnaround? People will more times than not do something for a positive reward than to avoid punishment. I remember reading about a psychology major in college conducting experiments on rats and finding out that the rats would run the maze faster and remember it better if there was cheese at the other end than if they were given an electrical shock for not running it. Try to give positive reinforcement. That's not to say a reprimand isn't called for now and then. But overall, you should encourage your child for achievement instead of punishing them for failure.

So, if your child eats his vegetables, give him a pass. If she isn't drinking cola for a day, give her two passes. You'll find it's a lot easier and effective than laying down the law.

To take this kind of approach a step further, check out "The Drew Bledsoe Foundation." Mac Bledsoe, the father of professional quarterback Drew Bledsoe, was a teacher for 29 years. Based on his experiences with children, he developed a program called "Parenting with Dignity," which has helped many parents turn difficult situations into positive gains. He says that it's important to give your child a certain amount of responsibility by allowing them to make some of their own decisions. For example: allow the child to decide what to wear; what to have or where to go for dinner on occasion; what to put on the grocery list, and so on. By allowing them to think for themselves, they'll be more likely to do so later in life and be able to resist peer pressure and other negative influences. Although I cannot go into these kinds of parenting skills here, I highly recommend you check out Mac's program. His strategies along with my recommendations, will help you raise amazingly healthy, well balanced, and happy children. You can contact "The Drew Bledsoe Foundation" at (508) 543-6543 or www.drewbledsoe.com.

Dietary and Lifestyle Recommendations

• Buy and eat as much organically raised food as possible.

Not only is it cleaner, it's more nutritious. Nutrient for nutrient, it is actually less expensive than conventionally grown foods – as was shown in Chapter XII. You may think you're paying more for it, but when you consider the added nutrition, you'll not need to eat as much (since your body will be satisfied sooner because it realizes it is getting fed better), and you'll be saving untold medical bills down the road. You and your kids will be less likely to get some degenerative diseases, since you'll be getting the extra nutrition. Your child needs as clean a diet as possible to improve. If he or she doesn't get it, improvements from other treatments will be much more difficult to realize. If you must buy nonorganic produce, soak it in a sink full of water with one-teaspoon hydrogen peroxide or apple cider vinegar added. Soak about 10 minutes and then rinse well. That will help remove pesticides and other impurities. Most people believe that fruits and vegetables are the main sources of pesticide contamination. This is not the case, since these impurities bioaccumulate down the food chain and animal foods have higher concentrations of pesticides than produce. So it's very important to obtain organically raised meat, poultry, eggs, and dairy products.

• Eat as much whole, natural, unprocessed food as possible.

Scientists believe that there is less than 1/100,000th of a difference between the metabolism of modern man and that of people 10,000 years ago. (1) But our diets would be unrecognizable to those ancestors. Our digestive system is just not made for and has not adapted to the 50,000 synthetic chemicals in our food supply and all the modern processing we do to our food. For best nutrition, we would best eat the same foods in similar fashion our ancestors did hundreds of years ago. Think of it this way: If our ancestors of 500 years ago didn't eat it, we shouldn't eat it either. That means no soft drinks, no Doritos, no white bread, pasteurized milk, and so on and so on. And children should consume animal products on a regular basis. The important thing here is to be sure the meat, dairy, and eggs are clean, organically raised and prepared properly (and often times raw). Your child can still have hot dogs, but buy them from a health food store. Serve them on whole wheat buns or Ezekiel bread (a special kid of "sprouted grain" bread at health food stores). Buy organic mustard, ketchup, relish, sauerkraut, and so on.

• Avoid irradiated foods.

Many fruits and produce now are irradiated in order to better preserve the food and increase shelf life (and profits). However, it's been shown that irradiation of our food can cause kidney damage, chromosomal damage, mutations, and heart damage. Extending shelf life is not a good trade-off for shortening human life. More on this subject can be found in the book *The Food That Would Last Forever: Understanding the Dangers of Food Irradiation* by Gary Gibbs, M.D. Shopping at health food stores and buying organically raised products will help you avoid buying this kind of food.

• Avoid genetically engineered (GE) foods (also known as genetically modified organisms or GMOs).

• Cook in the right cookware.

Cook *only* in glass, unchipped enamel, Corning, or stainless steel cookware. *Do not* use aluminum or nonstick cookware. The wrong cookware can introduce toxic chemicals into your food.

• Cook properly to preserve nutrients

Cook food as little as possible to preserve nutrients. Light steaming is the most preferable way of cooking vegetables, followed by boiling and quick frying. Meat and fowl are best slow-roasted or broiled. Poach, broil, or bake seafood and poach or soft-boil eggs.

• Eat a raw egg yolk a day.

Egg yolks are rich in many nutrients your child needs for development and growth. Include a raw egg yolk in your family's diet every day, preferably from fertile eggs from organically raised chickens. (An easy and nutritious breakfast with raw eggs is given below.) If you must cook, poach or soft-boil eggs rather than frying or scrambling them. Eggs contain sulfur, which binds with mercury, helping to eliminate it from the body.

• Eat a lot of raw food.

You should make it a goal to consume at least 50 percent to 70 percent of your food in an uncooked state. This includes animal products. Cooking destroys

The Truth About Children's Health

many nutrients and changes many others to unusable and sometimes harmful forms. Remember Pottenger's cats? The cats fed only cooked food degenerated and died out in just a few generations. Life begets life. You and your child need some uncooked food every day.

• Avoid canned vegetables, frozen dinners, and commercial fruit juices.

Canned vegetables are overcooked and usually contain salt or sugar. Frozen dinners are usually filled with preservatives, dyes, and other chemicals (including MSG), and are usually packaged in aluminum. Commercial fruit juices have too much sugar and have been shown to be harmful for kids. Make your own dinner, and make your own juice. Please note that even freshly prepared friut juices are high in sugar and may disrupt blood sugar levels. Other things to avoid are candy, pastry, jam, jelly, ice cream, crackers, cereals, catsup, soft drinks, coffee, tea (herbal is OK), and processed, canned, preserved or packaged foods.

• Eat on schedule.

You child needs structure in his or her life. Having meals on a regular schedule helps establish that order. Perhaps more important, it regulates blood sugar metabolism and other bodily functions – and discourages improper food choices by staving off hunger. Regular meals may be difficult to establish in this fast-paced society, but it's worth the effort. Plan for healthy between-meal snacks also.

• Soak all nuts, seeds and grains overnight, avoid roasted nuts and seeds.

All seeds and grains have substances called phytates which block absorption of iron, calcium, magnesium,copper, and zinc. Nuts, seeds, and grain also contain enzyme inhibitors that interfere with digestion. Both phytates and these enzyme inhibitors are inactivated by water. If you've had trouble digesting nuts or seeds, this is probably the reason. If you soak them overnight, they'll be easy to digest. Even rice and wheat should be soaked at least overnight and as long as a couple days. Only whole grain, brown rice should be consumed. Most vegetarians eat a lot of rice, yet I haven't met many that know this about phytates and rice. I think that this, along with the fact that many vegetarians eat a lot of soy products, is the reason you hardly ever meet a healthy vegetarian! Roasting nuts and seeds turns their fats rancid and alters their proteins and carbohydrates. It's best to buy your nuts and seeds raw (organic), and sprinkle some soy sauce over them. They are best stored in the refrigerator or freezer.

• An easy breakfast or protein smoothie.

Here's a simple, nutritious, fast, and delicious recipe to start your and your child's day off right. It's loaded with enzymes, protein, good fatty acids, vitamins, and minerals. One great thing about this meal is that it "sticks to your ribs." Since your body is getting a lot of wholesome nutrients, it realizes it's being well fed and doesn't get hungry. In fact, some days I don't get hungry until after lunch-time after I eat this for breakfast. Although you may be under the belief that the eggs are bad for your cholesterol and fat levels, since they are raw, the opposite is actually true. So you won't gain weight on this meal. In fact, you'll probably lose weight (if you need to) by eating this consistently since it's so

How to Prevent and Reverse Disease

"nutrient dense" without empty calories (such as the processed sugars found in breakfast cereals).

Ingredients (All ingredients should be raw and organically grown when possible):

3-6 raw eggs from free-roaming hens. Fertile eggs are preferable.

1 banana, 1/2 teaspoon unheated honey (see Resource Guide for the good brands), 1-2 tablespoons raw, unsalted butter or two to three ounces of raw cream.

Place all ingredients in a blender and blend on medium speed for several seconds until all ingredients are blended into a smoothie. You can put this in a container and eat it on the run, as I often do. Replacing your child's store-bought cereal with this all-natural meal will be like changing about 30 percent of their diet. It will go a long way in helping them get and stay healthy.

• Do not microwave your food or your baby's food.

Microwaving your food distorts the electrical integrity of the food. It's believed to alter fats, proteins and vitamins, making them more difficult to digest and assimilate. Eating microwaved food results in abnormal blood profiles, which are very similar to those found in the early stages of cancer. Please don't use a microwave to heat your baby's bottle since microwaved milk can be toxic to the liver and nervous system, especially for infants. (2) It also presents a burn risk since microwaving heats unevenly, potentially leaving pockets of heat you can't detect with a test drop on your wrist.

Yes, microwaved food is bad news for you and your child. In fact, mcirowaves are so potentially harmful the Soviet Union banned their use in 1976. Consistently eating microwaved food shorts out electrical impulses in the brain, causing permanent brain damage, loss of memory, concentration, and emotional stability. It can shut down or alter hormone production, cause immune system deficiencies, decrease intelligence, and cause intestinal cancerous growths. Minerals, vitamins, and other nutrients of all microwaved food are reduced and altered so the body gets little or no benefit or also absorbs altered compounds that it cannot break down. (3)

• Use only butter and extra virgin olive oil.

Avoid margarine and all commercial vegetable oils, including canola oil and corn oil and any products made with these in them. They're abundant in the wrong kinds of fats – trans-fatty acids – and contribute to weight gain, depression, cardiovascular disease and other health problems. Eat butter, preferably raw (i.e., not pasteurized), unsalted and organic from grass fed cows. No, it won't give you a heart attack. It has a valuable fatty acid (butyric acid) that is difficult to obtain from any other source. Butyric acid has antifungal and antitumor properties. If you're worried about cholesterol, again, please remember that the body needs cholesterol. Of course, if you have high cholesterol, it's best to get it under control. Making the dietary and lifestyle changes recommended here will go far in that regard. Why? Because you will be eating many fats in their raw and natural state, which does not raise your cholesterol, blood pressure or make you fat. It's the cooked fats that have been deranged and ruined that cause all the havoc in the body. And again, kids especially need the fat and they need the cholesterol for proper development of their nervous system.

- Eliminate all nonfoods and junk foods.

You will need to eliminate as much as possible from your child's diet (and hopefully your own) all of the following:

◊ All products made with soy unless it's fermented soy sauce; soy is bad food for you and your child. Soy has been shown to upset hormonal balances and tofu is loaded with aluminum.

◊ Give up all sugar.

Sugar in every way, shape, and form must be removed from the diet. No high-fructose corn syrup, added sucrose or fructose, or any other form of added sugar. Now they try to hide the added sugar by calling it "carbohydrates." Yes, sugar is a carbohydrate, so they're not lying, just being deceptive. The only way is to make sure the product says "No Sugar Added" on the label. That's supposed to ensure that no sugar was added. (In this day and age though, who knows.)

You'll find that by eliminating every kind of sugar and all its substitutes, you'll have cleaned up your child's diet by a huge degree. In fact, if you use just one dietary guideline, this would be it since sugar is in just about everything overprocessed and unhealthy. It has to be, or the product would taste bad. Read the labels. If in doubt, don't buy. Use raw, unheated honey instead. It's loaded with enzymes and minerals.

If you don't take your child off sugar, again, you're making improvement much more difficult and slow. Your child won't improve significantly until you remove this most toxic and injurious substance. Remember, sugar was once considered a drug and was snorted like cocaine is today. It was a rich man's luxury, which started the rich man's illnesses. All the counseling in the world and all the clinics and seminars and psychoanalysis, special learning programs, and so on, will not work nearly so well unless you first start to change the child's physical and mental makeup at the cellular level. Eliminating sugar will do this faster than just about anything.

For many of you new to the "health food" arena, this may seem like quite a stretch. That's OK; it is for everyone. Do the best you can. Some parents go all out and just throw away everything in their cupboards with sugar and start over from scratch. Others go gradually, using up what they have and replacing it with more wholesome products.

Usually, gradual dietary changes are best since the enzyme systems in your body take a little time to adjust to a new diet. In extremely critical situations, more drastic changes may be warranted. Use your judgment and do the best you can.

- Stop consuming all white flour products.

All white flour products are not only nutrient-deficient, but are poisoned from bleaching agents including cadmium and aluminum. They also, more often than not, contain some amount of sugar. Get them out of your diet as soon as possible.

That includes bagels, any pastries, most brown-looking bread at the regular grocery store (coloring the bread is another trick to make you think it's healthy, and one brand I examined actually had sawdust in it!), pizza, spaghetti, and so on.

Remember, white flour products have had the germ removed, which is the source of B vitamins in the wheat. Lack of B vitamins creates stress in the body. The best bread to buy is called "Ezekiel." You'll only find it at the health food stores. There are other whole-grain or sprouted grain products at the health food stores too. Once you eat them for a while, and then you taste regular bread again you'll see that regular white-flour products taste and feel like paste. I remember when I was in second grade, we made a map using flour, salt, and water. We mixed them up, slapped the goo on a board, formed mountains, streams, and so on, painted it with food coloring, and let it harden over night. The stuff became hard as rock. Nobody ever stopped to realize that this is essentially the recipe for bread and that this white-flour stuff may harden inside us too (like in our arteries and colon). You'll find that many whole grain and sprouted grain products are kept refrigerated. They have to be or they'll soon go rancid since they don't have preservatives and are real food.

The best pasta to buy is called "Vita-Spelt." It has significantly more protein and nutrients than other brands. Eating brown-looking spaghetti may seem weird at first, but you'll get used to it. Pasta made from kamut is good too. Whole-wheat pastas are OK, but not as good as spelt or kamut since the spelt and kamut grains have more nutrients in them to begin with. (Most regular wheat on the market is from hybridized plants that are not that nutrient dense.)

One of the biggest problems with wheat products is that many people are allergic to them. That's because of the high amount of gluten (the sticky stuff) in these products. Not so with the whole-grain and sprouted grain products. You may find a lot of your and your child's allergies diminishing when you switch to these more nutritious, less allergic foods.

• Avoid cereal products.

Especially those found in regular supermarkets. If you have to feed your child cereals, make sure they're whole-grain with no added sugar. Then, you can add your own sweetener (if you must). Use good old fashioned raw whole milk. Above all, stay away from the common supermarket milk. Soy-milk and soy products are second rate and not good foods – no matter how hard they advertise to the contrary.

• Avoid any and all products that contain aspartame.

This includes the brand names of Equal and Sweet 'n Low, among others. Avoid any other kind of artificial sweetener. Again, unheated honey is best sweetener. Others, in order of whole-food goodness, are stevia, powdered dates, Grade A or B dark amber maple syrup, blackstrap molasses, and succanate (unprocessed cane sugar).

A great-tasting, very nutritious and refreshing drink that will replace Kool-Aid and sodas in your child's diet is to squeeze a lemon or lime into a couple glasses of water, add a tablespoon or two of the dark amber maple syrup or unheated honey, and blend. Adjust ingredients to suit your and your child's taste.

- Eliminate all pasteurized milk and pasteurized milk based products, but use plenty of raw dairy.

If milk is raw and from cows fed organically, cow's milk is a great food for babies, children, and adults. Cow's milk also contains lactose, which most people cannot metabolize if the milk is pasteurized. But in it's raw state, the milk contains lactase, the enzyme necessary to digest this sugar. So those with lactose intolerance will not experience problems with raw dairy products. Remember, most cows raised at conventional dairies are injected with hormones to make them produce more milk faster (to make more money, of course). (Note: a century ago, a cow that produced 600 pounds of milk a year was considered a high producer. These days, that's not the case because the cows are treated with hormones so they will produce more and more milk. Of course, this milk is inferior and tainted. In 1972, an American cow named Hattie produced 44,019 pounds of milk in one year! This is very unnatural. Chickens are similarly treated so they will produce more and more eggs and farmers are now experimenting with new and different lighting systems to increase egg production to 400 or 500 eggs a year – up from the current (and forced) one egg a day. This also goes to show the importance of the role light can play in biological systems.) (4)

History proves that raw dairy has been a valuable food for many healthy and long-lived peoples. For example, many healthy populations throughout history have relied on dairy products (naturally produced) as a major part of their diet; The Swiss, Greeks and other inhabitants of the Mediterranean; Africans; Tibetans; the long-lived citizens of Soviet Georgia; the hearty Mongols of Northern China; Americans up to the first World War; and the long-lived people of Austria and Switzerland. (5)

These cultures consumed dairy products primarily in the cultured or fermented form. In Europe before industrialization, people consumed milk as yogurt, cheese, clabber or curds and whey. Fermentation, due to the lactic-acid-producing bacteria, preserves the milk for days or weeks, and in the case of cheese, for several years (this was before the invention of pasteurization). *Yogurt* comes from Bulgaria. The beverages *kefir* and *Koumiss* come from Russia, Scandinavians drink a cultured milk product called *longfil*. *Dahi*, a soured milk product is consumed in India with almost every meal.

Fermenting milk results in beneficial changes. For one, milk protein (casein) is broken down and essentially predigested. If you have a little one troubled by allergies, switching from regular dairy products to raw, cultured dairy products will go a long way in alleviating his or her suffering. Culturing increases the lactase content which helps digest lactose (milk sugar). Many traditional societies give fermented milk products to the sick, aged, and nursing mothers because they value their health-promoting properties. Vitamins B and C increase when milk is fermented, and cultured dairy provides beneficial bacteria and lactic acid to the digestive tract.

Can your child get enough calcium if he or she does not drink raw milk? Some researchers think not. Sally Fallon, in a personal commuincation, says, "Children cannot get adequate calcium from green vegetables (and adults can't either). The only two good sources of calcium in human diets are milk products and bone broths. In cultures where milk products are not used, bone broths are an essential part of the diet. Parents who cannot find decent milk products need to make bone broth and serve it at almost every meal... By the way, when children get plentiful calcium and fat-soluble activators in the diet they are well protected against many of the toxins in our food, including the toxic metals."

I would refrain from supplementing your diet with calcium pills. Most calcium supplements on the market have the wrong kind of calcium in them anyway (because it's the cheapest kind). Squeeze some fresh oranges or invest in a juicer and make vegetable juices (carrots, celery, cucumber, parsley, tomato, etc.) and have your child drink an 8-oz. glass a day with some cream, butter or milk (the fat in these help with vitamin and mineral absorption.) There's plenty of calcium in that one little glass of fresh, unpasteurized orange juice or vegetable juice. You can get a little hand-squeezer – the kind you twist an orange half on – for a couple dollars. Decent juicers can be found at most department stores..

• Drinking water.

Chemists consider water to be the "universal solvent." It dissolves just about anything, including bones and tissue. The purer the water is, the more it will dissolve. Distilled water, being devoid of all minerals, is very hungry, aggressive water that should not be drunk. And, if you are distilling water that has been treated with chlorine, a toxic byproduct of the distillation process called trihalomethanes will end up in the distilled water. If you do distill water, be sure there's a carbon filter attachment on the distiller to get rid of the trihalomethanes. Distilled water is bad enough for adults, but is catastrophic for kids. They don't need minerals leached out of their growing bodies

The only water that is tolerated by the body is mineral water from pure sources. The Hunzas, one of the longest lived people on earth, drink mineral-dense water from melting glaciers called "glacial milk." Water from natural springs, like Perrier water from France, is fine. Ideally you and your child should get most of the water you need from the food you eat, raw milk, and vegetable juices. Drinking large quantities of raw milk is fine and even healthful. (Please avoid fruit juices since they tend to dissolve and leach minerals out of the body.) Eating food in it's raw state will also help you stay hydrated since the water in this live food is very bioavailable and beneficial.

If you're craving a soft drink or glass of iced tea, have a glass of milk, juice or mineral water first. Drink juice, milk, or mineral water whenever you like, and you don't have to drown yourself with the prescribed eight glasses a day. Drink when you're thirsty – don't force yourself.

• Avoid salt.

If you must use salt, use only Celtic Sea Salt since it is unheated and has a good mineral balance.

• Get enough and the correct kind of fat.

Without the correct fats your child's nervous system and brain cannot develop properly. *Do not* put your child on a low-fat diet, even if he or she is overweight. A child can always slim down, but the window of nervous system development is short, and you may be doing him or her irreversible harm in restricting fats in their diets. A better alternative is to limit sugar and other high-carbohydrate foods (like pizza and pasta), since the excess sugar gets stored as unhealthy fat. Fat is so important for growing children, that they actually benefit from a diet that contains more calories as fat than as protein.

Again, a good practice is to have your child eat a raw egg yolk a day.. Egg yolks are a good source of eicosapentaenoic acid (EPA) and docasahexaenoic acid (DHA), which are not essential, but are often times difficult to manufacture by the body. Consuming egg yolks, liver and other organ meats, fish oils, and organically raised chickens will supply EPA and DHA. GLA can be found in borage oil and evening primrose oil, and AA is found in butter and organ meats. If you want a good supplement with DHA in it, I recommend Neuromins made by MMS. Neuromins is a purified form of DHA and has been clinically shown to be safe for infants, children, and pregnant and lactating women. There are other DHA products on the market made from fish oils that can be used also, but Neuromins is DHA from a plant source, which has been shown to have less contamination (especially mercury) than fish oil DHA.

Arachidonic acid (AA) and gamma-linolenic acid (GLA) are two other fatty acids that are often times difficult for the body to manufacture, so these must be obtained from the diet as well.

• Get enough vitamin A

Vitamin A is considered to be the catalyst on which all other biological processes depend, so it's important your child obtain enough of it daily. An egg a day will help, but they need more vitamin A than that. Some say that carotenes are metabolized into vitamin A, but please realize that carotenes can only be converted to vitamin A under optimal conditions. Cod liver oil, liver, butter, egg yolks, fresh cream, and shellfish are good sources of vitamin A. I also recommend getting a good supply of essential fatty acids – especially the omega 3s. You can find good sources at your health food store. You should look for ones that are cold-pressed from organic sources and kept in the refrigerator section. These oils can go rancid easily so you need to keep them refrigerated.

• Avoid most nutritional supplements.

Over the years I have researched and experimented with a variety of health supplements such as vitamin and mineral supplements. What I've discovered is that it's almost impossible to tell a good one from a bad one, and a vast majority of them are bad. Nor can we be sure whether we really need all or any of the ingredients. For one thing, most vitamin or mineral pills contain a host of impurities that can not only make their ingredients unusable by the body, but are health hazards in themselves. In recent years, for example, "colloidal mineral" products have become popular. They contain 70 or so minerals, some of which are known to be toxic. They are loaded with aluminum. I don't recommend them. If you have a good diet, with some raw fat and animal products, you'll be getting all the minerals and trace minerals you need. Most companies are in business to make money, and although there are many well-intentioned people in this business, the bottom line oftentimes wins out over quality. In addition, everyone's body and specific nutritional needs are different. So just taking a multivitamin/mineral pill may not be right for your biochemistry. You may not need more calcium or iron, for example, and yet they are in most multivitamin/mineral supplements.

The human body is designed to acquire its nutrition from foods, not from pills made in some laboratory. The vitamins, minerals, fatty acids, proteins, and carbohydrates in whole foods are in the right forms for your body to use as nourishment. This is why I emphasize eating organic food so strongly. If we ate nothing but wholesome, clean, and nutritious food, we wouldn't need supplements of any kind.

But, most of us can't eat only organic food. And even organic food is not as nutritious as food was hundreds or thousands of years ago because our soils have been depleted. That's why it's important to eat nutrient dense foods such as animal products. The only supplements I recommend taking, if you feel you need them are glandulars. They are dried and powdered forms of different glands of animals, usually cattle. They supply many nutrients that support the various glands of the body and have been helpful in restoring health. Good glandulars can be obtained from Dew's 21st Century Products at (940) 243-2178 or Health Excel (800) 690-1088.

• Eliminate as many toxins from your environment as possible.

Avoid using dishwasher powder you buy at the supermarket since it is extremely poisonous – there are more pure dishwasher powders available at health food stores. Avoid fluoridated toothpastes, tablets, gels, and all other fluoridated products. Fluoride is basically a pesticide since it works by poisoning the bacteria and plaque in your mouth. It is particularly unsafe for children since they tend to swallow much of the toothpaste they use. Avoid drinking fluoridated water. Eliminate using pesticides and herbicides in and around the house. Clean the toxins that tend to settle on floors, toys, and surfaces children play on and put in their mouths. Reduce or eliminate using deodorants, cosmetics, and nail polish since they are all laden with poisons and can get into the air you and your child breathe.

• Avoid EMF pollution — sleep grounded.

Do not sleep with electric blankets, or with a waterbed heater on. These disturb the electromagnetic fields of the body. In fact, electromagnetic pollution is becoming quite a problem in our highly technological society. EMF (electromagnetic fields) have been implicated in a wide variety of illnesses such as sleep disorders, stress-related and autoimmune diseases including arthritis, asthma, fibromyalgia, lupus, cardiovascular disease, and many more. The problem is that our bodies take on some of the electromagnetic charges around us, and we actually act like a battery and store some of these charges. Trouble is, our electrical system (our nervous system) operates on very low voltage. When we take on too much voltage from the environment, we get "overcharged" which leads to stress and overproduction of adrenaline and other stress hormones.

One solution is to be grounded. When we walk barefoot in the sand or on bare ground, the excess charge is pulled into the earth (the grounding agent). That's one of the reasons going to the beach is so realxing... we walk on the sand and have the excess electromagnetic charges disapated from us. So we sleep better, digest our food better and are happier. Our whole body functions better. But most of us can't go barefoot on the beach every day, and we all wear shoes with synthetic materials that don't allow grounding. So what can we do?

A researcher named Clint Ober discovered that if you are grounded at night while you sleep, you're body will "discharge" and consequently rest better. You'll get a deeper and more healing sleep, wake refreshed, and have more energy throughout the day. This lead him to invent a mattress pad that is grounded to the earth. You simply put this pad under your sheets and sleep as usual - you don't even know it's there. The results of people sleeping on this pad have been impressive: 85% of test subjects reported the time to fall asleep decreased: 100% woke feeling more rested: 82% had less muscle stiffness and pain: 78% reported an increase in general well being. Many subjects said they saw imporvements in back pain, arthritis, lupus, PMS, allergies, multiplesclerosis, and fibromyalgia.

Although Mr. Ober has not done any scientific testing on children, he says that children benefit immensely from sleeping on the pad. Since sleep is the time the body heals, if a child is not sleeping deeply, his or her body has no chance to make the proper repairs. All that electromagnetic pollution your child (and you) pick up duing the day has to be discharged, or we'll be "wired" all night. This can lead to many degenerative problems, physically, mentally, and emotionally.

I have personally used this mattress pad and have experienced a tremendouos improvement in my sleep as have others I know who have tried it. And consequently, I perform better during the day and are happier, more balanced and generally a nicer guy! Aren't you when you get a good night's sleep?

I highly, HIGHLY recommend you invest in this mattress pad for your child and yourself. You will see amazing improvements in your health and well being.

For more information or to order the mattress pad, call EarthTether at (800) 620-9912.

• Avoid exposing your child to smoke.

That means both tobacco smoke and marijuana smoke. Marijuana smoke contains nine times the amount of the toxic heavy metal cadmium of tobacco smoke. To protect your child from the effects of second hand smoke, consider doing the following:

◊ If you smoke, quit. If you do smoke, don't smoke where your child can see you. If otherwise your child may come to believe its healthy and OK. You are their primary role model.

◊ Don't smoke within the airspace of your child. Smoke out of doors and away from your child and avoid smoking in your car.

◊ Choose the day care you send your child to carefully. Make sure the day care providers don't smoke.

Children and especially infants are more vulnerable to the effects of pollutants than adults, since their organs of elimination are not fully developed yet. Protecting children from exposure to tobacco smoke is good preventative medicine.

• Exercise.

We all know that exercise is important. It increases circulation and improves overall cardiovascular health. It burns fat and increases your metabolism so you will burn fat even when you're not exercising. It's very helpful and sometimes a great cure for depression because when you exercise, serotonin and endorphins are produced – which make you feel good.

Exercise not only burns fat, but also burns amino acids known as branched-chain amino acids for fuel in your muscles. If these amino acids are not burned, they compete with tryptophan, so that tryptophan is less easily converted to serotonin. The less serotonin, the less of a good mood you'll be in. Make an effort to exercise for an hour at a time continuously. The duration is important to activate certain enzymes needed for weight control. Have your child go outdoors and play every day in the sunshine, with no sunblock on, for at least an hour. Take walks together, play a sport, go fishing, go camping, take up golf with them. Get involved with them as much as you can – outside. Turn off the TV and video games and get outside. Not only will you be raising a healthier child physically, but mentally and emotionally as well since he or she will not be spending as much time in front of mind-warping television shows, movies, and games.

• Love your kids.

The emphasis of this book has been on the physical, chemical, and psychological aspects of children's health. My belief is that if we are physically and mentally sound, we will naturally be loving and caring. And as your and your child's health improves, you'll find that arguments and conflicts arise less frequently and your life will become easier. But as physically and mentally healthy as we may become, we still need love.

Love makes things grow and brings joy into our lives. Children need that "warm and fuzzy" feeling more than anyone. Give your children a hug every day. Tell them you love them. Hold them close and whisper sweet nothings in their ears. For some, this may sound corny. To a child, it's the breath of life. Don't be ashamed to verbalize and demonstrate your love and make a habit of it. If you're afraid or ashamed to, it probably means you weren't raised in a loving atmosphere yourself, so break that chain and be brave! It doesn't hurt – really!

Show them you care by laying down the law when needed and making sure they understand you're doing it for their betterment. You don't need to be your child's best friend, but you do need to be a loving and caring steward, directing them with "gentle firmness" toward the truly good things in life.

If you're having trouble in your marriage, it's best to try and work it out – for the kids sake. Children from intact families are healthier and do better in school, sports, and socially. There's something to be said for the good old nuclear family. But you don't want to live in an untenable situation either and I am definitely not a marriage counselor but here's my advice anyway:

You as a family can take this book and make it a project. Husband and wife reading it and then working on it together as a team to improve your life and the life of your child. If your child is old enough, have him or her read it too. Analyze it and discuss it – maybe even do some research on your own. Read what's recommended in "Recommended Reading" below. Try putting some of the recommendations in this book to work and watch things change.

You'll see over time, that as you get healthier and closer to the "real you," personality conflicts will dissolve by themselves without any effort. You and your spouse will remember why you fell in love with each other, and you'll start feeling that magic feeling again. Not just emotionally, but physically as well. I guarantee that if you follow my recommendations, even your sex life will improve dramatically – especially if one or both of you are having any kinds of sexual dysfunction. (Aajonus Vonderplanitz, the raw animal-food eater, says, "I enjoy sex 1-6 hours, and maintain energy with only 5-6 hours sleep daily. I feel like I have finally achieved and chosen heaven on Earth.") (7)

Tell your spouse "I love you." Even if you have to fake it to start. Where the mouth leads, the body and mind often follow.

Have some fun along the way. Get some joke books out of the library and make it a family tradition to have someone tell a joke every evening before dinner. Laughter lifts the mood and helps digestion. To get you started, here are two of my favorite pretty bad golf jokes:

1. Man and wife sitting at the breakfast table eating toast and eggs - he reading a golf magazine as usual. She says, "Harry, all you think about is golf, golf, golf... You haven't even noticed this fine Sunday breakfast you're eating." "Sure I have dear," he replies. "Oh, and would you please pass the putter."

2. "Darling, remember the day we got married?" "Sure do," he replies, "Sank a 35-foot putt the day before!"

Don't make getting healthy a bore or a chore, but try to make it fun and an exploration. I know it's a complicated world and sometimes it seems overwhelming. Take one little step at a time and try not to worry. Take a break now and then. Go and treat yourself and your kids for a job well done, even if it means going out for pizza or ice cream every now and then. The healthier you and your kids become, the less you'll be attracted to junky foods. Once you start reversing the downward spiral and see some positive things happen, you'll be able to do more and more with less and less effort.

Give it some time, be patient, and don't give up. And tell your kids you love them.

• Get plenty of rest and sleep.

Allow your child to sleep as much as he or she likes. Sleep is the time when the body makes repairs, and processes new information, and it knows just how much time it needs make them. Adequate sleep is essential for learning. "A full night's sleep is one of the most important factors for learning and absorbing information," says Mark DiDea, M.D. Bruce D. Perry, M.D., agrees, "Sleep is probably the most important period of the day for processing new information. Children have many new concepts to learn in school. A good night's sleep not only lets them process what they learned but also helps them be alert in class." (8) It's best for children to go to bed early, say around 7:00 p.m. and 8:00 p.m. at the latest. This keeps the body in tune to the natural nocturnal rhythms of humans in general. Benjamin Franklin's advice "Early to bed and early to rise makes a man healthy, wealthy, and wise" is true, and especially important for youngsters. If your child is sleeping more than you think he or she should, or has changed his or her sleeping patterns, it may mean something else is wrong. Often times when the body starts healing, it will require more sleep. If you make some positive changes to your child's diet and lifestyle and he or she starts sleeping longer, this may be the reason. The body also needs adequate rest, and you should allow your child this downtime also. Lounging around the house and being lazy does not qualify! You may need to give your child a little pat on the fanny to get him up and active, especially in the beginning of your changes. They need the exercise... *then* they need to rest!

Tips for making sure your child gets enough sleep: maintain a regular bedtime; read a story before bedtime to wind down your child; don't serve chocolate, tea, or sodas with caffeine from late afternoon on (if at all); don't have a TV in the bedroom; give your child a snack before bed; keep your child away from bright light before bedtime. Consider getting an Earth Tether Mattress Pad (see above).

• Have your child get some sunshine every day.

That means real sun without any sunscreen or sunblock. It does not mean exposing them excessively so they burn. Sunlight is needed for proper vitamin D production and thus calcium absorption and hormonal regulation. Too much of anything is harmful. Be sensible and cautious, but have them get some sun!

• Take control of the TV.

The National Institute on Media and the Family makes the following recommendations on how to give you, the parent, control over television-watching in your home:

1. Avoid using TV as a babysitter.

2. Know what your kids are watching. The younger the child, the more impressionable he or she is. Emotional images may intrude upon and interrupt sleep.

3. Keep TV out of kids' bedrooms. It's hard to monitor what they're watching if they're watching it in their own rooms. Having their own private television also discourages participation in family activities and tempts them to watch it when they should be doing homework or sleeping.

4. Set guidelines about when and what your children watch. You can talk to them about the guidelines, but remember you have the final say.

5. Practice "appointment" TV watching. Decide in advance what's good and then watch it. Avoid "channel surfing."

6. Talk to your child about what he or she is watching. Ask them questions. Ask them why they like particular shows. Discuss the commercials and their perception of toys, cereals, and so forth.

7. Turn the TV off during meals. Revive family discussions.

8. Use the VCR. Tape shows that you want to watch and view them at more convenient times.

9. Put the family on a TV diet. Limit the time the TV is on. Schedule other things to do such as playing games, going for a walk, doing crafts etc. Watch TV with your kids.

10. Create a TV coupon system similar to the "Pass" system already discussed. But be sure you still have the final say on what they can watch.

11. Don't make the TV the focal point of the room. Make your children the focus of your attention, not the TV. Move it to a less obvious spot in the room. People watch less TV if it's not in the most prominent location in the room.

12. Express your opinions about the shows and commercials, but to the stations and networks carrying them. You could sit down with your kids and write letters to the TV stations with yours and their opinions.

Addressing Some Specific Problems

I. Lead

Check with your local health agency for more information on lead and abatement and corrective action programs. The following strategies are taken from the report "Lead In Your Home: A Parent's Reference Guide" (EPA 747-B-99-003, May 1999) (9), a report I recommend you get for yourself; you can do so by calling your regional EPA office or going to www.epa.gov/lead on the internet. But here are some highlights:

Although lead cannot be seen or felt, lead poisoning can be prevented. If your home was built before 1978 and you have children age six or younger, you should consider having your home tested for lead. A good time to do this is before you move into a home or when you have a baby coming. For a list of qualified lead inspectors or risk assessors contact:

National Lead Information Center
1025 Connecticut Ave., NW, Suite 1200
Washington, DC 20036
(800) 424-LEAD

There are labs that will test dust, paint chips, and scrapings from your home to determind if they contain high levels of lead. The test kits are around $20 and they're available from: Mets Laboratories (800) 604-1995 and HomeFree (800) 622-7522.

There's also a neat product available at health food stores that you can use to check surfaces to see if lead is present. It doesn't cost much and you get results immediately, so you don't need to send samples off to a lab. It's called "Lead Check" and it's made by Homax Products, (800) 729-9029. One word of caution here is that some say the home test kits are not as reliable as when you send the sample to a lab.

If your home was built with any materials containing lead, lead dust particles could be in the air inside your home and in the soil outside around your house. Lead breaks down into a fine, virtually invisible dust, which can enter children's bodies when they breathe or when they put their fingers in their mouths. Lead can also get into children when they drink water from pipes with lead in them.

To avoid having lead in your home, do the following: look for chipping; peeling or cracked paint which could contain lead; check for scraped or rubbed paint at doorways or windows; be sure to check painted trim around windows and doors for chipping; look for places where dust could settle; check all plumbing in your home for lead pipes and fixtures; look closely around the sides of the house for places where worn paint may have fallen off. If paint is missing, there could be lead dust nearby.

If you suspect lead in your home – especially if it was built before 1978 – the following actions can limit leads availability to your child:

- Thoroughly wash all surfaces and do this frequently in places where children spend a lot of time.
- Clean everything from countertops and window sills to children's toys.
- Create safe rooms for children where all inside surfaces are kept clean and are known to be lead-free.
- Use baby wipes often to help keep kid's hands and toys clean including stuffed animals and pacifiers. Remember that cloth can collect lead dust.
- Keep curtains and upholstery clean and carefully dispose of cloth rags.
- Keep a clean cloth with you to put infants' toys and pacifiers on.
- Buy pure water for drinking or cooking; if you use tap water, let it run a few seconds before you use in. Cold water is less likely to have lead in it.
- Good nutrition can help increase your child's resistance to lead poisoning – fruits and vegetables and foods rich in vitamin C and calcium are effective barriers against lead poisoning.
- A full stomach acts as a barrier to lead. Giving kids small snacks throughout the day can reduce the amount in lead they take in; avoid walking in bare soil.

The Truth About Children's Health

- You can cover bare spots on the ground with mulch, landscaping, or walkways and have children play in grassy, not bare areas.

- Create safe play areas by removing soil that may be contaminated and replacing it with dirt or sand that is lead-free.

- Never allow children to play under windows or around painted surfaces that often rub together or get bumped.

- Make children wash their hands after playing outside and before eating or going to bed.

- Keep children from chewing on painted surfaces such as window sills, cribs, or playpens.

- To keep lead out of your house, use the doormat before entering and change the doormats periodically. Better yet, take off you shoes and leave them at the door.

Since lead can cause birth defects, it is especially important for pregnant women to protect themselves and their fetus from lead.

If your child lives in or is consistently exposed to areas where they may be exposed to lead, check with a doctor. You may want to have them tested. The doctor will probably order a blood test. You can also get a tissue mineral analysis which will show the levels of lead over a longer term. You could find someone who does this in your area by calling a chiropractor or two. If they don't do it themselves, they could probably refer you to someone who does. A couple places to get a hair analysis performed are listed in the Resource Guide. However, it's best to get it done under the care of a qualified health professional so he/she can make an accurate interpretation of the lab results.

II. Mercury

- Vaccines, Amalgam Fillings, and Braces

Mercury is another heavy metal that is very toxic to life and can create all sorts of problems in the human body and mind. The best thing to do is to avoid mercury exposure as much as possible. There are hundreds if not thousands of products in today's society that contain mercury. A partial list is shown at the end of this section.

I cannot emphasize enough that most vaccines contain thimerosal and other trace amounts of mercury. Each dose of mercury is like a straw added to the back of your child. Eventually, the mercury builds up (since it accumulates in tissue), and your child could suffer.

If you would like to avoid having your child vaccinated, you can try to get him or her exempt for religious, medical, or philosophical grounds. You must know what the law says in your state to make sure you go about this correctly. You can find state code at your local library.

I recently talked with a mother of four who got the necessary exemptions and not one of her children received even one vaccine. They are all alive and well and she says they hardly ever get as much as a sniffle. She also feeds them well and keeps them off junk foods as much as possible, but their immune systems are stronger simply because they never received vaccines. I asked her how she got the exemptions, and she said she simply wrote letters saying she didn't believe in them. I don't know if this approach will work in every case, but it may be worth a try.

You may consider home-schooling your kids to avoid the requirements for vaccines. Call the National Vaccine Information Center (NVIC) at (800) 909-SHOT for more information or for help in getting your child out of getting vaccinated.

If you feed your child well and keep him or her off the junk food and junk baby food, then they won't get sick. A healthy child will not succumb to any bacteria or virus. Many childhood illnesses are due to us treating our babies without regard to the rules of nature. They, like us, need whole, natural foods. Not sugar, additives, and pesticide-laden and overprocessed foods. They don't need pasteurized milk, soy-milk, sugared infant formula, etc. Reread the section on baby foods. If you treat your baby right, he or she will be strong and healthy and won't need some man-made concoction of dead bacteria or viruses laced with toxic heavy metals and antibiotics (antilife) that is making the pharmaceutical companies rich and killing and maiming our kids. The authorities will tell you you're taking a big risk by not vaccinating your child. Tell that to the parents who's kids turned out dead or autistic or learning impaired because of vaccines.

Healthy things beget health. Dead and toxic things beget death and impairment. Even if your child does get the measles, mumps or whatever, if you are feeding and caring for them correctly, the case will be mild and will pass quickly. On the other hand, giving your child vaccines that have more mercury in them than the EPA daily allowable limit for adult, is certain to cause some kind of problem – either readily noticeable (like autism) or something that's harder to detect later on (like a lower IQ and increased aggression). As Congressman Dan Burton said, "How is it that mercury is not safe for food additives and OTC drugs, but is safe in vaccines and dental amalgams?" (10)

One more thing on vaccines: I have a friend who has her own dog-training business. I was telling her one day about the dangers of vaccines. She mentioned that a friend of hers who breeds dogs professionally has stopped giving the dogs shots because he noticed that the dogs themselves are not only healthier in the long run, but they give birth to healthier and heartier puppies. Since the unvaccinated dogs were not "sickened" on purpose by vaccines, which weaken their cellular constitution, that strength is passed on to the next generation. Likewise, cellular weakness is passed on too. This is "The Ancestry Factor" I discussed in Chapter XII.

Do not have any silver-mercury amalgams put into your teeth or the teeth of your child. Not only does the mercury leech into the bloodstream, but it also outgasses from the filling. And, as it interacts with the saliva, it creates significant electrical charges in the mouth that may interfere with the functioning of the nervous system. After all, the nervous system runs on subtle electrical currents.

334

If you or your child already have amalgams in your teeth, it's wise to get them removed as soon as possible. Your dentist will probably tell you there's no problem and that you're crazy for wanting to remove them. Don't listen. The state of California actually requires dentist to post a health warning about amalgam fillings. There are plenty of dentists who understand that mercury is a problem and will be happy to remove the fillings. The fillings need to be removed in a certain order, depending on their respective electrical discharges. You need to find a dentist who has the appropriate testing equipment and knows what he's doing.

To find a dentist near you who is qualified to remove amalgam fillings call "Dental Amalgam Mercury Syndrome, Inc." (DAMS, Inc) at (800) 311-6265.

There are plenty of good, new materials to use in your cavities rather that amalgams. Dentistry has come a long way in just the last couple decades. Most of the newer materials are non-toxic. However, they all may not be suited to your specific body chemistry. It's a good idea to get a "Compatibility Test" done. This is a test in which a sample of blood is drawn and analyzed for allergic-type reactions to the various dental materials on the market. The test will tell you which materials your body chemistry is compatible with. You can get your (new) dentist to have this test done. If your dentist does not know about this or says it's unnecessary, you need to get another dentist.

Anyway, don't waste your money having your amalgams replaced just to have it done with material your or your child's body will not be happy with. Do it right the first time.

Another thing to consider is the effect of braces. The metal itself not only corrodes to some degree in the acidic environment of the mouth, but the interaction of this metal and any other metals in the mouth (i.e., in fillings) sets up an electrical storm in the mouth. This can cause severe personality shifts and problems in the adolescent during a time when their hormones are giving them enough trouble as it is. For a detailed discussion on these effects, read the book *Uninformed Consent* by Dr. Hal Huggins.

Getting the Heavy Metals Out

• Foods and Supplements

Once you get the amalgams out of you and your child's teeth, it's best to detoxify your body from the mercury it's built up over time. Getting the Heavy Metals Out.

Although heavy metals have and tend to stay in the body a long time and, as you now know, can cause many problems, it *is* possible to eliminate them from your body using the right foods and juices. I do not recommend you use chelating agents or supplements claiming that they will remove heavy metals. Most of them are toxic in their own right and will, over the long haul, cause problems.

It's important to realize that heavy metals and other toxins in the body are eliminated by binding to fats in the diet. Butter, coconut oils and meat, olive oil, eggs, cream, and milk fats are excellent for this. In order to mobilize the toxins out of the tissues, certain vegetable juices can be consumed. Juicing fresh cilantro, parsley, celery, and zucchini, with some carrots mobilizes the toxins and nourishes the tissues as well. Then the toxins bind to the fats and get eliminated from the body. Be sure to consume some fat with the juice. Putting a couple ounces of raw cream in the juice will do nicely.

Some foods are believed to help with eliminating mercury from the body. These are foods high in sulfur, which is believed to bind with mercury. You may consider adding these foods to your diet on a regular basis: eggs (raw, soft boiled or poached), garlic, onions, cilantro, parsley, cabbage, and broccoli.

Things to Avoid to Prevent Further Mercury Contamination

(For a more complete list, see *It's All In Your Head* by Hal A. Huggins, D.D.S)

Note: Many of these items are fungicides and antiseptic preparations. The mercury is in them to preserve them and is sometimes the active ingredient that's in there to *kill* an offending organism. Mercury *kills*. Don't put it in or on your body and you'll live better and longer.

- Thimerosal in vaccines.
- Grains treated with methyl mercury fungicides – especially wheat.
- Large saltwater fish such as swordfish, shark, cod, etc.
- Shellfish, including shrimp, lobster, crab, oyster, etc.
- Tuna – canned or fresh.
- Hair dyes, mascara, skin lightening creams, many face creams, acne preparations and foot powders (fungicides).
- Mercurochrome, Mercoseptic, Benzocaine, Calomel, Calamine lotion, Lanacane, other ointments and lotions.
- Contact lens solutions, wetting solutions, Murine, other eye drops.
- Hemorrhoidal ointments and suppositories – Preparation H, Lanacane cream.
- Ear drops, nasal sprays, some throat lozenges.
- Vaginal jellies tablets and douches such as Vagisil.
- Bar soaps.
- Some veterinary preparations.
- Mildew retardants, wood preservatives, yellow, vermilion and cinnabar pigments of paints, dyes and inks. Many latex and oil-based paints. Mercury in the paints out-gasses and gets into the air in your living space. You may consider repainting your house with a mercury-free paint. If nothing else, repaint your child's room with it.
- Lead/mercury solder.

- Garden chemicals such as seed fungicides, protectants and disinfectants, plant fungicides, herbicides, insecticides.

- Tattoos.

- Floor waxes and polishes, batteries, air-conditioner filters, fabric softeners.

- Barber and hairdresser chemicals.

- Dental amalgams.

- Chemicals used by laboratory workers and morticians and nurses.

- Numerous industrial processes and operations.

III. Physical Therapies

- Neural Organization Technique (NOT)

This unique form of treatment was started in 1980 and has proven to be effective in helping kids with a number of problems including ADHD; dyslexia; head injuries; seizures; Down's Syndrome; allergies; Temporomandibular Joint problems; structural deficits in the skeleton; digestive problems; and immune system problems.

The theory behind NOT is that when the body has been through some sort of trauma (like a difficult birth, being vaccinated, emotional stresses, car accidents, surgeries, dental work, poor diet, etc.) it goes into what is called "fight or flight." This is a mode of operating the body uses to ensure basic survival. "Fight or flight" is fine for emergency situations, but when it becomes a regular state of being, we're headed for problems. The end result of a person getting stuck in "fight or flight" is that many systems in the body fail to function correctly. The adrenal glands become overtaxed from producing a continual supply of adrenaline, which eventually weakens them and makes hormonal reactions throughout the body imbalanced. Skull bones may shift and other subtle physiological changes may take place that effect the person's posture and gait, making him or her more prone to future accidents weaknesses.

As the endocrine system weakens because of the adrenal burnout, the body becomes less and less integrated and less and less responsive. Since the person cannot "feel" life as acutely, they then are drawn to substances and foods that give them a "lift." That explains why kids may get hooked on sugar and then soft drinks and then drugs. And it also explains why some children have a tough time learning since their minds are less integrated and responsive, and the information coming in just doesn't have as much of an impact as a child with normal sensory awareness.

NOT can unlock the tightness caused by the "fight or flight" response. This opens up neural pathways by organizing the central nervous system and makes the person (child or adult) more coherent, responsive and aware. They can then handle all the sensory input and process it correctly and they no longer have to "shut-down" or on the other hand, "act out."

If you're interested in seeing if NOT can help your child, you can contact:

Dr. Carl Ferreri
(718) 253-9702
www.notint.com

Ocea Wilkes, CMT
(434) 974-6610
email: echoocea@cstone.net

• Chiropractic Adjustments

If the spine is not aligned properly, the nerves coming from it and going to it (which comprise most every nerve in the body) will not function properly. Interference in the nervous system is known as a subluxation. Subluxations may occur as early in life as birth since the infant's skull and spinal column are compressed and distorted during the birthing process. Subluxations cannot normally correct themselves but can be by proper corrective adjustment by a licensed chiropractor. If not, they may have life-long consequences for the child that could include learning disabilities, personality problems, and problems in basic biological functioning. A properly trained chiropractor will be able to determine if this has happened.

Many chiropractors use X-rays to observe if the vertebrae are aligned properly. Although X-rays can be revealing, they are not necessary and may have adverse effects. It's also important to note that not all chiropractors practice or have been trained in the same methods of adjustments – and just picking a chiropractor out of the phone book may not be the best for you or your child. It is my opinion that for the best results, the chiropractor should be trained as an Upper Cervical Specialist. The cervical portion of the spine is the neck, and the upper part of it is where the neck joins the skull. This first bone (or vertebrae) below the skull is called the Atlas and it is most important that it be aligned properly so that the nerves are not pinched or distorted in any way. If they are, virtually every part of the body will be adversely effected. An Upper Cervical Specialist can perform a special adjustment known a an Upper Cervical Specific, which puts the Atlas back into the proper position.

The chiropractor that introduced me to this technique has had good results with children who have had learning disabilities and other problems. He told me of one nine-year-old girl who had never smiled, never ran, had been through the first grade three times, had difficulty eating and was severely underweight. Once he made the Upper Cervical Specific adjustment, she looked at him and smiled for the first time in her life. She got off the adjustment table and ran to the door, turned around, and ran into her parent's arms giggling. Her mom and dad shed tears of joy, as did the others who witnessed this amazing event. Now she knows when her body needs food and eats normally, is doing well in school and is leading a normal life for a child her age.

There are only a thousand chiropractors in the country that can perform the Upper Cervical Specific adjustment, and it requires a special adjustment table to be performed properly. To find one, contact:

Virginia Institute of Chiropractic
Chad Hawk, D.C.
P.O. Box 201
4916 Plank Road, Suite 201
North Garden, VA 22959
(434) 872-9440
info@Vachiropractic.com

• CranioSacral Therapy

John Upledger, D.C., a former advisor to the Office of Alternative Medicine at the National Institutes of health, is a pioneer in physical therapy called CranioSacral Therapy, a gentle yet powerful form of bodywork that directly influences the brain and spinal cord. It's used to treat pain, discomfort and trauma to the head or face, including Temporal Mandibular Joint (TMJ) or jaw-joint dysfunction and headaches. Most of the time it's used on adults, but children can and do benefit greatly from regular treatments. CranioSacral Therapy can also relieve physical and emotional trauma. In fact, Upledger has recently had success treating autisitic children and also achieved dramatic results in treating post-tramatic stress disorders in Vietnam veterans.

The reason this therapy works on the brain, and eventually on the whole body, is that it frees up the skull bones and meninges of the brain. Upledger says that he's consistently observed in autistic children that the intracranial membranes are very tight. The therapy decreases stress on these membranes and increases circulation and oxygenation to the brain. When these things happen, the person being treated experiences a great release of tension and his or her body feels like it's being flooded with joy.

Upledger says that the behavior oftentimes seen in autistic children of banging their heads against walls is an attempt to release a compressive force in the head that is quite painful for them. It is the child's attempt to change or correct physiological and/or anatomical dysfunctions that may be causing pain or discomfort. By adjusting the bones in the skull, the pressure is released and the head-banging stops. Chewing on the wrist or sucking on the thumbs to the point of causing injury can also be helped because the child no longer feels the need to inflict pain upon themselves. He says, "It was consistently observed that CranioSacral Therapy directed at alleviation of abnormal transverse (side to side) compression of the cranial vault resulted in the child immediately demonstrating love and affection. The child will often hug and kiss the therapist after the compression has been released. Subsequently, improved socialization is often demonstrated by showing love and affection to parents and caretakers, as well as beginning to interact with other children and adults, whereas previously their interactions were with inanimate objects. Additionally, during the CranioSacral Therapy session the child often releases a lot of emotion."

Upledger also suggests good nutrition to restore the vitality of the brain. Among those he suggests are B complex, B-12, docosahexaenoic acid (Neuromins), alpha lipoic acid. (11)

There are many CranioSacral body workers around today in just about every town in America. Be sure to check and see that they are qualified. To find one near you, call the Upledger Institute at (800) 233-5880, www.upledger.com.

• Neurocranial Restructuring (NCR)

Another therapy that works on the cranial bones is called Neurocranial Restructuring or NCR. It is said to be even more powerful than CranioSacral therapy because it works by moving the bones of the skull outward from inside the nasal cavity. This unlocks the bones of the skull, which are often times jammed together, and allows the meninges of the brain to function correctly. Louis Arrandt, D.C., N.D., says, "The approach of NCR is to improve the flow of cerebrospinal fluid (CSH) by changing the shape of the skull. As the cranium optimizes, the flow of CFS becomes more and more uniform, removing the problem of poor distribution of the fluids in the brain. This seem like such a simple solution to an aggravating problem, and it is. But clinically it provides better results than the medications." (12) This treatment also helps with problems with TMJ (Temporomandibular Joint) problems and has shown to be helpful in the treatment of Down's Syndrome, eye problems, insomnia, Alzheimer's, headaches, and concussions.

Louis Arrandt, D.C., N.D., is an expert in NCR. He can be reached at (305) 279-0850.

• Whole Brain Writing

This has been shown to help with learning disabilities and attention deficits. See the discussion in Chapter VI. Jeanetter Farmer can be reached at (303) 740-6161 or www.retrainthebrain.com..

Special Section on Sudden Infant Death Syndrome (SIDS)

SIDS, also known as crib or cot deaths, is the number one cause of death for infants one month to one year of age. It's estimated that eight babies a night die from SIDS. Most researcher and doctors say the cause is unknown. But as we've examined, many think that parental smoking and vaccines are major causes.

There is one other factor you need to know about that, when corrected, has shown to stop SIDS from occurring in a vast majority of cases. Dr. Jim Sprott, a New Zealand scientist says that crib death is caused by toxic gasses that emminate from the mattress. The fire retardants (including arsenic, antimony and phosphorus) used in the manufacturing of the mattress react with a fungus that typically grows in bedding materials to produce this toxic gas. If the baby breathes this gas at high enough levels, the central nervous system shuts down, stopping breathing and heart function A normal autopsy would not reveal any sign of this poisoning.

Dr. Sprott recommends that the mattress be sealed in a high-grade polyethylene (plastic) that stops the gas from getting into the air-space of the baby.. The New Zealand government listened to Dr. Sprott, and instituted a program of mattress wrapping seven years ago. Since then, *there has not been a single SIDS death reported among the over 100,000 New Zealand babies who have slept on a wrapped mattress!* During this same period, the number of crib deaths involving unwrapped mattresses was over 500!

Dr. Sprott also recommends using a pure cotton under blanket, with only cotton or poly-cotton sheets and woolen or cotton blankets over the baby.. No other bedding materials should be used, especially synthetic sheets or blankets, a duvet, sleeping bag or sheepskin. (13)

The initial research by Dr. Sprott was published in 1994, and the New Zealand mattress wrapping program has been going on for seven years with a 100 percent success rate. So why hasn't the United States instituted such a program? Well, this information is being suppressed because the mattress manufacutrers are required to use the fire retardants due to government regulations. They would have to change their manufacturing processes and admit that their mattresses were causing babies to die — leaving them open to major liability.. In addition, crib death research has been a major source of funding for medical researchers in the United States. They don't want their meal-ticket revoked. (SIDS research has just about stopped in New Zealand.)

You can order these plastic mattress covers (be sure you get the right ones) from BabeSafe, PO Box 58-245, Greenmount Auckland, NEW ZEALAND, Phone: 64-9-5231150, Fax: 64-9-5231150, sprott@iconz.co.nz.

Four Simple Steps for Health

Being healthy yourself and raising a healthy child is actually quite simple: All you have to do is live within the laws of nature! It's the complex world we've created that makes it difficult and confusing. I've already discussed many strategies for you to take, and here are the most important ones in a nutshell

1. Clean up and super-charge your and your child's diet.

- Eat as much organically raised food as possible.
- Be sure you and your child are getting enough and the right kind of fat and vitamin A – raw and from clean sources. An egg yolk a day will greatly help in this regard, as will a high quality cod liver oil.

2. Clean up their environment and keep toxins out of it the best you can.

- Do not use pesticides or toxic cleaning agents around the house.
- Don't smoke in the house or around your children.
- Reconsider vaccinations and avoid them.
- Eliminate EMF pollution by sleeping on an EarthTether mattress pad.

3. Love your kids.

- Give them a hug every day and tell them, "I love you."
- Love them by having their body checked out by a qualified upper-cervical chiropractor, CrainoSacral, NCR or Neural Organizational Technique expert.
- Love them by turning off the TV and playing with them.
- Learn successful parenting skills.

4. Be persistent, patient, and grateful. Never give up. Changes for the better take time. Nature moves slowly, surely, but correctly.

Epilogue

We live in a complicated world. Society, science, and technology are moving so fast it can make your head spin. But as complicated as things might get, there are some simple truths we as living organisms must adhere to in order to survive and thrive. These truths will never change for they are universal laws of physics and biology that all matter and every organism is subject to.

The human organism was created to exist as part of nature and has survived and thrived for millions of years with only the things nature has provided. But in the last couple hundred years or so, our intellect and ingenuity have produced things beyond even our own imaginations. With these discoveries and inventions we have created a world of comfort, convenience, and power. But along with these advances come new hazards – some readily recognizable and some which may not become apparent for years.

The objective of this book has been to show you things that may be affecting your and your child's health in unhealthy and unnatural ways. I wanted to demonstrate from a scientific viewpoint why health problems might arise. Sometimes we lose sight of the big picture – we "don't see the forest for the trees" – and go in directions that prove futile and harmful. It is my contention that science, technology, and greed have produced things totally unsuited to the human body and mind. These substances are effecting us and our children in ways that cause biological malfunctions. The malfunctions can be immediate, like a drug overdose, or take years and even generations to manifest, like the rising infertility rate.

Getting treatments without knowing the true cause of the problem will only cause more havoc. If we know the real cause, then taking the proper corrective actions will be simple. Often times it's a case of eliminating an offending substance from our environment or diet. Sometimes it's making sure we have the correct nutrition. Merely treating the symptom in the short run may provide comfort but it will do nothing to stop the symptom or other symptoms from eventually reappearing.

Some of the ideas in this book may at first seem quite outrageous. We like to think humankind is advancing toward some higher good and getting stronger and healthier. But if you look around, is that really what you see? Why have heart disease, diabetes, asthma, ADHD, and autism become "epidemics?" Why are children shooting each other? Is it because we're becoming enlightened? Or is something going wrong?

The next 30 years will be very interesting. Will we wise up and make wholesale changes to our environment and lives, eliminating toxic substances and cleaning up our food, water, and air? Or will we continue to stick our heads in the sand and deny that unnatural things beget unhealthy beings? Will science and politics, influenced by corporate profits, keep hiding behind sayings such as: "there is no observable effect" or "there is no real scientific evidence" when simple common sense tells us otherwise?

Will we see the continual decline in people's and children's health, with each generation getting sicker and weaker at younger and younger ages. Will aggression, violence, stupidity, perversity, divorce, and immorality keep rising? Or will we realize that the body and mind need to be treated in certain ways for harmony to exist? The saying "you are what you eat" has become "you are what you consume." If we continue to consume and subject ourselves to substances that cause biological discord (mercury, chlorine, fluoride, sugar, aspartame, etc.), we will continue to see discord and disease in our lives and our society. If we continue to consume with our mind television, video, and movie violence, we will continue to be influenced by it.

Sadly, I have little hope for the masses. Most people do not have the courage to think for themselves and question authority and the "experts." And since the toxic environment is affecting the intellect and reasoning powers of our population, people will be less and less able to separate truth from dogma. They will listen and follow until they can literally no longer hear and walk or reproduce. And along the way, man and society will get more violent, barbaric, and immature.

But as in ages past, some of you will recognize cause and effect and have the courage and energy to take a different path. Going against the grain is never easy, but for those of you, who recognize the truth, there will be no other choice.

Yes, on one hand, it will be hard. But the rewards of health and happiness will be well worth the struggle. And you can rest easy knowing you are not only improving your own life and the life of your child, but the lives of those of future generations.

For there will arise out of these ashes of twisted bones, twisted minds, and twisted values a nation. Not a nation bound by rivers or mountains or geographical lines on a map – but a nation of people bound together by knowledge and truth. A truth that will enable them to overcome their confusion, greed, and malice and develop into the species they were meant to be – one of grace, compassion, and courage. A group of individuals devoted to becoming more and more and reaching higher and higher, not just for themselves, but for their progeny. For each of *their* generations will become greater and greater, stronger and stronger, more and more compassionate, until compassion is rarely needed. They will build on the strength of those enlightened ones before them so that they may become more enlightened. And the earth may become the paradise it once was, and even more.

This is your challenge and your charge. To heed the voice of truth and follow it the best you can. For the truth is not relative. It is absolute, bound by the laws of physics and nature. And the truth will not only set you free, but also allow you and yours to become more than you ever imagined.

Struggle against decay is never easy. For you are the first of this small but powerful wave, and your struggle against the lies and misinformation is greater due to the inertia it has developed over the decades and even centuries. But stem that tide you must – *as best you can.* For we are not supermen, superwomen, and superkids... yet. And our flesh and will are sometimes weak and compromised.

Future generations will look back and call you their forefathers and their heroes. Forefathers of the humans we were meant to be. Heroes because you were brave, resilient, and insightful. Recognizing the truth and acting on it: that is your greatness and your genius. Good luck, and Godspeed.

Resource Guide

Organic Food

You can find organically raised foods at most health food stores. A couple national chains are Whole Foods and Wild Oats. You can also obtain them through mail order. You can get a directory of organic sources, the National Organic Directory, at (800) 852-3832.

Jaffe Bros.
P.O. Box 636
Valley Center, CA 92082-0636
(760) 749-1133
Wide variety of nuts, seeds, oils, dried
fruit, pastas, grains, dates, etc.

Starr Organic Produce
P.O. Box 561502
Miami, FL 33256-1502
(305) 262-1242

Diamond Organics
P.O. Box 2159
Freedom, CA 95019
(800) 922-2396
www.diamondorganics.com
Wide variety of organic food
including produce and dairy.

D'Artagnan
399-419 St. Paul Ave.
Jersey City, NJ 07306
(800) DAR-TAGN
Organic meat and poultry.

Community Mill & Bean
267 Rt. 89 South
Savannah, NY 13146
(800) 755-0554
Organic baking mixes, whole grains and beans.

Raw Milk and Dairy Products

You can check with local dairy farmers to see if they sell raw dairy products. Finding one may be difficult, so I suggest you contact The Weston A. Price Foundation who publishes listings of providers of unpasteurized dairy products. You will have to sign up for their quarterly magazine, but it is well worth the price in many ways.

The Weston A. Price Foundation
PMB 106-380
4200 Wisconsin Ave., N.W.
Washington, D.C., 20016
(202) 333-HEAL; www.westonaprice.org.

Another place you can find sources of raw milk products is:

www.realmilk.com.

Unheated Honey

Both of the brands below can be found at most health-food stores.

Y.S. Organic Bee Products
(815) 496-9416

Really Raw Honey Company
(800) REAL- RAW

Oils

These oils are pressed below 96 degrees F, which preserves their nutrients. They can usually be found at health food stores, but if not, here are phone numbers. You can get extra virgin olive oil, coconut oil, coconut butter, flax seek oil etc. from these sources.

Flora, Inc.
(800) 446-2110

Omega Nutrition
(800) 661-3529

Eggs

To obtain raw, fertile eggs from free range hens, check at your healthfood store.

Essential Fatty Acid Products

These can be found at most health food stores (be sure they're refrigerated) or by contacting:

Omega Nutrition (Arrowhead brand)
(800) 661-3529

Flora, Inc. (Udo's Choice brand)
(800) 446-2110

Salt

Salt should be avoided. But, if you are going to eat it, you and your child should eat only Celtic Sea Salt. You can find it at most health food stores or by calling:

Grain & Salt Society
(800) 867-7258

Radiant Life
(888) 593-8333

Marine Salt Traders
(800) 903-SALT

Enzymes and Personalized Nutritional Counseling

Dr. Maile Pouls
517 Liberty Street
Santa Cruz, CA 95060
www.yournutrition.com
(831) 423-7554

David Getoff, CCN, CNC, FAAIM
P.O. Box 803
Jamul, CA 91935
www.naturopath4you.com

Glandular Products

Dew's 21st Century Products
(940) 243-2178
Sells a good multiglandular called
"VitalGlands"

Health Excel
Offers a variety of good glandulars.
(800) 323-3842
www.healthexcel.com

Water

Use Perrier water or other good mineral water. For a good, inexpensive water filter or "the best" spring water call:

PRI, Inc.
(434) 263-8256

DHA (docasahexaeonoic acid)

Get Neuromins (purified plant based DHA) from MMS Pro by calling:

Emerson Ecolgics
(800) 654-4432

Martek Corp.
6480 Dobbin Road
Columbia, MD 21045
(800) 662-6339
www.dhadepot.com

Lead Inspection

Contact the National Lead Information Center (800) 424-LEAD. For a list of lead-inspection and -abatement renovators in your area:www.leadlist.org

For test kits to determine if your home is contaminated:

Homax Products
(800) 729-9029

Mets Laboratories
(800) 604-1995

HomeFree
(800) 622-7522

Hair Analysis

(Note: Please consult a qualified health care practitioner first.)

Great Smokies Lab
(800) 522-4762
www.gsdl.com

Analytical Research Lab
(800) 528-4067
www.arltma.com

Doctor's Data
(800) 323-2784
www.doctorsdata.com

Nontoxic Household Products

Most health food stores now carry a wide variety of nontoxic household products from soaps and cleansers to flea collars and carpet cleaners. Seventh Generation products are good. A good all purpose cleaner is called "Ultra-Safe Solution." You can get it by calling (800) 301-9111 or www.solutions-4-you.com. A manufacturer of nontoxic carpeting is:

Earth Weave Carpet Mills, Inc.
P.O. Box 6120
Dalton, GA 30722
(706) 278-8200
earthweave@earthweave.com

Two good books to read concerning nontoxic products are:

Nontoxic, Natural, & Earthwise by Debra Lynn Dadd

Better Basics for the Home: Simple Solutions for Less Toxic Living by Annie Berthold-Bond

Electromagnetic Pollution Protection

EarthTether mattress pad and other EMF fighting products.

(800) 620-9912 or www.earthtether.com

Vaccine Information

For information concerning vaccinations and alternatives to getting them, contact:

National Vaccine Information Center (NVIC)
(800) 909-SHOT

Mercury Fillings Removal

To find a qualified dentist in your area who will remove your and your child's amalgam fillings correctly, contact:

Dental Amalgam Mercury Syndrome (DAMS, Inc.)
(800) 311-6265

Successful Parenting Skills

For a successful, practical program to teach you how to be an effective parent, order "Parenting with Dignity" from: (Do not overlook this! It will make changes come a lot easier!)

"The Drew Bledsoe Foundation"
(508) 543-6543; www.drewbledsoe.com.

Therapies

Neural Organization Technique (NOT)

Dr. Carl Ferreri
(718) 253-9702
www.notint.com

Ocea Wilkes, CMT
(434) 974-6610
email: echoocea@cstone.net

Upper Cervical Specialist Chiropractors

Chadwick Hawk, D.C.
Virginia Institute of Chiropractic
P.O. Box 201
4916 Plank Road, Suite 201
North Garden, VA 22959
(434) 872-9440
info@VAchiropractic.com

CranioSacral

To find a practitioner near you contact:
The Upledger Institute
(800) 233-5880
www.upledger.com

Neurocranial Restructuring (NCR)

The Wellness Center
10651 N. Kendall Dr., Ste. 222
Miami, FL 33176
Dr. Louis Arrandt
(305) 279-0850

Touch & Movement

Sensory Integration Therapy
Oregon Hope and Help Center, Inc.
152 Arthur St., P.O. Box 406,
Woodburn, OR 97071
(503) 981-0635

Handwriting Therapy

www.retrainthebrain.com or call Jeanette Farmer at (303) 740-6161

Recommended Reading

The Complete Children's Safety and Protection Kit, with 14 Days to a Safer Child Day-Planner Lesson Plan, by PRI Publishing. Teaches children how to avoid abductions, getting lost, injuries, and more. Doctor approved. Includes colorful children's book, CD with songs and book narration, Sterling the Safety Seal beany toy, Parents' and Teachers' Instruction Guide, fun stickers, 14 days of detailed lesson plans, quizzes, final exam, diploma. Call PRI Publishing at (434) 263-8858.

We Want to Live by Aajonus Vonderplanitz. Published by Carnelian Bay Castle Press, P.O. Box 66663, Los Angeles, CA 90066. To order call (800) 247-6553.

Health & Healing Wisdom Journal. Published by the Price-Pottenger Nutrition Foundation, P.O. Box 2614, La Mesa, Ca 91943. To order call (800) 366-3748.

The Crazy Makers by Carol Simontacchi. Published by Penguin Putnam, Inc., 375 Hudson St., New York, NY, 10014. Available through the Price-Pottenger Nutrition Foundation, (800) 366-3748.

Vaccination, Social Violence, and Criminality by Harris L. Coulter, Published by North Atlantic Books, Berkeley California.

A Shot in the Dark by Harris L. Coulter and Barbara Loe Fisher. Published by Avery Publishing, NY, NY.

The Consumer's Guide to Childhood Vaccines by Barbara Loe Fisher. Published by the National Vaccine Information Center, 512 W. Maple Ave., Suite 206, Vienna, VA, 22180. To order call (800) 909-SHOT.

For Tomorrow's Children – A Manual for Future Parents. Published by Preconception Care, Inc., P.O. Box 357, Blooming Glen, PA 18911. To order call Price-Pottenger Nutrition Foundation at (800) 366-3748.

The Curse of Louis Pasteur – Why Medicine is Not Healing a Diseased World by Nancy Appleton. Published by Choice Publishing, P.O. Box Santa Monica, CA 90403. To order call Price-Pottenger Nutrition Foundation at (800) 366-3748.

Sugar Blues by William Dufty. Published by Warner Books, Inc., 1271 Avenue of the Americas, New York, NY 10020. Available at most book stores.

Uninformed Consent – The Hidden Dangers in Dental Care by Hal A. Huggins and Thomas E Levy. Published by Hamption Roads Publishing Company, Inc, 1125 Stoney Ridge Road, Charlottesville, VA 22902. To order call (800) 766-8009.

It's All in Your Head – The Link Between Mercury Amalgams and Illness by Hal A. Huggins. Published by Avery Publishing Group, Inc., Garden City Park, NY.

Nourishing Traditions by Sally Fallon. Published by NewTrends Publishing, Inc., Washington, D.C. To order call (877) 707-1776.

Wise Traditions Newsletter. Published quarterly by The Weston A. Price Foundation, PMB 106-380, 4200 Wisconsin Ave., N.W., Washington, D.C., 20016. To order call (202) 333-HEAL.

The Recipe for Living Without Disease, by AajonusVonderplanitz, Published by Carnelian Bay Castle Press, P.O. Box 66663, Los Angeles, CA 90066. To order call (800) 247-6553.

Training the Brain to Pay Attention the Write Way by Jeanette Farmer. To order call (303) 740-6161, www.retrainthebrain.com.

Bibliography

Introduction

1. Buttram, Harold, Richard Piccola. *Who is Looking After Our Kids? A Guide for Parent's to Protect Their Children From Environmental Hazards.* Foresight America Foundation, Quakertown, PA . December 1997. And www.healing.org/Child-intro.html.

2. Schettler, Ted, M.D., M.P.H., and Jill Stein, M.D. In Harm's Way: *Toxic Threats to Child Development.* Boston: Greater Boston Physicians for Social Responsibility, 2000.

3. Fallon, Sally, and Mary G. Enig, Ph.D. *Nourishing Traditions,* Washington, DC: New Trends Publishing, Inc. 1999.

Chapter I — Children of the USA

1. Federal Interagency Forum on Child and Family Statistics. "America's Children: Key National Indicators of Well-Being." 2001.

2. American Psychological Association. "Is Youth Violence Just Another Fact of Life?" 2000.

3. Federal Bureau of Investigation. "Juveniles and Violence." 1995.

4. New York Times, "Homicide Rate Up For Young Blacks." A26. December 7, 1990.

5. Landrigan, Philip J., et al. National Research Council. *Pesticides in the Diets of Infants and Children.* National Academy Press: Washington, DC, 1993, p. 61.

6. Wiles, Richard, et al. "Pesticides in Children's Food." Washington, DC: Environmental Working Group, June 1993. www.ewg.org.

7. Landrigan, Op cit. p. 43.

8. Carlson, Elisabeth, et al. "Evidence for Decreasing Quality of Semen During Past 50 Years." *British Medical Journal* 305: 609-613 (1992).

9. Gray, J.R., and Leon Earl. "Chemical-Induced Alterations of Sexual Differentiation: A Review of Effects in Humans and Rodents." In *Advances in Modern Environmental Toxicology*, edited by M.A. Mehlman. Princeton, NJ: Princeton Scientific Publishing Co. Inc., 1992, pp. 203-230.

10. *Infant Risks From Pesticides,* Washington, DC: Environmental Working Group, 2001. www.ewg.org.

11. Peto, R., et al. "Effects on 4080 Rats of Chronic Ingestion of N-Nitrosodiethylamine or N-Nitrosodimethylamine: A Detailed Dose-Response Study." *Cancer Research* 51 (1991): 6415-51.

12. McConnell, Ernest. *Comparative Responses in Carcinogenesis Bioassays as a Function of Age at First Exposure. Similarities & Differences Between Children and Adults.* Washington, DC: ILSI Press, 1992, pp. 66-78.

13. Snodgrass, Wayne R. "Physiological and Biochemical Difference Between Children and Adults As Determinants of Toxic Response to Environmental Pollutants." In *Similarities and Differences between Children and Adults: Implications for Risk Assessment,* edited by Philip S. Guzelian, Carol J. Henry, and Stephen S. Olin. Washington, DC: International Life Sciences Institute, 1992, pp. 35-42.

14. Landrigan, Philip J., et al. Op cit.

15. Ibid.

16. Ibid.

17. Ries, L., et al. *Cancer in Children, SEER Cancer Statistics Review, 1973-1990.* Washington, D.C.: U.S. Department of Health and Human Services, 1993.

18. Masters, Roger D., Brian Hone, and Anil Doshi. "Environmental Pollution, Neurotoxicity and Criminal Violence." In *Environmental Toxicology,* edited by J. Rose. New York: Gordon and Breach Publishers, 1997.

19. Executive Order. *Protection of Children From Environmental Health Risks and Safety Risks.* The White House, Office of the Press Secretary. April 21, 1997.

20. *Preventing Child Exposures to Environmental Hazards: Research and Policy Issues.* Children's Environmental Health Network/California Public Health Foundation. 1994.

Chapter II - Hazards Our Children Face

1. Landrigan, Philip J. "Commentary: Environmental Disease – A Preventable Epidemic." *American Journal of Public Health* 82 (July 1992): 941-943.

2. Environmental Protection Agency. "Lead in Your Home: A Parent's Reference Guide." EPA 747-B-99-003. May 1999.

3. Committee on Environmental Health, American Academy of Pediatrics. "Lead Poisoning: From Screening to Primary Prevention." *Pediatrics* 92 (July 1993): 176-183.

4. Montague, Peter. "Dumbing Down the Children — Part 3," *Rachel's Environmental & Health Weekly.* Environmental Research Foundation. March 2, 2000.

5. Landrigan, Philip J. Op cit.

7. Agency for Toxic Substances and Disease Registry. "Toxicological Profile for Lead." July 1999, pp. 26-29.

8. Lanphear, Bruce P. "The Paradox of Lead Poisoning Prevention." *Science* 281 (September 11, 1998): 1617-18.

9. Montague, Peter. Op cit.

10. Environmental Protection Agency. Drinking Water Standards Program. "Lead & Copper." Office of Water, Ground Water and Drinking Water. www.epa.gov/safewater/leadcop.html.

11. Needleman, Herbert L., et al. "Bone Lead Levels and Delinquent Behavior." *Journal of the American Medical Association* 275, no. 5 (1996): 363-369.

12. de la Burde, Brigitte, and McLin S. Choate. "Early Asymptomatic Lead Exposure and Development at School Age." *Journal of Pediatrics* 87, no. 4 (1975): 638-642.

13. Bellinger, David, et al. "Pre- and Postnatal Lead Exposure and Behavior Problems in School-Aged Children." *Environmental Research* 66 (1994): 12-30.

14. Marlowe, Mike, and John Errera. "Low Lead Levels and Behavior Problems in Children." *Behavioral Disorders* 7 (1982): 163-172.

15. Montague, Peter. "Toxins Affect Behavior." *Rachel's Environmental & Health Weekly.* Environmental Research Foundation. January 16, 1997.

16. Byers, Randolph K. and Elizabeth E. Lord. "Late Effects of Lead Poisoning on Mental Development." *American Journal of Diseases of Children* 66, no. 5 (November 1943): 471-494

17. Masters, Roger D., Brian Hone, and Anil Doshi. "Environmental Pollution, Neurotoxicity, and Criminal Violence." In *Environmental Toxicology,* edited by J. Rose. New York: Gordon and Breach Publishers, 1997.

18. Environmental Protection Agency. *Lead in Your Home: A Parent's Reference Guide.* EPA 747-B-99-003. May 1999.

19. National Research Council. *Measuring Lead Exposure in Infants, Children, and Other Sensitive Populations.* Washington, DC: National Academy Press, 1993.

20. Flegal, Russell A., and Donald R. Smith. "Lead Levels in Preindustrial Humans." *New England Journal of Medicine* 326 (1992): 1293-1294.

21. Masters, Roger D., Brian Hone, and Anil Doshi. Op cit.

22. Motluck, Alison. "Pollution May Lead to a Life of Crime." *New Scientist* 154, no. 2084 (1997): 4.

23. Montague, Peter. "Dumbing Down the Children — Part 3," Op cit.

24. Pear, Robert. "States Called Lax on Tests for Lead in Poor Children." *New York Times*, August 22, 1999, p. A-1.

25. Montague, Peter. Op cit.

26. Lanphear, Bruce P. "Racial Differences in Urban Children's Environmental Exposures to Lead." *American Journal of Public Health* 86, no. 10 (1996): 1460-1463.

27. Schulte, A., et al. "Urinary Mercury Concentrations in Children With and Without Amalgam Restorations." *Journal of Dental Restoration* 73, no. 4 (1994): A-334.

28. Abraham, J.E., C.W. Svare, and C.W. Frank. "The Effect of Dental Amalgam Restorations on Blood Mercury Levels." *Journal of Dental Restoration* 663, no. 1 (1984): 71-73.

29. Associated Press. "Mercury Poses Health Risk." November 8, 1990.

30. Schettler, Ted, M.D., M.P.H., and Jill Stein, M.D. *In Harm's Way: Toxic Threats to Child Development*. Boston: Greater Boston Physicians for Social Responsibility. 2000.

31. Spyker, Joan, Sheldon B. Sparber, and Alan M. Goldberg. "Low Level Mercury Causes Behavior Problems During Pregnancy." *Science* (August 1972): 621-623.

32. Huggins, Hal A. *It's All in Your Head: The Link Between Mercury Amalgams and Illness*. Garden City Park, NY: Avery Publishing Group, Inc. 1993.

33. Bartolome, George, and Patricia Trepanier. "Dopamine Uptake in Brain Cells Changed by Methylmercury." *Toxicology and Applied Pharmacology* 65 (1982): pp. 92-99.

34. Pressinger, Richard W. "Mercury Exposure During Pregnancy—Links to Learning Disabilities, ADD, and Behavior Disorders." 2000. www.chemtox.com.

35. Siblerad, Robert L., John Moti, and Eldon Kienholz. "Psychometric Evidence That Mercury From Silver Dental Fillings May be an Etiological Factor in Depression, Excessive Anger, and Anxiety." *Psychological Reports* 74 (1994).

36. "Mercury Amalgam & Mental Illness." www.whale.to

37. Lichtenberg, H.J. "Elimination of Symptoms by Removal of Dental Amalgam From Mercury Poisoned Patients, as Compared With a Control Group of Average Patients." *Journal of Orthomolecular Medicine* 8 (1993) 145-148.

38. Huggins, Hal A. Op cit., pp. 32-33.

39. Huggins, Hal A. "Birth Defects." 2000. www.whale.to or www.hugnet.com.

40. Huggins, Hal A. *It's All in Your Head, The Link Between Mercury Amalgams and Illness*. Op cit., p. 33.

41. DAMS, Inc. www.dams.cc or www.amalgam.org. or (800) 311-6265.

42. Huggins, Hal A. Op cit., pp. 35, 54,150.

43. Huggins, Hal A. "Politics of Medicine—The Struggle for Freedom of Medical Choice. California Dentists Forced Out of State of Denial." *Alternative Medicine* 41 (May 2001): 114-117.

44. "Mercury Inducing Disease in Animal Experiments." 2000. www.whale.to.

45. Jacobson, Joseph L., and Sandra W. Jacobson. "Intellectual Impairment in Children Exposed to Polychlorinated Biphenyls in Utero." *New England Journal of Medicine* 335, no. 11 (1996): 783-789.

46. Jacobson, Joseph L., and Sandra W. Jacobson. "Dose-Response in Perinatal Exposure to Polychlorinated Biphenyls (PCBs): The Michigan and North Carolina Cohort Studies." *Toxicology and Industrial Health* 12, nos. 3/4 (1996): 435-445.

47. Fein, Greta G., et al. "Prenatal Exposure to Polychlorinated Biphenyls: Effects on Birth Size and Gestational Age." *The Journal of Pediatrics* 105 (August 1984): 315-320.

48. Jacobson, Sandra W., et al. "The Effect of Intrauterine PCB Exposure on Visual Recognition Memory." *Child Development* 56 (1985).

49. Jacobson, Joseph L., et al. "Effects of In Utero Exposure to Polychlorinated Biphenyls and Related Contaminants on Cognitive Functioning in Young Children." *Journal of Pediatrics* 116 (January 1980): 38-45.

50. Jacobson, Joseph L., et al. "Effects of Exposure to PCBs and Related Compounds on Growth and Activity in Children." *Neurotoxicology and Teratology* 12 (1990): 319-326.

51. Jacobson, Joseph L., et al. "Effects of Prenatal PCB Exposure on Cognitive Processing Efficiency and Sustained Attention." *Developmental Psychology* 28, no. 2 (1992): 297-306.

Bibliography

52. Daly, Helen B. "The Evaluation of Behavioral Changes Produced by Consumption of Environmentally Contaminated Fish." In *The Vulnerable Brain and Environmental Risks,* edited by Robert L. Isaacson and Karl F. Jensen. New York: Plenum Press, 1992, pp. 151-171..

53. Montague, Peter. "PCB Exposure Linked to Low IQ," *Rachel's Environmental & Health Weekly.* Environmental Research Foundation. September 19, 1996.

54. Schuld, Andreas. "Fluoride—Worse Than We Thought." *Wise Traditions* 1, no. 3 (Fall 2000). Weston A. Price Foundation.

55. "The Effect of Fluorine on Dental Caries." *Journal of the American Dental Association* 31 (1944): 1360.

56. "Did Government Approve Citizens as Toxic Waste Sites? Are We Being Poisoned?" *The Winds.* 1998, p. 12. www.thewinds.org.

57. Schuld, Andreas. Op cit.

58. Centers for Disease Control and Prevention. "Achievements in Public Health, 1900-1999— Fluoridation of Drinking Water to Prevent Dental Caries." *Morbidity and Mortality Weekly Report* 48(41) (1999): 933-940.

59. Green, Jeff. "Just What is Fluoride?" *Health & Healing Wisdom, the Journal of the Price-Pottenger Nutrition Foundation* 23, no. 1 (Spring 1999): 5.

60. Borne, Gregory. "Phosphoric Acid Waste Dialogue, Report on Phosphoric Wastes Dialogue Committee, Activities and Recommendations; Southeast Negotiation Network." *EPA Stakeholders Review.* September 1995.

61. "Did Government Approve Citizens as Toxic Waste Sites? Are We Being Poisoned?" Op cit., p. 11.

62. National Research Council, Committee on Toxicology, Board on Environmental Studies and Toxicology, Commission on Life Sciences, Subcommittee on Health Effects of Ingested Fluoride. *Health Effects of Ingested Fluoride.* August 1993, p. 59.

63. *Fluorides and Human Health.* World Health Organization. 1970, p. 239.

64. Carton, R.J., and J.W. Hirzy. "Applying the NAEP Code of Ethics to the Environmental Protection Agency and the Fluoride in Drinking Water Standard." *Proceedings of the 23rd Annual Conference of the National Association of Environmental Professionals.* GEN 51-61 (June 1998): pp. 20-24.

65. Carton, Robert J. "Corruption and Fraud at the EPA." *The Winds.* July 28, 1995. www.thewinds.org

66. "Did Government Approve Citizens as Toxic Waste Sites? Are We Being Poisoned?" Op cit.

67. Mullenix, Phyllis. "Neurotoxicity of Sodium Fluoride in Rats." *Journal of Neurotoxicology and Teratology* 17, no. 2 (1995).

68. Ibid. See also, Joel Griffiths and Chris Bryson's "Fluoride Teeth and the Atomic Bomb," 1997, an article originally commissioned by the *Christian Science Monitor* but never published in it. You can find it at www.winds.org.

69. "Did Government Approve Citizens as Toxic Waste Sites? Are We Being Poisoned?" Op cit., p. 10.

70. Bennett, J.V., et al. "Infectious and Parasitic Diseases." In *Closing the Gap: The Burden of Unnecessary Illness,* edited by R. Amler and H.B. Dull. Oxford, England: Oxford University Press. 1987. (The figure cited is not an official CDC estimate, though it was informally developed by CDC scientists.)

71. Morris, R., and R. Levin. "Estimating the Incidence of Waterborne Infectious Disease Related to Drinking Water in the United States." In *Assessing and Managing the Health Risks From Drinking Water Contamination,* edited by E. Richard. London: International Association of Hydrological Sciences, 1996.

72. "40 CFR Parts 9,141,132." *Federal Register* 63, no. 241 (December 16, 1998).

73. Thornton, Jacqui. "Chlorinated Tap Water Linked to Birth Defects." *The Electronic Telegraph,* February 20, 2000.

74. Klotz, Judith B., and Laurie A. Pyrch. *Case-Control Study of Neural Tube Defects and Drinking Water Contaminants.* Atlanta, GA: Agency for Toxic Substances and Disease Registry. January 1998.

75. Cantor, Kenneth P. "Drinking Water and Cancer—Epidemiologic Research on Cancer Risk and Chlorination By-Products in Drinking Water." *Cancer Causes and Control* 8 (1997).

76. Waller, Kirsten, et al. "Trihanomethanes in Drinking Water and Spontaneous Abortion." *Epidemiology* 9, no. 2 (March 1998): 134-140.

77. Cantor, Kenneth P. Op cit.

78. Betts, Kellyn S. "Miscarriages Associated With Drinking Water Disinfection Byproducts, Study Says." *Environmental Science & Technology* (April 1, 1998): 169A-170O.

79. Zaslow, Sandra A., and Glenda M. Herman. "Health Effects of Drinking Water Contaminants." North Carolina Cooperative Extension Service, publication he-393 (May 1992).

80. Durant, John L., et al. "Elevated Incidence of Childhood Leukemia in Woburn, Massachusetts: NIEHS Superfund Basic Research Program Searches of Causes." *Environmental Health Perspectives* 103: Supplement 6 (September 1995).

81. Physicians for Social Responsibility. "Physicians Give Failing Grade to Congress on Child Health Issues." August 26, 1998. www.psr.org/reportcard.htm.

82. Physicians for Social Responsibility. www.atsdr.cdc.gov/toxhazsf.html.

83. Zaslow, Sandra A., and Glenda M. Herman. Op cit.

84. Natural Resources Defense Council. "Clean Water and Oceans: Drinking Water: In Brief: FAQs. Arsenic in Drinking Water." June 30, 2000. www.nrdc.org/water/drinking/quarsenic.asp

85. Watersafe™. "Pocket Guide—Have You Tested Your Drinking Water Lately?" Silver Lake Research, Monrovia, CA.

86. Self, James R., and Reagan M. Waskom. "Nitrates in Drinking Water." Colorado State University Cooperative Extension Service. June 1992.

87. Natural Resources Defense Council. "Clean Water and Oceans: Drinking Water: In Brief: FAQs. Bottled Water: Pure Drink or Pure Hype?" April 29, 1999. www.nrdc.org/water/drinking/nbw.asp.

88. Landrigan, Philip J., et al. National Research Council. *Pesticides in the Diets of Infants and Children.* National Academy Press: Washington, D.C., 1993.

89. "A Short History of Pesticides." *Simplelife.* 1995/96. www.simplelife.com.

90. Needham, Larry L., et al. "The Priority Toxicant Reference Range Study: Interim Report." *Environmental Health Perspectives* 103, supplement 3 (April 1995).

91. Landrigan, Philip J. "Commentary: Environmental Disease—A Preventable Epidemic." *American Journal of Public Health* 82 (July 1992): 941-943.

92. "Pesticide Exposure During Pregnancy." www.chem-Tox.com/pregnancy/pregpest.htm.

93. "Pesticide Statistics." *Simplelife.* 1995/96. www.simplelife.com

94. Pearce, Fred, and Debora Mackenzie. "It's Raining Pesticides: The Water Falling From Our Skies is Unfit to Drink." *New Scientist:* 23 (April 3, 1999). www.newscientist.com.

95. Montague, Peter, "Pesticides in the News." *Rachel's Environmental & Health Weekly.* Environmental Research Foundation. July 22, 1999.

96. Schmidt, Charles W. "Childhood Cancer: A Growing Problem." *Environmental Health Perspectives* 106, no. 1 (1998): A18-A23.

97. Burros, Marian. "High Pesticide Levels Seen in U.S. Food." *New York Times,* February 19,1999. (n.p.—see http://-archives.nytimes.com.)

98. Pogoda, Janice M., and Susan Prestonu-Martin. "Household Pesticides and Risk of Pediatric Brain Tumors." *Environmental Health Perspectives* 105, no. 11 (1997): 1214-1220.

99. Montague, Peter. "Children's Cancer and Pesticides," *Rachel's Environmental & Health Weekly.* Environmental Research Foundation. March 5, 1998.

100. Lewis, R.G., et al. "Measuring Transport of Lawn-Applied Herbicide Acids from Turf to Home: Correlation of Dislodgeable 2,4-D Turf Residues with Carpet Dust and Carpet Surface Residues." *Environmental Science and Technology* 30, no. 11 (2000): 3313-3320.

101. Fenske, Richard A., Kathleen Black, and Kenneth P. Elkmer. "Home Pesticide Flea Treatments Cause Illegally High Air Levels." *American Journal Public Health* 80, no. 6 (1990): 689-693.

102. Hayes, Howard M., et al. "Case-Control Study of Canine Malignant Lymphoma: Positive Association with Dog Owner's Use of 2,4-Dichlorophenoxyacetic Acid Herbicides. *Journal of the National Cancer Institute* 83 (September 4, 1991): 1226-31.

103. Montague, Peter. "Pet Dogs Get Cancer From Week Killers." *Rachel's Environmental & Health Weekly.* Environmental Research Foundation. September 11, 1991.

104. Aschengrau, Ann, and Richard R. Monson. "Paternal Military Service in Vietnam and the Risk of Late Adverse Pregnancy Outcomes." *American Journal of Public Health* 80 (October 1990): 1218-24.

105. Fenske, Richard and Todd Sternbach. "Indoor Air Levels of Chlordane in Residences in New Jersey." *Bulletin Environmental Contamination Toxicology* 39 (1987): 903-910.

106. Ozonoff, David, et al. "Leukemias and Blood Dyscrasias Following Exposure to Chlordane and Heptachlor." *Teratogenesis, Carcinogenesis and Mutagenesis* 7 (1987): 527-540.

107. Kliburn, Kaye H. and John C. Thornton. "Chlordane Causes Neurological Disorders ADD Symptoms in 216 Adults Tested." *Environmental Health Perspectives* 103 (1995) 690-694.

108. Montague, Peter. "Children's Cancer and Pesticides." *Rachel's Environmental & Health Weekly.* Environmental Research Foundation. March 5, 1998.

109. Barich, Bob. "Hedging Your Bets." Greatlife. January, 2001, p10.

110. Nordstrom, M., et al. "Occupational Exposures, Animal Exposure and Smoking as risk Factors for Hairy Cell Leukaemia Evaluated in a Case-Control Study." *British Journal of Cancer* 77 (1998): 2048-2052.

111. Hardell, Lennart, and Mikael Eriksson. "A Case-Control Study of Non-Hodgkin Lymphoma and Exposure to Pesticides." *Cancer.* 85, no. 6 (1999): 1353-60.

112. Buckley, J.D., et al. "Pesticide Exposure in Children with Non-Hodgkin Lymphoma." *Cancer* 89, no.11 (2000).

113. Montague, Peter. "Pesticides and Aggression." *Rachel's Environmental & Health Weekly.* Environmental Research Foundation. April 29, 1999.

114. Guillette, Elizabeth A., et al. "An Anthropological Approach to the Evaluation of Preschool Children Exposed to Pesticides in Mexico." *Environmental Health Perspectives* 106, no. 6 (1998): 347-353.

115. Koop, C.E., and G.D. Lundberg. "Violence in America: A Public Health Emergency." *Journal of the American Medical Association* 267, no. 22 (1992): 3075-3076.

116. Cummins, Ronnie, Being Aware of Gene-Altered Foods. *Well Being Journal* 10, no. 3 (Summer 2001): 26.

117. Ibid.

118. Montague, Peter. "Pet Dogs Get Cancer From Week Killers." Op cit.

119. Montague, Peter. "Hazardous Waste is Legally 'Recycled' into Pesticides and Labeled 'Inert.'" *Rachel's Environmental & Health Weekly.* Environmental Research Foundation. November 6, 1991.

120. Davis. Devra L. Testimony of Devra Lee Davis, Ph.D., M.P.H., F.A.C.E., before Congress of the United States Human Resources and Intergovernmental Relations Subcommittee of the Committee on Government Operations Hearing on Breast Cancer. December 11, 1991

121. Westin, Jerome B., and Elihu Richter. "The Israeli Breast-Cancer Anomaly." In *Trends in Cancer Mortality in Industrial Countries,* edited by Devra L. Davis and David Hoel. New York: Academy of Sciences, 1990, pp 259-268.

122. Montague, Peter. "Breast Cancer Epidemic Continues; Prevention Philosophy is Ignored," *Rachel's Environmental & Health Weekly.* Environmental Research Foundation. December 25, 1991.

123. Davis, Devra L., et al. "Medical Hypothesis: Xenoestrogens as Preventable Causes of Breast Cancer." *Environmental Health Perspectives* 101 (October 1993): 372-377.

124. Montague, Peter. "Chemicals and Health—Part 1." *Rachel's Environmental & Health Weekly.* Environmental Research Foundation. December 23, 1993.

125. Montague, Peter. "Human Breast Milk is Contaminated," *Rachel's Environmental & Health Weekly.* Environmental Research Foundation. August 8, 1990.

126. Foster, Warren, et. al. "In Utero Exposure of the Human Fetus to Xenobiotic Endocrine Disrupting Chemicals." Presented at the Endocrine Society's 81st Annual Meeting in San Diego, CA, June 14, 1999.

127. You, L., et. al. "Impaired Male Sexual Development in Perinatal Sprague-Dawley and Long-Evans Hooded Rats Exposed in Utero and Lactationally to p,p'-DDE." *Toxicological Sciences* 43, no. 2 (1998): 162-173.

128. Loeffler, I.K., and R.E. Peterson. "Interactive Effects of TCDD and p,p'-DDE on Male Reproductive Tract Development in Utero and Lactationally Exposed Rats." *Toxicology and Applied Pharmacology* 154, no. 1 (1999): 28-39.

129. Mitchell, J.A., and S.F. Long. "The Behavioral Effects of Pesticides in Male Mice." *Neurotoxicology and Teratology* 11 (1989): 45-50.

130. Landrigan, Philip J. "Commentary: Environmental Disease—A Preventable Epidemic." Op cit., pp. 941-943.

131. Davis, Geoff. "Household Cleaners: Part 2-Dirty Little Secrets." Natural Home. www.gaiam.com.

132. www.epa.gov.

133. SafeScience. "The Need for Chemically Safe Cleaners." 2000. www.safescience.com.

134. Davis, Op cit.

135. Ibid.

136. Prochko, Judy. "The Air You Breathe-Part 2." The League of Women Voters of the Fairfax Area. www.lwv-fairfax.org.

137. American Journal of Industrial Medicine. 39 (2001): 121-132.

138. *Targeting Tobacco Use: The Nation's Leading Cause of Death, At-A-Glance*. Atlanta, GA: Centers for Disease Control and Prevention. November 2, 2000. www.cdc.gov/tobacco.

139. American Heart Association. "Cigarette Smoking and Cardiovascular Diseases." 2000. www.americanheart.org.

140. "Targeting Tobacco Use: The Nation's Leading Cause of Death, At-A-Glance." Op cit.

141. American Heart Association. "Cigarette Smoking Statistics." 2000. www.americanheart.org.

142. American Heart Association. "Cigarette Smoking and Children." 2000. www.americanheart.org.

143. Gidding, Samuel S., et al. "Active and Passive Tobacco Exposure: A Serious Pediatric Health Problem." American Heart Association: AHA Medical/Scientific Statement. June 16, 1994.

144. American Heart Association. "Clean Indoor Air Laws." 2000. www.americanheart.org.

145. diFranza, Joseph, and Robert Lew. "Morbidity and Mortality in Children Associated with the Use of Tobacco Products by Other People." *Paediatrics* 97 (1996): 560-568.

146. DeNoon, Daniel J. "Parents' Smoking Gives Children Asthma, Wheezing." *WebMD Medical News*. Healtheon/WebMD Corporation. December 2, 1999.

147. "Smoking Around Children." Michigan Department of Public Health. Lansing, MI. 2000.

148. Action on Smoking and Health. "Parents Are Deliberately Making Their Kids Sick: At What Point Does It Become Child Abuse or Endangerment?" 2001. http://ash.org.

149. Tobacco Free Kansas Coalition. "Impact of Smoking: Children's Health." 1999. www.tobaccofreekansas.org.

150. Gilliland, Frank. "Smoking During Pregnancy Impairs Child's Future Lung Function." *Thorax* 55, no. 4 (2000): 271-276.

151. Frost, Pam. "Environmental Tobacco Smoke Harms Non-Smoking Children for Years." Environment News Service (ENS). 1999.

152. "Smoking During Pregnancy Damages Children's Lungs." 2000. www.antenna.nl/nietrokers/e/n/14030.html.

153. National Clearinghouse on Tobacco and Health. "Youth and Tobacco: Smoking Around Children and During Pregnancy." 2001. www.cctc.ca.

154. Gidding, Samuel S., et al. "Active and Passive Tobacco Exposure: A Serious Pediatric Health Problem." American Heart Association: AHA Medical/Scientific Statement. June 16, 1994.

155. Ibid.

156. *The Health Consequences of Smoking for Women: A Report of the Surgeon General*. Rockville, MD: U.S. Department of Health and Human Services, 1981.

157. Stathis, Stephen L., et al., "Study Links Maternal Smoking During Pregnancy to Children's Ear Troubles." American Academy of Pediatrics electronic pages. 104 (2):e16, August, 1999.

158. Kleinman, J.C., et al. "The Association of Maternal Smoking With Age and Cause of Infant Death." *American Journal of Epidemiology* 128 (1988): 46-55.

159. Centers for Disease Control and Prevention. "Ingestion of Cigarettes and Cigarette Butts by Children – Rhode Island, January 1994-July 1996." *Morbidity and Mortality Weekly Report* 46, no. 6 (1997): 125-128.

160. Gidding, Samuel S., et al. "Active and Passive Tobacco Exposure: A Serious Pediatric Health Problem." American Heart Association: AHA Medical/Scientific Statement. June 16, 1994.

161. Tobacco Free Kansas Coalition. Op cit.

162. Milberger, S., et al. "Is Maternal Smoking During Pregnancy a Risk Factor for Attention Deficit Hyperactivity Disorder in Children?" *The American Journal of Psychiatry* 153 (1996): 1138-1142.

163. Brennan, Patricia, et al. "Study Shows Smoking During Pregnancy Can Affect Behavior of Children." *Archives of General Psychiatry.* March 1999.

164. Marcus, Adam. "In Teens, Smoking and Sleep Don't Mix." *HealthScout.* August 7, 2000. www.healthscout.com.

165. Henningfield, J.E., R. Clayton, and W. Pollin. "Involvement of Tobacco in Alcoholism and Illicit Drug Use." *Br. J. Addit* 85 (1990): 279-291.

166. Food and Drug Administration. "President's Plan to Reduce Children's Use of Tobacco." Press release. January 5, 2001. www.wellweb.com.

167. American Heart Association. "Tobacco Industry's Targeting of Youth, Minorities and Women." www.americanheart.org.

168. American Heart Association. "Smoking Cessation." 2000. www.americanheart.org.

169. Centers for Disease Control and Prevention, "Nutrition and Physical Activity." 2000.

170. Mokdad, Ali, et al. "The Spread of the Obesity Epidemic in the United States, 1991-1998." *Journal of the American Medical Association* 282, no. 16 (October 1999).

171. Hale, Ellen. "Youths Untouched by Health Trends: Obese Young People Invite Heart Disease with Unhealthy Diets." *Iowa Press-Citizen.* December 18, 1986.

172. Centers for Disease Control and Prevention, Improving Child and Adolescent Health Through Physical Activity, 1999.

173. Horlick, Mary. Endocrine Society's 2000 annual conference, 2000.

174. Hale, Ellen. Op cit.

175. "Media Education," *Pediatrics* 104, no. 2 (August 1999).

176. Robinson, Thomas N. "Reducing Children's Television Viewing to Prevent Obesity; A Randomized Controlled Trial," *Journal of the American Medical Association* 282, no. 6 (October 1999).

177. "Media Education." Op cit.

178. Ibid.

179. "Children, Adolescents and Advertising." *Pediatrics* 95, no. 2 (February 1995).

180. "Violence on Television" (brochure). American Psychological Association, 2001.

181. National Coalition on Television Violence.

182. "Violence on Television," Op cit.

183. Marks, Alexandra. "What Children See and Do: Studies on Violence on TV." *Christian Science Monitor,* April 17, 1998.

184. "Violence on Television." Op cit.

185. Ibid.

186. FactSheets (tm), "TV Professional Wrestling and Children." National Institute on Media and the Family, 2000.

187. Krugman, H.D. "Brain Wave Measurements of Media Involvement," *Journal of Advertising Research* 11:1, Feb. 1971.

188. Setzer, Valdemar W. "TV and Violence: A Perfect Marriage." 2001. www.ime.usp.br/~vwsetzer.

189. Ott, John N. *Health and Light.* New York: Pocket Books, 1973.

190. 21CFR1030.10. (Code of Federal Regulations, Title 21, Volume 8, Part 1030. "Performance Standards for Microwave and Radio Frequency Emitting Products." Section .10, Revised as of April 1, 2001)

191. Naisbitt, John. *High Tech, High Touch: Technology and Our Search for Meaning.* London: Nicholas Breadley. 2000.

192. Setzer, Valdemar, W. "The Risks to Children Using Electronic Games." 2001. www.ime.usp.br/~vwsetzer.

193. McCormac, Patricia. "Role of Light In Health." *Los Angeles Times,* February 17, 1980, p. 9,10.

194. Ott, John N. *Light, Radiation, & You,* New York: Devin-Adair Publishers, 1985.

195. Hollwich, F., and B. Dieckhues. "The Effect of Natural and Artificial Light Via the Eye on the Hormonal and Metabolic Balance of Animal and Man," *Opthalmologica* 180, no. 4 (1980).

196. Mughal, Zulf, M.D. "Air Pollution May Cause Vitamin D Deficiency," *Proceedings, 22nd Meeting of the American Society for Bone and Mineral Research,* 2001.

197. Ibid.

108. Waldie, K.E., et al. "The Effects of Pre- and Post-natal Sunlight Exposure on Human Growth: Evidence from the Southern Hemisphere." *Early Human Development* 60: 35-42. (November 1, 2000).

199. Kime, Zane R. M.D., M.S. *Sunlight,* Penryn, CA: World Health Publications, 1980.

200. Ott, John N. *Health and Light.* Op cit.

201. Blum, H.F. *Carcinogenesis by Ultraviolet Light.* Princeton NJ: Princeton University Press, 1959.

202. Sissonn, Thomas R., M.D., et al. "Retinal Changes Produced by Phototherapy," *Journal of Pediatrics* 77, no. 2: 221-227

203. Ott, John N. *Health and Light,* op cit.

Chapter III — Cancer

1. *Dorland's Pocket Medical Dictionary.* W.B. Saunders Company, Philadelphia: Harcourt Brace Jovanovich, Inc., 1989.

2. U.S. Bureau of the Census, *Statistical Abstract of the United States: 1955.* (Seventy-sixth edition.) Washington, D.S., 1955.

3. Landrigan, Philip J. "Commentary: Environmental Disease — A Preventable Epidemic." *American Journal of Public Health* 82 (July 1992): 941-943.

4. Ries, L.A.G., et al., eds. *Cancer Incidence and Survival among Children and Adolescents: United States SEER Program 1975-1995,* National Cancer Institute, SEER Program. NIH Pub. No.99-4649 (1999): 1.

5. Schmidt, Charles W. "Childhood Cancer: A Growing Problem." *Environmental Health Perspectives* 106, no. 1 (1998): A18-A23.

6. Ries, L.A.G., et al., eds. *SEER Cancer Statistics Review, 1973-1995.* National Cancer Institute, http://www.seer.ims.nci.nih.gov (1998).

7. Kosary, C.L., et al. eds. *SEER Cancer Statistics Review, 1973-1992: Tables and Graphs,* National Cancer Institute. NIH Pub. no. 96-2789 (1995): 455.

8. Miller, B.A., et al. eds. *SEER Cancer Statistics Review 1973-1990.* NIH Publ. no. 93-2789 (1993).

9. Ries, L.A.G. Op cit. p. 5.

10. Schmidt, Charles W. Op cit.

11. Montague, Peter. "Children's Cancer and Pesticides." Environmental Research Foundation. *Rachel's Environment & Health Weekly,* no. 588: 1 (March 5, 1998).

12. Lichtenstein, P., et al. "Environmental and Heritable Factors in the Causation of Cancer — Analyses of Cohorts of Twins from Sweden, Denmark, and Finland." *New England Journal of Medicine* 343, no. 2: 28-85 (2000).

13. *Preventing Child Exposures to Environmental Hazards: Research and Policy Issues.* Children's Environmental Health Network/California Public Health Foundation. Emeryville, CA. 1994,1995. www.cehn.org.

14. Barich, Bob. "Hedging Your Bets." Greatlife. January, 2001, p10.

15. Li, Frederick P., et al. "Cancer Mortality Among Chemists." *Journal of the National Cancer Institute* 43: 1159-1164 (1969).

16. Walrath, Judy, et al. "Causes of Death Among Female Chemists." *American Journal of Public Health* (August 1985): 883-885.

17. Thomas, Terry L., and Pierce Decoufle. "Mortality Among Workers Employed in the Pharmaceutical Industry: A Preliminary Investigation." *Journal of Occupational Medicine* 21: 619-623 (September 1979).

18. Arnetz, Bengt B. "Mortality Among Petrochemical Science and Engineering Employees." *Archives of Environmental Health* 46: 237-248 (July/August 1991).

19. Sinclair, Wayne. "Chemicals and Pesticides. Environmental Causes of Child Cancers and Remission Information." 2000. www.chem-tox.com./cancerchildren/default/htm.

20. U.S. Food and Drug Administration. "Food Additives" (brochure). FDA/IFIC. January 1992.

21. U.S. Food and Drug Administration, Center for Food Safety & Applied Nutrition. "'Everything' Added to Food in the United States (EAFUS)." Office of Premarket Approval. June 8, 2001.

22. "Adverse Effects of 'Inactive' Ingredients." www.feingold.org/effects.html (Sources: The American Academy of Pediatrics Committee on Drugs in Pediatrics in October 1985 "E is for Additives"; *Health Letter* by Public Citizen Health Research Group, March/April 1985)

23. U.S. Food and Drug Administration. January 1992.

24. Strubbe, B. "Killing Me Sweetly." ECHO Magazine 4, no. 10 (November 2000).

25. Gold, M.D. "The Bitter Truth About Artificial Sweeteners," *Nexus Magazine* 2, no. 28 (October-November 1995); 3, no.1 (December 1995-January 1996).

26. Ibid.

27. "Cover Story Interview with Mary Nash Stoddard," *Nutrition & Healing* 2, issue 11 (November 1995).

28. Ibid.

29. Blaylock, R.L., M.D. *Excitotoxins: The Taste That Kills.* Santa Fe, NM: Health Press, 1997.

30. Ibid.

31. Gold. M.D., 1996. Op cit.

32. Blaylock, R.L., 1997. Op cit.

33. Mullarkey, Barbara. "How Safe Is Your Artificial Sweetener?" *Informed Consent Magazine,* September/October 1994.

34. "Cover Story Interview with Mary Nash Stoddard." Op cit.

35. Walton, R.G., M.D. "Analysis Shows Nearly 100% of Independent Research Finds Problems With Aspartame." www.holistickmed.com/aspartame/100.html. October 17, 1996.

36. Schiffman, S.S., et al. "Aspartame and Susceptibility to Headache." *New England Journal of Medicine* 317, no. 19: 1181-1185.

37. Camfield, P.R., et. al. "Aspartame Exacerbates EEG Spike-Wave Discharge in Children with Generalized Absence Epilepsy: A Double-Blind Controlled Study." *Neurology* 42, issue 5: 1000-1003 (1992).

38. Rowen, J.A., et al. "Aspartame and Seizure Susceptibility: Results of a Clinical Study in Reportedly Sensitive Individuals." *Epilepsia* 26, no. 3:270-275 (1995).

39. Woodrow, M.C. "Aspartame: Methanol and the Public Health." *Journal of Applied Nutrition* 36, no. 1: 42-53.

40. Gold, Mark D. "Scientific Abuse in Methanol/Formaldehyde Research Related to Aspartame." Aspartame Toxicity Information Center. 2000. www.holisticmed.com/aspartame/abuse/seizures.html.

41. Gold, Mark D. "Aspartame is Dangerous For Everyone." Aspartame Toxicity Information Center. 2000. www.holisticmed.com/aspartame/abuse/seizures.html.

42. Congressional Record SID835: 131 (August 1, 1985)

43. National Cancer Institute SEER Program Data.

44. Olney, J.W., et al. "Diet Drinks Suspected for Increasing Brain Cancer Risks." *Journal of Neuropathology & Experimental Neurology* 55, no. 11: 1115-1123 (1996).

45. Roberts, H.J. *Aspartame (NutraSweet), Is it Safe?* City: The Charles Press, Publishers, 1992.

46. Ibid.

47. Walton, R.G., Robert Hudak, Ruth Green-Waite. "Adverse Reactions to Aspartame: Double Blind Challenge in Patients from a Vulnerable Population." *Biological Psychiatry* 34: 13-17 (1993).

48. Mullarkey, Barbara. Op cit.

49. Gold, M.D. "Aspartame (NutraSweet)." Aspartame Toxicity Information Center. 1996. www.holisticmed.com/aspartame/aspart2.txt.

50. Ibid.

51. Mullarkey, B., ed. "Bittersweet Aspartame—A Diet Delusion." *Health Watch Book*, April 1992.

52. Gold, Mark D. "Aspartame is Dangerous For Everyone." Aspartame Toxicity Information Center. 2000. www.holisticmed.com/aspartame/abuse/seizures.html.

Chapter IV –Diabetes

1. National Institute of Diabetes and Digestive and Kidney Diseases, "Diabetes Statistics." National Diabetes Information Clearinghouse, National Institutes of Health. 2000. www.niddk.nih.gov.

2. National Institutes of Health. *Conquering Diabetes: A Strategic Plan for the 21st Century, A Report of the Congressionally Established Diabetes Research Working Group.* NIH Publication no. 99-4398. 1999.

3. Montague, Peter. "Diabetes is Increasing," *Rachel's Environmental & Health Weekly.* Environmental Research Foundation. August 7, 1997.

4. Christian, Henry A. *The Principles and Practice of Medicine,* 16th Edition, p. 582. New York: D. Appleton-Century, 1947.

5. Coulter, Harris. "Childhood Vaccinations and Juvenile-Onset (Type 1) Diabetes." Testimony before the Congress of the United States, House of Representatives, Committee on Appropriations, Subcommittee on Labor, Health and Human Services, Education, and Related Agencies. April 16, 1997. (Available from the National Vaccine Information Center, www.909shot.com)

6. Centers for Disease Control and Prevention. CDC's Diabetes Program, 1990-1998. 2000. www.cdc.gov.

7. Pinhas-Harniel, Orit, et al. "Increased Incidence of Non-Insulin-Dependent Diabetes Mellitus Among Adolescents, Part I." *The Journal of Pediatrics* 128, no. 5: 608-615. May 1996.

8. National Institutes of Health. "Conquering Diabetes, A Strategic Plan for the 21st Century: A Report of the Congressionally Established Diabetes Research Working Group." NIH Publication no. 99-4398. 1999.

9. Ibid.

10. Ibid.

11. LaPorte, Ronald E., Masato Matsushima, and Yue-Fang Chang. *Diabetes in America, 2nd Edition,* National Diabetes Data Group, NIH Publication No. 95-1468. 1995.

12. Pinhas-Harniel, Orit, et al. Op cit.

13. Langer, Stephen E. and James F. Scheer. *Solved: The Riddle of Illness.* New Canaan, CT: Keats Publishing, Inc. 1984, p. 92

14. Ibid.

15. Ibid, p. 94.

16. Ibid, p. 96.

17. Notkins, Abner L. "Environmental Etiology of Type 1 Diabetes: Viruses and Other Factors. Environmental Etiology Workshop Final Report," NIDDK, National Institutes of Health. September 1998.

18. Henriksen, Gary L., et al. "Serum Dioxin and Diabetes Mellitus in Veterans of Operation Ranch Hand." *Epidemiology* 8, no. 3: 252-258 (May 1997).

19. Kohlmeier, Lenore, and Martin Kohlmeier, "Adipose Tissues as a Medium for Epidemiologic Exposure Assessment." *Environmental Health Perspectives Supplements* 103, Supplement 3: 99-106 (April 1995).

20. Consumption of soft drinks and calorie intake were obtained or calculated from U.S. Department of Agriculture surveys—Continuing Survey of Food Intakes of Individuals, 1994-96 (Data Tables 9.4, 9.7, 10.4 10.7); 1987-88 (Report no. 87+1, Tables 1.2-1 and -2; 1.7-1 and -2); Nationwide Food Consumption Surveys, 1977-78 (Tables A1.2-1 and -2; A1.7-1 and -2).

21. Valentine, Judith. "Soft Drinks—America's Other Drinking Problem." *Wise Traditions in Food, Farming, and the Healing Arts.* Summer 2001.

22. Ibid.

23. National Soft Drink Association. "Soft Drinks and Nutrition." Washington, DC. Undated

24. Associated Press. "Consumer Group Attacks Artificial Sweetener." August 1, 1996.

25. Jacobson, Michael F. "Liquid Candy—How Soft Drinks are Harming Americans' Health." Center for Science in the Public Interest. October 1998.

26. Center for Science in the Public Interest. "Soft Drinks Undermining Americans' –Teens Consuming Twice as Much 'Liquid Candy' as Milk." CSPI News Release, October 1998.

27. Valentine, Judith. Op cit.

28. Nakamura, David. *The Washington Post.* "Schools Hooked on Junk Food." February 27, 2001, p. A1, A8.

29. Center for Science in the Public Interest. Op cit.

30. Jacobson, Michael F. Op cit.

31. Federal Register. 44:37212-37221. 1979.

32. Baldwin, J.L., A.H. Chou, and W.R. Solomon. "Popsicle-induces Anaphylaxis Due to Carmine Dye Allergy." *Allergy Asthma Immunology* 79 (1997): 415-419.

33. National Osteoporosis Foundation. Fast Facts on Osteoporosis. www.nof.org/stats.html.

34. Analyses by Environment Inc. based on USDA CSFII 1994-1996 two-day data. September 1998.

35. Wyshak, Grace. "Teenaged Girls, Carbonated Beverage Consumption, and Bone Fractures." *Pediatrics & Adolescent Medicine* 154, no. 6 (June 2000).

36. Wyshak, G., and R.E. Frisch, "Carbonated Beverages, Dietary Calcium, the Dietary Calcium/Phosphorus Ration, and Bone Fractures in Girls and Boys." *Journal of Adolescent Health* 15, no. 3: 210-215 (1994).

37. Center for Science in the Public Interest. Op cit.

38. "Caffeine: The Inside Scoop—Osteoporosis." *Nutrition Action Healthletter.* December 1996. Center for Science in the Public Interest. www.cspinet.org.

38. Jacobson, Michael F. Op cit.

39. Barger-Lux, M.J., and R.P. Heaney. "Caffeine and the Calcium Economy Revisited." *Osteoporosis Intern* 5, no. 2: 97-102 (March 1995).

40. Ismail, A.I, et al. "The Cariogenicity of Soft Drinks in the United States." *Journal of the American Dental Association* 109, no. 2: 241-245 (1984).

41. Valentine, Judith. Op cit.

42. Ibid.

43. Freedman, David S., et al. "The Relationship or Overweight to Cardiovascular Risk Factors Among Children and Adolescents: The Bogalusa Heart Study." *Pediatrics* 103: 1175-1182 (1999).

44. National Institute of Diabetes and Digestive and Kidney Diseases. www.niddk.nih.gov.

45. Shuster, J., et al. "Soft Drink Consumption and Urinary Stone Recurrence: A Randomized Prevention Trial." *Journal of Clinical Epidemiology* 45, no. 8: 911-916 (1992).

46. Jacobson, Michael F. Op cit.

47. Center for Science in the Public Interest. "Label Caffeine Content of Foods, Scientists Tell FDA." Press Release. July 31, 1997. www.cspinet.org.

48. "Caffeine: The Inside Scoop—Birth Defects & Miscarriages." *Nutrition Action Healthletter.* December 1996. Center for Science in the Public Interest. www.cspinet.org.

49. Ibid.

50. Nehlig, Astrid, "Consequences on the Newborn of Chronic Maternal Consumption of Coffee During Gestation and Lactation: A Review." *Neurotoxicology and Teratology* 6: 531-43 (1994).

51. *Nutrition Action Healthletter.* Op cit.

52. Nehlig, Astrid. Op cit.

53. Gordon, Serena. "One in Five Kids May Have Mental Problem. Psychological Disorders in Kids Almost Tripled in Last 20 Years." *HealthScout Newsletter,* 2000. www.healthscout.com

54. 40CFR 261.22 (Code of Federal Regulations, Title 40, Volume 22, Part 261 – "Identification and Listing of Hazardous Waste." Revised as of July 1, 2001.)

55. Dufty, William. *Sugar Blues.* New York: Warner Books, Inc., 1975.

56. Martin, W.C., "When is a Food a Food—and When a Poison?" *Michigan Organic News,* March 1957, p. 3.

57. Dufty, William. Op cit.

58. Ibid.

59. Ibid.

60. Pauling, Linus. "Orthomolecular Psychiatry." *Science* 160: 265-271 (April 19, 1968).

61. Hoffer, Abram. "Orthomolecular Approach to the Treatment of Learning Disabilities." Synopsis of reprint article issued by the Huxley Institute for Biosocial Research, New York.

62. Tintera, John W. *Hypoadrenocorticism.* Mt. Vernon, NY: Adrenal Metabolic Research Society of the Hypoglycemia Foundation, Inc., 1969.

63. Fallon, Sally, and Mary G. Enig, Ph.D. *Nourishing Traditions,* 2nd ed. Washington, DC: New Trends Publishing Inc. 1999.

64. Dufty, William. Op cit.

65. Ibid.

66. Ibid.

67. Ibid.

68. Center for Science in the Public Interest. "America: Drowning in Sugar." Press release. www.cspinet.org. August 3, 1999.

69. Center for Science in the Public Interest. "FDA Weighing Sugar Labeling." Press release. www.cspinet.org. June 26, 2000.

Chapter V - Asthma

1. Sheffer, A.L., and V.S. Taggart. "The National Asthma Education Program: Expert Panel Report Guidelines for the Diagnosis and Management of Asthma. *Med Care* 31(suppl) (1993): MS20-MS28.

2. Fulwood, R., et al. "Asthma-United States, 1980-1987." *Morbidity and Mortality Weekly Report* 39, no. 29 (1990): 493-497.

3. Sly, Michael R. "Mortality From Asthma, 1979-1984." *Journal of Allergy and Clinical Immunology* 82, no. 5 (1988): 705-717.

4. Mannino, David M., et al. "Surveillance for Asthma—United States, 1960-1995." *Morbidity and Mortality Weekly Report* 47(SS-1) (April 24, 1998): 1-28.

5. U.S. Department of Health and Human Services. "Action Against Asthma—A Strategic Plan for the Department of Health and Human Services." May 2000. http://aspe.hhs.gov/sp/asthma/

6. Montague, Peter. "Asthma is Increasing Among U.S. Children," *Rachel's Environmental & Health Weekly*. Environmental Research Foundation. January 30, 1991.

7. U.S. Department of Health and Human Services. "Action Against Asthma—A Strategic Plan for the Department of Health and Human Services." May 2000. http://aspe.hhs.gov/sp/asthma/

Chapter VI - ADHD

1. Montague, Peter. "ADHD and Children's Environment," *Rachel's Environment & Health Weekly*, no. 678 (December 2, 1999): 2. Environmental Research Foundation.

2. "CHADD Facts." Children and Adults with Attention-Deficit/Hyperactivity Disorders (CHADD). 1996. www.chadd.com.

3. Ibid.

4. "Focus: Reading, Writing, 'Rithmetic, and Ritalin." *Education Reporter.* July 1996. www.eagleforum.org.

5. Montague, Peter. Op cit., p. 1.

6. Ibid.

7. "CHADD Facts." Op cit.

8. LeFever, G.B, K.V. Dawson, and A.L. Morrow. "The Extent of Drug Therapy for Attention Deficit-Hyperactivity Disorder Among Children in Public Schools." *American Journal of Public Health* 89 (1999): 1359-1364.

9. Bellanti, Joseph A., William G. Crook, Richard E. Layton, eds. *ADHD Attention Deficit Hyperactivity Disorder, Causes and Possible Solutions: Conference Syllabus of Presentation Papers, November 4-7, 1999, Arlington, VA.* Alexandria, VA: International Research Consultants. November 1999.

10. American Academy of Neurology. "Brain Abnormalities Found in Children with ADHD." Press release. April 19,1999. (This can be found at the CHADD website www.chadd.com.)

11. Montague, Peter. Op cit.

12. Ibid.

13. Ibid.

14. Jacobson, Michael F., and David Schardt. *Diet, ADHD & Behavior; A Quarter-Century Review.* Washington, DC: Center for Science in the Public Interest. November 1999. www.cspinet.org. (Also see: "Food Additives," brochure. U.S. Food and Drug Administration [FDA/IFIC], January 1992.)

15. Shaywitz, Bennett A. "Food Colorings Given Following Birth Generate Attention Deficit Disorder Symptoms." *Neurobehavioral Toxicology* 1, no. X (year): 41-47.

16. Reif-Lehrer, Liane. "Infant Seizures Improve After MSG Removal." *Federation Proceedings* 1, no. 11 (1976): 2205-2212.

17. Pressinger, Richard W. "MSG & Aspartame During Pregnancy." www.chem-tox.com.

18. Olney, John W. "MSG & Aspartate Cause Brain Damage Following A Single Low Level Dose." *Nature* 227 (August 8, 1970).

19. Olney, John W. "Obesity-Shorter Growth-and Reproduction Problems from MSG Intake." *Science* 164 (1969): 719-721.

20. Ibid.

21. Reif-Lehrer, Liane, Op cit.

22. Schettler, Ted, M.D., M.P.H., and Jill Stein, M.D. *In Harm's Way: Toxic Threats to Child Development.* Boston: Greater Boston Physicians for Social Responsibility, 2000.

23. Ibid.

24. Ibid.

25. Weintraub, Skye. Natural Treatments for ADD and Hyperactivity. P. 187. Pleasant Grove, UT: Woodland Publishing, Inc. 1997.

26. Wilson, Lawrence. "Evidence for Traditional Diets From Hair Mineral Analysis." *Health & Healing Wisdom, the Journal of the Price-Pottenger Nutrition Foundation* 23, no. 31 (Spring 1999): 9.

27. Weintraub, Skye. *Natural Treatments for ADD and Hyperactivity*. Pleasant Grove, UT: Woodland Publishing, Inc., 1997, p. 187.

28. Ibid.

29. Wilson, Lawrence. Op cit.

30. Jacobson, Michael F., and David Schardt. Op cit.

31. Rudlin, Donald. *The Omega-3 Phenomenon, The Nutrition Breakthrough of the 80s*. New York: Rawson Associates, 1989.

32. Evans, Lara, "Life in the Fat Lane." *Delicious Living*, December 2000, p. 28.

33. Weintraub, Skye. Op cit.

34. Ibid.

35. Wilson, Lawrence. Op cit.

36. Weintraub, Skye. Op cit.

37. Ibid.

38. Evans, Lara. Op cit.

39. Enig, Mary G., Ph.D., *Know Your Fats. The Complete Primer for Understanding the Nutrition of Fats, Oils & Cholesterol*. Bethesda, MD: Bethesda Press, 2000.

40. Kane, Patricia C. "Lifting Depression." *Alternative Medicine Digest*, issue 22: 64-70.

41. Weintraub, Skye. Op cit.

42. Evans, Lara. Op cit.

43. www.allergyconnection.com.

44. Weintraub, Skye. Op cit.

45. Ibid.

46. *For Tomorrow's Children*. Blooming Glen, PA: Preconception Care, Inc. 1990.

47. Whitaker, Julian. "Nature's Perfect Food? A Second Opinion!" *Health & Healing, Tomorrow's Medicine Today* 8, no. 10 (October 1998).

48. Vonderplanitz, Aajonus. "What Started Pasteurization?" *Right to Choose Healthy Food*. 1999. ww.odomnet.com/rawmilk.

49. Vonderplanitz, Aajonus, "Micro-Phobia Destroys the Nutrients in our Food and, in Turn, Destroys our Health." *Right to Choose Healthy Food*. 1999. ww.odomnet.com/rawmilk

50. "Milk: Why is the Quality so Low?" *Consumer Reports*, January 1974, pp. 70-76.

51. Vonderplanitz, Aajonus, Micro-Phobia Destroys the Nutrients in our Food and, in Turn, Destroys our Health." Op cit.

52. Cousens, Gabriel, *Conscious Eating*. Patagonia, AZ: Essene Vision Books, 1992.

53. Ibid.

54. Pouls, Maile. Personal communication.

55. Fallon, Sally, and Mary G. Enig, Ph.D. *Nourishing Traditions*, Washington, DC: New Trends Publishing, Inc. 1999, p. 35.

56. Weintraub, Skye. Op cit.

57. Ibid.

58. Ibid.

59. Ibid.

60. Tucker, Priscilla. "More Kids Are Hyper and Sad Inside." *HealthScout*. 2000. www.healthscout.com.

61. Gordon, Serena. "One in Five Kids May Have Mental Problem." *HealthScout*. 2000. www.health-scout.com.

62. Ibid.

63. National Institute of Mental Health, "Depression in Children and Adolescents, A Fact Sheet for Physicians." NIH Publication no. 00-4744. 2000. www.nimh.nih.gov.

64. Ibid.

65. Ibid.

66. Ibid.

67. Weintraub, Skye. Op cit.

68. Eberstadt, Mary. "Why Ritalin Rules." Policy Review, The Heritage Foundation, April & May 1999, no. 94.

69. Diller, Lawrence H. *Running on Ritalin: A Physician Reflects on Children, Society, and Performance in a Pill.* Bantam Books, 1998.

70. Hollowell, Edward M., and John Ratey. *Driven to Distraction, Recognizing and Coping with Attention Deficit Disorder from Childhood Through Adulthood.* New York: Pantheon Books, 1994.

71. Eberstadt, Mary. Op cit.

72. Breggin, Peter R., and Ginger Ross Breggin. "The Hazards of Treating 'Attention-Deficit/Hyperactivity Disorder' with Methylphenidate (Ritalin)." *The Journal of College Student Psychotherapy* 10, no. 2 (1995): 55-72.

73. Ibid.

74. Eberstadt, Mary. Op cit.

75. Golden, G.S. "Role of Attention Deficit Hyperactivity Disorder in Learning Disabilities." *Seminars in Neurology* 11, no. 1 (1991): 3541.

76. Children and Adults with Attention-Deficit/Hyperactivity Disorders (CHADD) "CHADD Facts." 1996. www.chadd.com.

77. Langer, Stephen E., and James F. Scheer. *Solved: The Riddle of Illness.* New Canaan, CT: Keats Publishing, Inc., 1984.

78. Mason, Nathan, *The New Psychiatry.* New York: Philosophical Library, Inc., 1959, p. 21.

79. Elwood, Cathryn. *Feel Like a Million.* New York: Devin-Adair Co., 1956, p. 235.

80. Holmes, J.M. "Cerebral Manifestations of Vitramin B12 Deficiency." *British Medical Journal* (1956) 2:1394-1398.

81. Langer, Stephen E., and James F. Scheer. Op cit.

82. Breggin, Peter R. and Ginger Ross Breggin. Op cit.

83. Ibid.

84. Chira, Susan. "Is Small Better? Educators Now Say Yes for High School." *New York Times,* July 14, 1993, Section A, Page 1.

85. Breggin, Peter R. and Ginger Ross Breggin. Op cit.

86. Montague, Peter. Op cit.

87. "Focus: Reading, Writing, 'Rithmetic, and Ritalin." *Education Reporter.* July 1996. www.eagleforum.org.

88. Eberstadt, Mary. Op cit.

89. Ibid.

90. Montague, Peter . Op cit.

91. Gibbs, Nancy, "The Age of Ritalin." *Time,* November 30, 1998, p. 94.

92. Ibid, p. 96.

93. Ibid, p. 90.

94. Ibid, p. 92.

95. Weintraub, Skye. Op cit.

96. Ibid.

97. Eberstadt, Mary. Op cit.

98. Ibid.

99. American Psychiatric Association, *Treatments of Psychiatric Disorders – A Task Force Report of the American Psychiatric Association, Volume 2.* Washington, DC, American Psychiatric Association, (1989, p. 1221.)

100. Goodman, A.G., et al. *The Pharmacological Basis of Therapeutics,* 8th Edition. New York: Pergamon Press. 1991.

101. Spotts, J.V., and Spotus, C.A. (eds.), *Use and Abuse of Amphetamine and its Substitutes.* Rockville, MD: National Institute on Drug Abuse. DHEW Publication no. (ADM) 80-941. 1980.

102. "Focus: Reading, Writing, 'Rithmetic, and Ritalin." Op cit.

103. Eberstadt, Mary. Op cit.

104. Ibid.

105. Hollowell, Edward M., and John Ratey. Op cit.

106. Gibbs, Nancy. Op cit.

107. Breggin, Peter R. and Ginger Ross Breggin. Op cit.

108. Ibid.

109. Jacobson, Michael F. and David Schardt. Op cit.

110. Eberstadt, Mary. Op cit.

111. Gibbs, Nancy. Op cit., p. 94.

112. Eberstadt, Mary. Op cit.

113. Ibid.

114. Diller, Lawrence H. Op cit.

115. Shalin, Leonard. *The Alphabet versus the Goddess.* New York: Penguin/Compass, 1999.

116. Barkley, Russell, *ADHD and the Nature of Self-Control.* New York: Guilford Press, 1997.

117. Farmer, Jeanette. *Training the Brain to Pay Attention the Write Way.* Denver, CO: WriteBrain Press. 1995.

118. Ibid.

119. Ibid.

120. Hannafore, Carla. *Smart Moves: Why Learning is Not All In Your Head.* Arlington, VA: Great Ocean Publishers, Inc. 1995.

121. Farmer, Jeanette. Op cit.

122. McGinness, Diane. *Why Our Children Can't Read and What We Can Do About It.* New York: Simon & Schuster. 1997.

123. Joseph, R. *The Right Brain and the Unconscious, Discovering the Stranger Within.* New York: Plenum Press, 1992.

124. Farmer, Jeanette. Op cit.

125. Ibid.

126. Beckett, Cheryl. *Growing Up Inside Out.* Fort Collins, CO: Higher States Publishing. 1994.

Chapter VII - Birth Defects

1. March of Dimes, Birth Defects Information, 1999. www.modimes.org.

2. Centers for Disease Control and Prevention, "Birth Defects and Pediatric Genetics." CDC, 2000. www.cdc.gov.

3. National Research Council of the National Academies, "Major Advances in Biology should be Used to Assess Birth Defects From Toxic Chemicals." Press Release. June 1, 2000. www.books.nap.edu/catalog/9871.

4. U.S. Bureau of the Census, *Statistical Abstract of the United States, 1955* (76th edition.), Washington, DC, 1955, p. 71; and 83rd edition, 1962, p. 66; and 101st edition, p. 90, 1980; and 121st edition, 2000.

5. *National Vital Statistics Reports.* Table 30, 47, no. 19. June 30, 1999.

6. Edmonds, Larry D. "Temporal Trends in the Prevalence of Congenital Malformations at Birth Based on the Birth Defects Monitoring Program, United States, 1979-1987." *Morbidity and Mortality Weekly Report, CDC Surveillance Summaries* 39, no. SS-4 (December 1990): 19-23.

7. Skjaerven, Rolv, et al. "A Population-Based Study of Survival and Childbearing among Female Subjects with Birth Defects and the Risk of Recurrence in Their Children." *The New England Journal of Medicine* 340, no. 14 (1999): 1057-1062.

8. Lie, Rolv T., Allen J. Wilcox, and Rolv Skjaerven. "Survival and Reproduction Among Males With Birth Defects and Risk of Recurrence in Their Children." *Journal of the American Medical Association* 285, no. 6 (2001).

9. Montague, Peter. "Birth Defects — Part 2: Why Birth Defects Will Continue To Rise," Environmental Research Foundation. *Rachel's Environment & Health Weekly,* no. 411 (October 13, 1994).

10. March of Dimes. "Birth Defect Information, Thalidomide." www.modimes.org.

11. March of Dimes. "Folic Acid Fact Sheet." www.modimes.org.

12. Centers for Disease Control and Prevention. "Folic Acid Now." CDC, 2000. www.cdc.gov.

Chapter VIII - Infertility

1. National Women's Health Information Center. "Infertility." Office on Women's Health, Department of Health and Human Services. 2000. www.4woman.gov.

2. Wright, Lawrence. "Silent Sperm." *New Yorker.* January 15, 1996.

3. Pinchbeck, Daniel. "Downward Motility." *Esquire.* January 1996.

4. Montague, Peter. "Sperm in the News," Environmental Research Foundation. *Rachel's Environment & Health Weekly,* no, 477, January 18, 1996.

5. Herman-Giddens, Marcia E. "Secondary Sexual Characteristics and Menses in Young Girls Seen in Office Practice: A Study from the Pediatric Research in Office Settings Network." *Pediatrics,* 99 no. 4 (1997): 505-512.

6. Sinclair, Wayne, and Richard W. Pressinger. "Environmental Causes of Infertility." 2000. www.chem-tox.com.

7. Wright, Lawrence. Op cit.

8. Giwercman, Aleksander, et al. "Sperm Counts Decline Since 1940s, Testicle Abnormalities Increase." *Environmental Health Perspectives* 101, no. 2 (1993): 65-71.

9. Sherman, J.K. "Lower Sperm Count Increases Risk of Miscarriage, University of Arkansas Study." *Washington Star,* January 7, 1979.

10. Furuhjelm, Mirjam, Birgit Jonson, and C.G. Lagergren. "Miscarriages Linked to Men With Low Sperm Counts." *International Journal of Fertility* 7, no. 1: 17-21.

11. Giwercman, Aleksander, et al. Op cit.

12. Carlson, Elisabeth, et al. "Evidence for Decreasing Quality of Semen During Past 50 Years." *British Medical Journal* 305: 609-613 (1992).

13. Wright, Lawrence. Op cit.

14. Ibid.

15. Pressinger, Richard. "Damaged Sperm & Common Chemical Exposure." 2000. www.chem-tox.com.

16. Ibid.

17. Little, Ruth and Charles Sing. "Father's Drinking Lowers Birth Weight of Babies." *Miami Herald,* June 19, 1986, p. 24A.

18. Strohmer, H., Andrea Boldizsar, and Barbara Plockinger. "Low Sperm Counts and Infertility More Common in Agricultural Workers." *American Journal of Industrial Medicine* 24 (1993): 587-592.

19. Omura, M., M. Hirata, and M. Ahao. "Pesticide Causes Testicle Damage, Reduces Sperm Counts." *Bulletin of Environmental Contamination Toxicology* 55 (1995): pp. 1-7.

20. Scott, Patricia P. J.P. Greaves, and M.G. Scott. "Surprising Testicle/Sperm Abnormalities Appear After Consumption of Chemically Grown Foods." *Journal of Reproductive Fertility* 1 (1960): 130-138.

21. Vine, Marilyn. "Smokers Have Lower Sperm Counts." *Fertility Sterility Journal* 6 no. 1 (1994): 35-43.

22. Joffee, Michael, and Zhimin Li. "Male and Female Factors in Fertility." *American Journal of Epidemiology* 140, no. 10 (1994): 921-928.

23. "Tolerance Develops to the Disruptive Effects of Delta-9 Tetrahydrocannabinol on Primate Menstrual Cycle." *Science* 219, no. 4591 (March 25, 1983).

24. Pressinger, Richard. "Environmental Causes of Infertility." 2000. www.chem-tox.com.

25. Ibid.

26. National Women's Health Information Center. "Infertility." Office on Women's Health in the Department of Health and Human Services. 2000. www.4woman.gov.

27. Pressinger, Richard. Op cit.

28. Ibid.

29. Ibid.

30. Center For Science in the Public Interest. "Caffeine: The Inside Scoop, Infertility." *Nutrition Action Newsletter*, December 1996. www.cspinet.org.

31. Ibid.

32. Pressinger, Richard. Op cit.

33. Baird, Donna D., and Allen J. Wilcox. "Cigarette Smoking Associated with Delayed Conception." *Journal of American Medical Association* 253, no. 20 (1985): 2979-2983.

34. Pizzi, William J., et al. "Reproductive Dysfunction in Male Rats Following Neonatal Administration of Monosodium L-Glutamate." *Neurobehavioral Toxicology* 1(1) (Spring 1979): 1-4.

35. *Harvard Health Letter*. October 1992.

36. Pressinger, Richard. Op cit.

37. "Chemical Caution: Miscarriages Are Linked to Two Solvents Used on Microchips." *Time*. October 26, 1992, p. 27.

38. Baranski, Boguslaw. "Conference of the Impact of the Environment and Reproductive Health Held in Denmark September 4, 1991." *Environmental Health Perspectives* 101 (suppl 2) (1993): 85.

39. Ibid.

40. Montague, Peter. "Warning on Male Reproductive Health." *Rachel's Environmental & Health Weekly*, Environmental Research Foundation. April 20, 1995.

41. Pressinger, Richard. Op cit.

Chapter IX — Pregnancy

1. Streissguth, Ann P., et al. "Aspirin and Acetaminophen Use by Pregnant Women and Subsequent Child IQ and Attention Decrements." *Teratology* 35 (1987): 211-219.

2. Ibid.

3. West, James R. and Daniel J. Bonthius. "Aspirin Augments Alcohol in Restricting Brain Growth in the Neonatal Rat." *Neurotoxicology and Teratology* 11 (1989): 135-143.

4. Pressinger, Richard W. "Summary of 1997 Graduate Student Research Project Conducted at the University of South Florida." www.chem-tox.com.

5. Ibid.

6. Jones, K.L., et al. "Outcome in Offspring of Chronic Alcoholic Women." *Lancet* 1:1076. 1974.

7. Clarren, S., et al. "Severe Child Brain Damage Due to Mother's Alcohol Drinking." *Journal of Pediatrics* 92, no. 1: 64-67.

8. Sulik, Kathleen, K., Malcolm C. Johnston, and Mary A Webb, "Fetal Alcohol Syndrome (FAS) Occurs After One Binge Drinking Episode." *Science,* November 20, 1981.

9. Hanson, James W. "Fetal Alcohol Syndrome Occurs at Moderate Alcohol Levels." *Journal of Pediatrics* 92, no. 3: 457-460.

10. Streissguth, Ann P., Helen M. Barr, and Paul D. Sampson. "Attention Deficit & Distractibility Increase when Mothers Consumed Alcohol During Pregnancy." *Neurobehavioral Toxicology and Teratology* 8 (1986): 717-725.

11. Pressinger, Richard W. Op cit.

12. Dumas, Ruth. "Early Memory Loss Occurs When Offspring's Mother Exposed to Alcohol." *Neurotoxicology & Teratology* 16 (1994): 283-289.

13. Coles, Claire D. "Reading Test Scores Lower in Children Whose Mothers Drank Alcohol During Last Trimester of Pregnancy." *Neurotoxicology & Teratology* 13 (1991): 357-367.

14. Shaywitz, Sally E. and Donald J. Cohen. "Hyperactivity-ADD and Behavior Disorders Linked With Alcohol Exposure." *Journal of Pediatrics* 96 (1990): 978.

15. Gusella, Joanne, and P.A. Fried. "Language Skills Damage Easily from Light Social Drinking." *Neurobehavioral Toxicology & Teratology* 6 (1984): 13-17.

16. Ravenhkolt, R.T. "Tobacco's Global Death March." *Population Dev. Reviews* 16 (1990): 213-240.

17. Denson, R. J. L. Nanson, and M. A. McWatters. "Smoking Mothers More Likely To Have Hyperactive (ADHD) Children." *Canadian Psychiatric Association Journal* 20 (1975): 183-187.

18. Henderson, D.K. and R.D. Gillespie. *A Textbook for Psychiatry for Students and Practitioners,* 6th Edition. London: Oxford University Press, 1944, p. 647.

19. Kanner, L. *Child Psychiatry,* 2nd Edition. Springfield: Charles C. Thomas. 1948, p. 418.

20. Wender, P.H. *The Hyperactive Child.* New York: Crown Publishers, 1973, pp.3-31.

21. Dufty, William. *Sugar Blues.* New York: Warner Books, Inc., 1975.

22. Denson, R. J., L. Nanson, and M.A. McWatters. Op cit.

23. Butler, R., and H. Goldstein. "Smoking in Pregnancy and Subsequent Child Development." *British Medical Journal* 4 (1973): 573-575.

24. McCartney Joel S., and Peter A. Fried, "Central Auditory Processing in School-Age Children Prenatally Exposed to Cigarette Smoke." *Neurotoxicology and Teratology* 16, no. 3 (1994); 269-276.

25. Makin, Judy, and Peter A. Fried. "A Comparison of Active and Passive Smoking During Pregnancy: Long-Term Effects." *Neurotoxicology and Teratology* 13, no. 1. (1991): 5-12.

26. Roy, T.S. "Effects of Prenatal Nicotine Exposure on the Morphogenesis of Somatosensory Cortex." *Neurotoxicology and Teratology* 16, no. 4 (1994): 411-422.

27. Weitzman, M., S. Gortmaker, and A. Sobol. "Maternal Smoking and Behavior Problems of Children." *Pediatrics* 90 (3) (September 1992): 342-349.

28. Wakschlag, Lauren S., Benjamin B. Lahey, and Rolf Loeber. "Smoking During Pregnancy Increases Conduct Disorders." *Archives General Psychiatry* 54 (July 1997): 670-676.

29. Department of Public Health, University of Oulu (Finland). "1,819 Mothers Who Smoked During Pregnancy." 1981.

30. Nehlig, Astrid. "Consequences on the Newborn of Chronic Maternal Consumption of Coffee During Gestation and Lactation: A Review." *Neurotoxicology and Teratology* 16, no. 6 (1994): 531-43.

31. Ibid.

32. Ibid.

33. Watkinson B., and P.A. Fried,. "Maternal Caffeine Use Before, During and After Pregnancy and Effects Upon Offspring." *Neurobehavioral Toxicology and Teratology* 7 (1995): 9-17.

34. Machera, K. "Hydrocephaly and Cleft Palate Birth Defects Occur After Pesticide Exposure." *Bulletin of Environmental Contamination Toxicology* 54 (1995): 363-369.

35. Olney, John W. "Obesity-Shorter Growth- and Reproduction Problems From MSG Intake." *Science* 164 (1969): 719-721.

36. Life Sciences Research Office, "Safety of Amino Acids," FASEB, FDA Contract no. 223-88-2124 Task Order no. 8. (See also Mark D. Gold's "The Bitter Truth About Artificial Sweeteners," *Nexus Magazine* 2, no. 28, October-November 1995, and 3, no. 1, December 1995 - January 1996.

37. Federation of American Societies for Experimental Biology. "Safety of Amino Acids Used in Dietary Supplements." FDA. July 1992.

38. Hande, Prakash. "Ultrasound During Pregnancy Suggest Routine Exams Not as Safe as Once Thought." *Neurotoxicology and Teratology* 17, no. 2 (1995): 179-188.

Chapter X - Breastfeeding

1. American Academy of Pediatrics. "Breastfeeding Policy Statement: Breastfeeding and the Use of Human Milk." RE9729.

2. Granju, Katie Allison. "The 411 On Baby Formula." Family.com. 1997. www.family.go.com.

3. Granju, Katie Allison. "Mothers Who Think: Formula for Disaster." Salon.com. 2000. www.salon.com.

4. Stehlin, Isadora B. "Infant Formula: Second Best but Good Enough." U.S. Food and Drug Administration. www.fda.gov.

5. Walker, M. "A Fresh Look at the Risks of Artificial Infant Feeding." *The Journal of Human Lactation.* 9(2) (June, 1993): 97-107.

6. Stehlin, Isadora B. Op cit.

7. Granju, Katie Allison. "Mothers Who Think: Formula for Disaster." Op cit.

8. Ibid.

9. Douglass, William Campbell. *The Milk Book.* Atlanta: Second Opinion Publishing, 1984.

10. Granju, Katie Allison. Op cit.

11. Ibid.

12. "Raising Kids, What Are the Health Risks?" Family.com. 1997. www.family.go.com.

13. Granju, Katie Allison. "Mothers Who Think: Formula for Disaster." Op cit.

14. Batten, W., J. Hirschman, and C. Thomas. "Impact of the Special Supplemental Food Program on Infants." *Journal of Pediatrics* 117 II (1990): S101-109.

15. Granju, Katie Allison. "Mothers Who Think: Formula for Disaster." Op cit.

16. Ibid.

17. Uvnas-Moberg, Eriksson. "Breastfeeding: Physiological, Endocrine, and Behavioral Adaptations Caused by Oxytocin and Local Neurogenic Activity in the Nipple and Mammary Gland." *Acta Paediatrica* 85, no. 5 (1996): 525-530.

18. Granju, Katie Allison. "Mothers Who Think: Formula for Disaster." Op cit.

19. Burby, Leslie. "101 Reasons to Breastfeed Your Child." ProMoM, Inc. 2000. www.promom.org/101/.

20. Granju, Katie Allison. "Mothers Who Think: Formula for Disaster." Op cit.

21. Ibid.

22. Burby, Leslie. Op cit.

23. Granju, Katie Allison. "Mothers Who Think: Formula for Disaster." Op cit.

24. Ibid.

25. Fallon, Sally, and Mary G. Enig, Ph.D. *Nourishing Traditions*, 2nd ed. Washington, DC: New Trends Publishing, Inc., 1999, p. 237.

26. Douglass, William Campbell. "A Substance Found in Breast Milk Helps Depression, Alzheimer's." *Second Opinion* XI, no. 3 (March 2001).

27. Stehlin, Isadora B. Op cit.

28. Morrow-Tlucak, M, R.H. Haude, and C. B. Ernhart. "Breastfeeding and Cognitive Development in the First Two Years of Life." *Soc. Sci Med.* 26 (1988):. 635-639.

29. Baumgartner, C. "Psychomotor and Social Development of Breast Fed and Bottle Fed Babies During Their First Year of Life." *Acta Paediatrica Scientiarum Hungarica.* 25(4):409-17 (1984).

30. Granju, Katie Allison. "Mothers Who Think: Formula for Disaster." Op cit.

31. Ibid.

32. BabyCentre, "Signs That Your Baby Is Getting Enough Milk." Babycentre.com.

33. Gerstein, H.C., "Cow's Milk Exposure and Type 1 Diabetes Mellitus." Diabetes Care, Vol. 17, No. 1, pp. 13-19. 1994.

34. Seppa, N., *Science.* 155, no. 26, (January 26, 1999).

35. Mubntoni et al., *The American Journal of Nutrition.* 71 (2000): 1525-9.

36. Hypponen et al., *Diabetes Care.* December, 1999.

37. *Cow's Milk Allergy in Children.* Children's Center. www.nutramed.com/children/kidsmilk.htm.

38. Sun, Zhongjie, and Robert Cade. "A Peptide Found in Schizophrenia and Autism Causes Behavioral Changes in Rats." *Autism* 3 (1999): 85-95.

39. Panksepp, J., "A Neurochemical Theory of Autism." *Trends in Neuroscience* 2 (1979):174-177.

40. Wing, Lorna, ed. *Aspects of Autism: Biological Research* , London: Gaskell/National Autistic Society, 1988, pp. 31-37.

41. Chan, June M., et al. "Plasma Insulin-Like Growth Factor-I and Prostate Cancer Risk: A Prospective Study." *Science* 279, (January 23, 1998): 563.

42. Hankinson, Susan E., et al."Circulating Concentrations of Insulin-Like Growth Factor-I and Risk of Breast Cancer." *Lancet* 351 (May 9, 1998): 1393.

43. Yu, He, et al. "Plasma Levels of Insulin-Like Growth Factor-I and Lung Cancer Risk: a Case-Control Analysis." *Journal of the National Cancer Institute* 91(2) (1999):151-156.

44. Stehlin, Isadora B. Op cit.

45. Gerber, Michael. "Infant Soy Formula: A Safe Replacement for Mother's Milk?" *Alternative Medicine*, Issue 41 (May 2001): 104-106.

46. Stehlin, Isadora B. Op cit.

47. Gerber, Michael, Op cit.

48. Herman-Giddens, Marcia E., et al. "Secondary Sexual Characteristics and Menses in Young Girls Seen in Office Practice: A Study from the Pediatric Research in Office Settings Network." *Pediatrics*, 99(4):505-512 (April, 1997).

49. Gerber, Michael. Op cit.

50. Fitzpatrick, Mike. *Soy Isoflavones: Panacea or Poison?* Washington, DC: The Weston A. Price Foundation. www.westonaprice.org/isoflavones.htm.

51. *Soy Infant Formula: Better Than Breastmilk?* Washington, DC: The Weston A. Price Foundation. www.westonaprice.org/isoflavones.htm.

52. Ibid.

53. Fallon, Sally, and Mary G. Enig, Ph.D. "Tragedy & Hype." *Nexus Magazine* 7 no. 3 (April-May 2000).

54. Ibid.

55. Ibid.

56. Goodman, David. "Soy Alert! Manganese Madness." *Wise Traditions* 2, no. 3 (Fall 2001).

57. Fallon, Sally, and Mary G. Enig, Ph.D. Op cit.

58. Mercola, Joseph. "Link Between High Soy Diet During Pregnancy and Nursing and Eventual Developmental Changes In Children." *Optimal Wellness Health News*, Issue 126, (November 7, 1999). http:mercola.com.

59. Ibid.

60. Ibid.

61. Gerber, Michael. Op cit.

62. Granju, Katie Allison. "Mothers Who Think: Formula for Disaster."

63. "FDA Recalls of Baby Formula." www.breastfeeding.com. 1998. (See also FDA Recall Enforcement Area of www.fda.gov.)

64. Granju, Katie Allison. "Mothers Who Think: Formula for Disaster."

65. FDA Recalls of Baby Formula. www.breastfeeding.com. 1998. Also see FDA Recall Enforcement Area of www.fda.gov.

66. "Be On the Lookout For Recalls." Family.com. 1997. www.family.go.com.

67. Fallon, Sally, and Mary G. Enig, Ph.D. Op cit., p. 522.

68. Ibid, p. 598.

69. Laign, Jeffrey, *Good Food for Babies and Toddlers.* Boca Raton, FL: AMI Health Library, 2001.

70. Ibid.

71. Fallon, Sally, and Mary G. Enig, Ph.D. Op.cit. p. 601.

72. Ibid, pp. 602-604.

73. "Feeding Infants & Toddlers: Got Goat's Milk?" 2000. www.askdrsears.com.

74. Gilbert, Sue. "Goat's Milk as Supplement to Breastmilk?" 2001. www.parentsplace.com.

75. "Feeding Infants & Toddlers: Got Goat's Milk?" Op cit.

76. Fallon, Sally, and Mary G. Enig, Ph.D. Op cit.

77. Ibid.

78. Ibid.

79. Laign, Jeffrey. Op cit.

80. Ibid.

81. "Sampling Plan and Testing Methods." In *Pesticides in Baby Food.* Washington, DC: Environmental Working Group. 2001. www.ewg.org.

82. "Forward." In *Pesticides in Baby Food.* Washington, DC: Environmental Working Group. 2001. www.ewg.org.

83. Ibid.

84. "Introduction." In *Pesticides in Baby Food.* Washington, DC: Environmental Working Group. 2001. www.ewg.org.

85. Laign, Jeffrey. Op cit.

86. Ibid.

87. Cousens, Gabriel. *Conscious Eating.* Patagonia, AZ: Essene Vision Books, 1992, p. 322.

88. Fallon, Sally, and Mary G. Enig, Ph.D. Op cit., p. 45.

89. Ibid, p. 48.

90. Batmanghelikj, F. *Your Body's Many Cries For Water.* Falls Church, VA: Global Health Solutions, Inc., 1992.

91. Jensen, Bernard. "The Hidden Hazards of Dehydration." *Health & Healing Wisdom Journal* 23, no. 1 (Spring 1999): 13.

92. Biser, Sam. *Using Water to Cure.* Charlottesville, VA: The University of Natural Healing, 1993, p. 21.

93. Ibid, p. 35.

94. Fallon, Sally, and Mary G. Enig, Ph.D. Op cit.

1. www.909shot.com – website of the National Vaccine Information Center

1a. Coulter, Harris L. and Barbara Loe Fisher. *A Shot in the Dark: Why the P in DPT Vaccination May be Hazardous to Your Child's Health.* Garden City Park, NY: Avery Publishing Group, 1991.

2. McBean, Eleanor. *Poisoned Needle.* Mokelumne Hill, CA: Health Research.

3. Fisher, Barbara Loe. *Shots in the dark, Discussion group on… Attempts at eradicating infectious diseases are putting our children at risk.* www.nextcity.com

4. "The Case For Vaccination." Healthwell. www.healthwell.com. December 3, 2000.

5. World Health Organization, Parents' Forum. Op cit.

6. Douglass, William Campbell. *Lethal Injections: Why Immunizations Don't Work and the Damage They Cause.* Atlanta: Second Opinion Publishing, Inc., 2000.

7. World Health Organization, Parents' Forum. Op cit.

8. "Vaccine Facts." www.access1.net.

9. "Vaccines: The Truth Revealed." www.odomnet.com.

10. Office of Special Programs. "National Vaccine Injury Compensation Program Monthly Statistics Report," U.S. Department of Health and Human Services, Health Resources and Services Administration, January 31, 2002. www.hrsa.gov/osp/vicp.

11. Cassel, Ingri. "Vaccinations - Do They Even Work and At What Price?" Vaccination Liberation Conference, Coeur d'Alana, ID. February 8, 2000. www.whale.to/vaccines/cassel.

12. Ostrom, Neenyah. "First Do No Harm, Barbara Loe Fisher and the National Vaccine Information Center Work to Prevent Vaccine-Related Injuries and Deaths by Educating the Public About Rights and Responsibilities." 2000. www.shronicillnet.org.

13. "Vaccine Facts." Op cit.

14. www.909shot.com

15. Balkan, Michael. "Shoot First and Ask Questions Later." Presented at the 2nd International Public Conference on Vaccination 2000. Arlington, Virginia. October 22, 2000. www.mercola.com.

16. Schlafly, Phyllis. "Congressional Hearing Exposes Conflicts of Interest." June 28, 2000. www.chem-tox.com.

17. Ibid.

18. Balkan, Michael. Op cit.

19. "Vaccine Facts." Op cit.

20. Coulter, Harris, L. *Vaccination, Social Violence, and Criminality: The Medical Assault on the American Brain.* Berkeley, CA: North Atlantic Books, 1990.

21. Ibid.

22. Ibid.

23. Cowart, V.S. "Attention-Deficit Hyperactivity Disorder: Physicians Helping Parents Pay More Heed." *Journal of American Medical Association* 259, no. 18 (May 13, 1988): pp. 2647-2652.

24. Coulter, Harris, L. Op cit.

25. Coulter, Harris L. and Barbara Loe Fisher. Op Cit.

26. Coulter, Harris, L. Op cit.

27. Cowart, V.S. Op cit.

28. Coulter, Harris, L. Op cit.

29. Ibid.

30. Ibid.

31. Workman-Daniels, K.L., et al. "Childhood Problem Behavior and Neuropsychological Functioning in Persons at Risk for Alcoholism." *Journal of Studies on Alcoholism* 43, no. 3 (1987): 187-193.

32. *Diagnostic and Statistical Manual of Mental Disorders, 3rd Ed., Revised.* Washington, DC: American

Psychiatric Association,1987, pp. 36-37.

33. Schettler, Ted, M.D., M.P.H. and Jill Stein, M.D. *In Harm's Way: Toxic Threats to Child Development.* Boston: Greater Boston Physicians for Social Responsibility, 2000.

34. Yazbak, Edward F. "Autism 99, A National Emergency." 1999.www.garynull.com.

35. Balkan, Michael. Op cit.

36. Mendelsohn, Robert. *How To Raise A Healthy Child... In Spite of Your Doctor.* Chicago: Contemporary Books, 1984.

37. Keusch, Gerald T. "Vitamin A Supplements—Too Good Not to Be True." *New England Journal of Medicine.* 323, no. 14 (October 4, 1990): 985-987.

38. Coulter, Harris. "Childhood Vaccinations and Juvenile-Onset (Type-1) Diabetes." Testimony before the Congress of the United States, House of Representatives, Committee on Appropriations, Subcommittee on Labor, Health and Human Services, Education, and Related Agencies. April 16, 1997.

39. "Juvenile Diabetes and Vaccination: New Evidence for a Connection." National Vaccine Information Center. 1996. www.909shot.com.

40. Coulter, Harris L. Op cit.

41. Yazbak, Edward F. Autism in the United States: a Perspective. *Journal of American Physicians and Surgeons.* Vol. 8, No. 4. Winter 2003.

42. Ibid.

43. Ibid.

44. Ibid.

45. Coulter, Harris, L. Op cit.

46. Ibid.

47. Ibid.

48. Yazbak., Edward F. Autism in the United States: a Perspective. Op cit.

49. Groves, Bob. "CDC Says Vaccine to be Mercury-Free." The Record Online. Bergen Record Corp. June 16, 2000. www.bergen.com.

50. "Thimerosal." www.whale.to/vaccines/thimerosal.htm.

51. Ibid.

52. Halsey, Neal A. "Limiting Infant Exposure to Thimerosal in Vaccines and Other Sources of Mercury [Editorial]." *Journal of the American Medical Association* 282, no. 18 (1999):1763-1765.

53. Groves, Bob. Op cit.

54. "Thimerosal." Op cit.

55. Halsey, Neal A. Op cit.

56. American Academy of Pediatrics. "AAP Addresses FDA Review of Vaccines."

Press Release, July 14, 1999. www.aap.org.

57. Halsey, Neal A. Op cit.

58. "Calculation of Mercury Content in Thimerosal-Containing Vaccines." October 26, 2001. www.whale.to/vaccines/thimerosal3.html.

59. Halsey, Neal A. Op cit.

60. www.whale.to/whaley.htms.

61. Ibid.

62. Burton, Dan. "Autism: Present Challenge, Future Needs—Why the Increased Rates?" Opening Statement, Government Reform Committee, U.S. House of Representatives. April 6, 2000.

63. Schettler, Ted, M.D. M.P.H. and Jill Stein, M.D. In Harm's Way: Toxic Threats to Child Development. Boston: Greater Boston Physicians for Social Responsibility, 2000.

64. Healy, Jane M. Endangered Minds: Why Our Children Don't Think. New York: Simon & Schuster, Inc. 1990.

65. Yazbak, F. Edward, and Kathy L. Lang-Radosh. "Adverse Outcomes Associated with Postpartum Rubella or MMR Vaccine." Medical Sentinel 6, no. 3 (2001): 95-99, 108.

Bibliography

66. Yazbak, F. Edward. Personal communication.

67. Yazbak, F. Edward, and Kathy L. Lang-Radosh. Op cit.

68. Yazbak, F. Edward. "Autism 99, A National Emergency." Op cit.

69. Harkins, Don. "Comprehensive, Independent Study Proves MMR Vaccine Link to Nation's Autism Epidemic." Idaho Observer. 4(3) (June 2000), p. 11.

70. Mendelsohn, Robert S. *How to Raise a Healthy Child... In Spite of Your Doctor.* Contemporary Books, Inc, Chicago, Illinois, 1984.

71. Coulter, Harris L. "Childhood Vaccinations and Juvenile-Onset (Type-1) Diabetes." Testimony before the Congress of the United States, House of Representatives, Committee on Appropriations, subcommittee on Labor, Health and Human Services, Education, and Related Agencies. April 16, 1997.

72. Ibid.

73. Juvenile Diabetes and Vaccination: New Evidence for a Connection. Op cit.

74. Ibid.

75. Ibid.

76. Coulter, Harris L. and Barbara Loe Fisher. Op cit.

77. Ibid.

78. Appleton, Nancy. *Rethinking Pasteur's Germ Theory.* Frog, Ltd., Berkely, CA. 2002.

79. Coulter, Harris L. and Barbara Loe Fisher. Op cit.

80. Mendelsohn, Robert S. *Immunizations: The Terrible Risks Your Children Face That Your Doctor Won't Reveal.* Atlanta: Second Opinion Publishing,1993.

81. Mendelsohn, Robert, "The Medical Time Bomb of Immunization Against Disease." *East West Journal.* November 1984. www.whale.to/vaccines/mendelsohnlhtm.

82. Coulter, Harris L. and Barbara Loe Fisher. Op cit.

83. Mendelsohn, Robert S. *How to Raise a Healthy Child... In Spite of Your Doctor.* Contemporary Books, Inc, Chicago, Illinois, 1984, p228. Also, Baraff, Larry, Pediatric Infectious Disease, January, 1983.

84. Torch, W.C., American Academy of Neurology 34th Annual Meeting: Diphtheria-pertussis-tetanus (DPT) Immunization: A Potential Cause of the Sudden Infant Death Syndrome (SIDS). Neurology, Vol. 32, No. 4. Pt. 2.

85. "Vaccine Facts." Op cit.

86. Ostrom, Neenyah. Op cit.

87. Coulter, Harris L. and Barbara Loe Fisher. Op cit.

88. "Vaccine Facts." Op cit.

89. Mendelsohn, Robert S. *How to Raise a Healthy Child... In Spite of Your Doctor.* Contemporary Books, Inc, Chicago, Illinois, 1984.

90. Funk & Wagonells New Encyclopedia., 1971. Funk & Wagonells, Inc. N.Y., Vol 19, pp 228-229.

91. Ibid.

92. Mendelsohn, Robert S. *How to Raise a Healthy Child... In Spite of Your Doctor.* Contemporary Books, Inc, Chicago, Illinois, 1984.

93. Ibid.

94. www.whale.to/v/sandler.html, and, Sandler, Benjamin P. "Diet Prevents Polio." The Lee Foundation for Nutritional Research. 1951.

95. McBean, Eleanor. *Poisoned Needle.* Op cit.

96. Intensive Immunization Programs, Hearings before the Committee on Interstate & Foreign Commerce, House of Representatives, 87th Congress, 2nd Session on H.R. 10541, Washington, DC, May 1962, Pp 96-97.

97. Los Angeles County Health Index Morbidity & Mortality, Reportable Disease. and; Kent, C, Gentempo P. *Immunization: Fact, Myth, and Speculation.* International Review of Chiropractic, Nov/Dec 1990.

98. Ibid.

99. Bayly, M. Beddow. *The Case Against Vaccination*. London: William H. Taylor & Sons, Ltd., June, 1936.

100. "Vaccine Law." www.whale.to.vaccines/law.html (click on Barbara Loe Fisher).

101. www.whale.to/v/shawl.htm.

102. Nathan Seppa. "The Dark Side of Immunizations? A Controversial Hypothesis Suggests That Vaccines May Abet Diabetes, Asthma." *Science News* 152, no. 21 (November 22, 1997): 332. November 22, 1997.

103. "Plagued by Cures." *The Economist* 344, no. 8044 (1997), p. 95.

104. Prevots, Rebecca D., et al. "Outbreaks in Highly Vaccinated Populations: Implications for Studies of Vaccine Performance." *American Journal of Epidemiology* 146, no. 10 (1997): 881.

105. Tomaselli, Kathleen Phalen. More Parents Refusing to Get Kids Vaccinated. *American Medical News*, Vol. 7, No. 6., Feb 9, 2004.

106. Schultze, Richard. "Cold and Flu Special Report: Influenza Facts." *Get Well Newsletter*. November 2000.

107. Mendelsohn, Robert, "The Medical Time Bomb of Immunization Against Disease." *East West Journal*. November 1984. www.whale.to/vaccines/mendelsohnlhtm.

108. National Vaccine Information Center, Opening Statement by Barbara Loe Fisher, Workshop on Risk Communication and Vaccination, May 13, 1996.

109. National Vaccine Information Center, "Statement on Vaccine Safety Research Needs— Perspective From Parents," April 1, 1996. National Vaccine Information Center. 1996.

110. Verner, J.R., et al. *Rational Bacteriology*, 2nd ed. New York: H. Wolff, 1953.

111. Vonderplanitz, Aajonus. "What Started Pasteurization?" Right to Choose Healthy Food, 1999. www.odomnet.com/rawmilk.

112. Appleton, Nancy. *The Curse of Louis Pasteur—Why Medicine is Not Healing A Diseased World*. Santa Monica, CA: Choice Publishing, 1999.

113. Shelton, Herbert M. *Human Life, Its Philosophy and Laws, An Exposition of the Principles and Practices of Orthopathy*, Mokelumne Hill, CA: Health Research, 1979, p. 194.

114. Ibid, p. 189.

115. Hume, Douglas E. *Bechamp or Pasteur*. Mokelumne Hill, CA: Health Research,

116. Appleton, Nancy. *Rethinking Pasteur's Germ Theory*. Frog, Ltd., Berkely, CA. 2002.

117. Shelton, Herbert M. Op cit, p. 188.

118. Appleton, Nancy. Op cit.

119. Ibid.

120. Nightingale, Florence. Notes on Nursing (1859). Reprint. Philadelphia: J.B. Libbincott Company, 1946.

121. Shelton, Herbert M. Op cit., p. 188.

122. Ibid., p. 193.

123. "Ten Things You Need to Know About Immunizations." National Immunization Program. Centers for Disease Control and Prevention. March 28, 2000. www.cdc.gov.

124. Shelton, Herbert M. Op cit., p. 191.

125. Ibid, p. 192.

126. Ibid, p. 193.

127. www.whale.to/vaccines/marchini.html.

128. Shelton, Herbert M. Op cit. p. 194.

129. www.whale.to/v/shawl.htm.

Chapter XII - The Ancestry Factor

1. Montague, Peter. "Chemicals and Health — Part 1," *Rachel's Environmental & Health Weekly,* Environmental Research Foundation. December 23, 1993.

2. Pottenger, Francis M. *Pottenger's Cats: A Study in Nutrition.* La Mesa, CA: Price-Pottenger Nutrition Foundation, Inc. 1983, p. 10.

3. Ibid, p. 11.

4. Price-Pottenger Nutrition Foundation, Resource Catalog, Spring/Summer 1999.

5. Pottenger, Francis M. Op cit., p. 11.

6. www.beyondveg.com.

7. Redmon, George S. "Minding the Minerals." *Healthy & Natural,* October 2000, p. 92

8. Ibid.

9. Buttram, Harold. Personal communication.

10. Baer, Firman, Stephen J. Toth, and Arthur L. Prince. "Variation in Mineral Composition of Vegetables." *Soil Science Society of America* 13, 1949.

11. Smith, Bob L. "Organic Foods vs. Supermarket Foods: Element Levels." *Journal of Applied Nutrition* 45, no. 1 (1993).

12. Pottenger, Francis M. Op cit. p. 13.

Chapter XIII — Alternative Health Land Mines

1. O'Shea, Tim. "Soy: Con, Soy is Not a Health Food." *Alternative Medicine,* no. 41 (May 2001): 51-65.

2. Ibid.

3. Ibid.

4. Ibid.

5. Abrams, Leon H. "Vegetarianism: An Anthropological/Nutritional Evaluation." *Journal of Applied Nutrition* 32, no. 2 (1980).

6. Ibid.

7. Kiple, Kenneth F, and Krienhild Conee Ornelas, eds. *Vegetarianism: Another View. Cambridge World History of Food, vol. 2.* Cambridge: Cambridge University Press, 2000, pp. 1564-1571.

8. Page, Melvin E., and H.Leon Abrams, Jr. *Your Body is Your Best Doctor!* New Canaan, CT: Keats Publishing, Inc., 1972, p. 215.

9. Ibid, p. 216.

10. Ibid, p.215.

11. Fallon, Sally, and Mary G. Enig, Ph.D. *Nourishing Traditions,* Washington, DC: New Trends Publishing, Inc. 1999, p. 47.

12. Bass, Stanley S., "Interview with Aajonus Voderplanitz." *Super Nutrition & Superior Health.* Jan, 2000. www.drbass.com.

13. Ibid.

14. Ibid.

15. Kiple, Kenneth F. and Krienhild Conee Ornelas, eds. Op cit., pp.1564-1571.

16. Ibid.

17. Fallon, Sally, and Mary G. Enig, Ph.D. Op cit. p. 28.

18. Langer, Stephen E. and James F. Scheer. *Solved: The Riddle of Illness.* New Canaan, CT: Keats Publishing, Inc. 1984, p. 52.

19. Ibid, p. 77.

20. Fallon, Sally and Mary G. Enig, Ph.D. Op cit., p. 28.

21. Ibid, p. 250.

22. Ibid, p. 245.

23. Ibid, pp. 253, 288.

24. Ibid, p. 113.

25. Ibid, p. 10.

26. Ibid, pp. 11,19.

27. Ibid, p. 20.

Chapter XIV — How to Prevent and Reverse Disease

1. *The H.O.P.E. Report.* p. 1-b-11. Health Excel, Inc.

2. Fallon, Sally and Mary G. Enig, Ph.D. *Nourishing Traditions.* 2nd ed. Washington, DC: New Trends Publishing, Inc. 1999, p. 68.

3. Wayne, Anthony, and Lawrence Newell. The Christian Law Institute. http://lawgiver.org.

4. PPNF News, "Food for Thought, But Not for Humans." *Health & Healing Wisdom, Journal of the Price-Pottenger Nutrition Foundation* 22, no. 4 (Winter 1998): 17

5. Ibid, p. 19.

6. Fallon, Sally and Mary G. Enig, Ph.D. Op cit., p. 80.

7. Bass, Stanley S., "Interview with Aajonus Voderplanitz." *Super Nutrition & Superior Health.* Jan, 2000. www.drbass.com.

8. Owens, Darryl. "Lack of Sleep Hurts Child's Grades." *Orlando Sentinel.* As quoted in *Caring for Your School-Age Child: Ages 5 to 12, Rev. Ed.* edited by Edward L. Schor, M.D. New York: Broadway Books, 1999.

9. EPA, *Lead In Your Home: A Parent's Reference Guide. EPA 747-B-99-003, May 1999.*

10. Brewitt, Barbara, and H. Hynn Amsbury, "MMR Vaccine and Autism." *Well Being Journal* 10, no. 3 (Summer 2000): 1.

11. Upledger, John E. *An Etiologic Model for Autism.* Committee on Government Reform, Rep. Dan Burton Chairman. www.house.gov/reform/hearings/healthcare/00.06.04/upledger.htm.

12. Arrandt, Louis. The Wellness Center. www.yourhealthdoctor.com.

13. Sprott, T.J. *The Cot Death CCover-Up?* Auckland, New Zealand: Penguin Books., 1996. Also see www.healthychild.com

Index

bacon 230
bacteria 281, 283
baked goods 223
bananas 139, 229
barbiturates 157
bassinets 151
BDMP 172
Bechamp, Antoine 279
bed wetting 127
Beech-Nut 230
behavioral problems 68
Benevia 85
Bernard, Claude 278, 279
Binge drinking 190
biological sensitivity 4
Bipolar Disorder 149
birth defects 21, 31, 32, 34, 36, 87, 90, 96, 107, 171, 172, 173, 177, 178, 183
Birth Defects Monitoring Program 172
birth weight 53, 107, 197
stillbirths 53, 182
blood lead levels 12
blood tests 144
blood-brain barrier 35, 87, 130, 132
blood-lead standard 17
blue baby syndrome 6, 34
bone fractures 104
bottle-fed 206, 211
bottle-feeding 205
braces 333, 335
brain allergy 139
breast milk 24, 44, 201, 202, 203, 212
breastfeeding 201, 203, 211, 212
bronchitis 40
bubonic plague 116
butter 137, 209, 222, 229, 233, 237, 240, 314, 320
butterfat 213
butyric acid 314

C

cadmium 128, 133, 134, 173, 183, 234
caffeine 102, 105, 106, 107, 148, 182, 195, 196, 223, 244
calcium 9, 16, 84, 104, 105, 111, 112, 134, 136, 142, 213, 215, 217, 234, 235, 324
calcium deficiency 16
calories 234
cancer 6, 7, 48, 50, 58, 66, 73, 74, 78, 81, 217, 305
cancer, brain 37, 38, 76, 79
cancer, breast 43, 78, 206, 211, 215, 216
cancer, causes of 78

cancer, childhood 76
cancer, kidney 76
Canderel 85
canola oil 312, 313
cardiovascular disease 138
Carnation 220, 221
carotene 241
carpeting 48
cartoons 63
casein 213, 214
casomorphin 214
cavities 27, 310
CBDRP 172
celery 239
Celtic Sea Salt 245
Center for Science in the Public Interest 103
Centers for Birth Defects Research and Prevention 172
Centers for Disease Control 12, 52, 55, 57, 59, 175, 252
ceramics 15
cereal 228
CFIDS 85
cheese 139
chemical fertilizers 180, 297
chemical solvents 183
chemical warfare 26
Chemicals 78, 180, 182
chicken broth 227
Children and Adults with Attention-Deficit/Hyperactivity Disorder 160
chinese restaurant syndrome 197
chiropractic adjustments 338
chlordane 36, 40
chloride 239
chlorinated chemicals 177
chlorine 30
chlorpyrifos 38, 39
chocolate 139, 238
cholesterol 110, 111, 138, 211, 218, 312
chromium 98, 111, 239
chromosomal damage 318
chronic fatigue and immune deficiency syndrome 85
Ciba-Geigy 160
cigarette consumption 181
cigarette smoke 134
cigarette smoking 191
cigarettes 192
clay 234
cleft palate 197
Coca-Cola 103, 244
cocaine 157, 177

Eskimo 310
essential fatty acid (EFA) 134, 135, 138
Essential Fatty Acid Products 349
estrogen 69, 216
ETS 52
evening primrose oils 137
Exercise 150, 328
extinction 297
Ezekiel bread 318, 322

F

farmers 40
FAS 188, 189
fast foods 59, 136
fat 135, 136, 137, 147, 211, 312, 325
fatal shock 83
father-figure 154
fatigue 69, 113, 127, 134, 138
fats 218, 232
FBI 17
Federal Food, Drug, and Cosmetic (FD&C) Act 80
fertility drugs 182
Fetal Alcohol Syndrome 188
fiber 233
fight or flight 169
fish 25, 133, 147
fish eggs 222
fish oils 137
fleas 38
floor and furniture polish 48
flu shots 275
fluorescent lighting 68
fluorescent lights 69
fluoridated water 30
fluoride 25, 26, 128
folate 175
folic acid 175, 228, 242
food additives 80, 129
food allergies 138
Food and Drug Administration (FDA) 14, 36, 80, 82, 83, 84, 85, 86, 89, 90, 92, 107, 117, 121, 129, 130, 157, 173, 195, 202, 204, 210, 218, 220, 221, 259, 295
food colorings 136
food labels 117
food supply 79
food, Chinese 130
food, organic 78, 180
formaldehyde 48, 51, 89, 90, 139, 251, 252
formula recalls 220
formula-fed 208, 211
formulas 201, 202

free radicals 313
fruit 146
fruit juices 90, 229
functionally sterile 177

G

galactose 218
gall stones 111
gamma-linolenic acid 137
gateway drug 157
GE 42, 318
Generally Recognized As Safe (GRAS) 121, 220
generation 297
genetic engineering 42
genetic modification 42
genetically engineered 318
genetics 172
genistein 219, 220
Gerber 42, 230
German measles 257
germs 279, 280, 282, 286
GLA 137
glandual products 350
glucose 110, 146
glucose tolerance test 113, 145
glutamate 87
GM 42
GMOs 318
Goat's milk 225, 227, 228
goiter 216
goitrogens 216
GTT 113
Guillian-Barre Syndrome 275

H

hair analysis 350
handwriting 163, 167
Harvard Medical School 269, 289
hay fever 274
head circumference 190
headache 86
headaches 40, 47, 69, 90, 106, 134, 213, 237
heart disease 106
heart palpitations 239
Heath High School 4
Heinz 230
hemoglobin 202, 234
hepatitis B 254
Hindus 308
histamine 138
Holocaust 172
hot dog 147

Lou Gehrig's disease 313
love 328
low birth weight 1
lung cancer 56, 215

M

Mad Hatter's Disease 18
magnesium 217, 238
manganese 16, 218, 240
Manhattan Project 26
March of Dimes 175, 183
margarine 209, 210, 223, 307, 313
marijuana 177, 181
maternal smoking 54, 191, 193, 194
Maximum Contaminant Level (MCL) 27
MCS 41, 47
Mead Johnson 220
measles 248, 274
measles vaccine 255
measles, mumps, rubella 264
meat 137, 147
melatonin 69
memory 153
men who smoke 181
Mendelsohn, Robert 257
mercury 18, 20, 22, 128, 132, 133, 173, 183,
252, 259
mercury fillings 351
mercury vapor 21
metals toxicity 17
methanol 86, 88, 89
methemoglobinemia 34
methionine 304
methyl mercury 19
methylparathion 37
methylphenidate 157
methylphenidate hydrochloride 155
microorganisms 278
microwave 320
microzymas 280
middle ear infections 53
migraines 138
milk 80, 103, 136, 139, 140, 144, 236
milk allergies 227
mineral deficiencies 297
mineral supplements 234
minerals 234
minimal brain dysfunction 125, 255
miscarriage 31, 107, 178, 182, 183
miscarriages 107, 177
MMR 257, 264
monosodium glutamate (MSG) 87, 129, 131,
183, 197

Monsanto 42, 86, 89
morning sickness 174
morphine 157
mothballs 48
mottled teeth 25
movement 150
Mozart 168
MSG, baby foods 130
multiple births 182
multiple chemical sensitivity 41, 47
multiple pesticides 5
multiple sclerosis 207
mumps 248, 257
myelin 217, 255
myelin sheath 136, 222

N

N, P, K 135
Ralph Nader 67
nail polish 139
National Academy of Sciences (NAS) 33,
35, 130, 231, 248
National Cancer Institute 76
National Childhood Vaccine Injury Act 250,
266, 276
National Committee on Radiation
Protection 67
National Immunization Program 251
National Institute of Dental Research 26
National Institute of Diabetes and
Digestive and Kidney Diseases 106
National Institute of Health Sciences 36
National Institute of Mental Health 62, 149
National Institutes of Health 103, 152
National Research Council 14, 15
National Soft Drink Association 88, 102
National Vaccine Information Center 250,
267, 276
National Vaccine Injury Act 273
National Vital Statistics 171
Natural Resources Defense Council 33
Nazis 172
NCI 76
NCR 340
neomycin 251
nephropathy 97
Nestle 220, 221
Neural Organization Technique 337
neural tube 31
neural tube defect 175
Neurocranial Restructuring 340
Neuromins 210
niacin 242

water, bottled 34
water, drinking 14
water, ground 37
wheat 139, 144, 228
whey 225
white flour 80, 223, 271
Whole Brain Writing 340
Whole grains 147
whooping cough 268
wine 139
Withdrawal symptoms 158
World Health Organization (WHO) 39, 201,
   208, 211, 248, 249, 259
Wyeth Nutritional 208, 220

X

X-rays 173, 199
xenoestrogens 44, 184

Y

Yazbak, R. Edward 264
yogurt 225

Z

zinc 16, 22, 111, 133, 134, 202, 217, 234, 236,
   304
Zoloft 92, 159
zucchini 239

Notes

Notes

Notes

To order more copies of the *The Truth About Children's Health –
Understanding, Preventing and Reversing Disease,* call
PRI Publishing at 434-263-8858 or email proreach@aol.com.
Quantity discounts available.

Check out our other fine titles below.

14 Days To A Safer Child
The Complete Children's Safety Kit

"The Most Complete Program for Children's Protection Available."
Did you realize that according to FBI statistics, every 41 seconds another child disappears? Abductions, kidnappings, and getting lost are real dangers for kids these days! Even worse, every year 6,700 children die and another 50,000 are seriously injured because of accidents and every day mishaps!

Protect your child to the fullest with the most gentle, effective, fun, and doctor approved methods that ensure your child's safety. The *Safety First Please Protection Kit* uses a unique 'multi-modal' approach to teaching your child how to recognize dangerous situations and avoid them. For ages 3-12. Each kit includes:

- CD (or tape) with safety songs, book narration, and sound tracks
- Fingerprinting kit, DNA sample kit, and Dental chart
- 14-day lesson plan with quizzes, fun activities, final exam, and diploma
- Folder for recent photo, personal/medical information, and important phone numbers
- Twenty-four *I'm a Safety Seal Kid* stickers – kids love them!
- Plush beany toy of *Sterling the Safety Seal*
- Critically acclaimed full color children's book *Safety First Please* (8½ x 11 hardcover)
- Teachers/Parents Instruction and Resource Manual

$29.95 + $5 S&H / Book only–$15.95 + $5 S&H / Book & CD only – $19.95 + $5 S&H

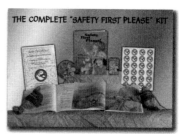

THE COMPLETE "SAFETY FIRST PLEASE" KIT

"As a child psychiatrist, I am always interested in new ways to help children be safe. The Safety First Please Kit is an excellent program that covers a lot of very important issues that all come down to keeping our children safe. I like the way it asks children what they would do... Using a multi-modal approach of reading, hearing, seeing, singing, rhyming, etc. will help this information 'sink in' and avoids the 'fear factor.' Thanks for your efforts."
— J Ronald Heller, M.D.

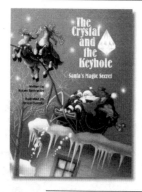

The Crystal and the Keyhole and Santa's Magic Secret

What child hasn't wondered how the presents get under the tree if there is no chimney for Santa? Well, little Jackie is no different and he's determined to find out! While waiting under the Christmas tree on Christmas Eve, he's surprised by a bright rainbow of light that explodes through the keyhole of his front door. Two cute and ambitious elves, Katie and Ben, grow out of the light and commence putting presents under the tree. Jackie befriends them, and learns that with the help of their magic crystal, they can get into houses that Santa cannot... "When there is no chimney, we elves save the day!" ...and Santa is up on the roof waiting for his elves to return from doing their job.

When they get ready to leave, Katie pulls out the magic crystal, and she and Ben say the magic words... "And together they said three times in a hush, Merry Christmas to all, and to all peace and love." Magic ensues, as Jackie watches and learns the whole secret about the elves, Santa Claus and Christmas without a chimney.

This heart-warming tale will enchant young and old alike with its sincere message, brilliant illustrations and surprising ending. And it will finally answer your youngsters' questions about how the presents are delivered when there is no chimney! 8½" x 11" full color hardcover.
$15.95 + $5 S&H

The Golfer's Night BeFORE! Christmas

The Christmas story every golfer has been waiting for is finally here! *The Golfer's Night BeFORE! Christmas* reveals the truth about Santa's love for the game of golf – and a problem with his golf swing! Dressed in red knickers, green thermal golf shirt and golf shoes, Santa pauses on his rounds to hit a few practice shots off of a fellow golf enthusiast's roof. But there's a problem! Santa just can't stop hitting a slice! His new golfing buddy comes to his rescue by offering a few tips and giving Santa a golf lesson right there on the roof on Christmas Eve! He tells Santa, "And keep your head steady, you don't want to sway... That belly of yours sometimes gets in the way!" Soon, Santa gets in the groove... "His backswing was slower, his wrists cocked a little... And this time he nailed that ball

straight down the middle!"

Filled with golf language, traditions, humor, and class, this book will make every golfer smile and rejoice in golfing satisfaction. You will not only see Santa's jolly golf swing, but also learn the amazing and magical secret of where his golf balls end up after he hits them off the roof.

The Par-fect gift and stocking-stuffer for any golfer on your Christmas list! Be a good caddy and get *The Golfer's Night BeFORE! Christmas* for the golfer you love!

"And I heard him call out as he swung back around... Merry Christmas FORE! all and FORE! all a good round!"
7" x 10" full color hardcover.

$11.95 + $5 S&H

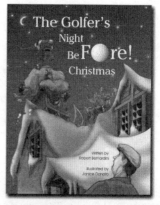

The Golfer's Night BeF**O**re! Christmas

PRI Publishing   P.O. Box 74, Clifford, VA 24533   Phone: (434) 263-8858   Fax: (434) 263-5797   email proreach@aol.com
Distributor & Bookstore discounts available.